Endoscopy in Small Bowel Disorders

Richard Kozarek • Jonathan A. Leighton
Editors

Endoscopy in Small Bowel Disorders

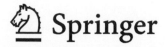 Springer

Editors
Richard Kozarek
Virginia Mason Medical Center
Digestive Disease Institute
Seattle, WA, USA

Jonathan A. Leighton
Division of Gastroenterology
  and Hepatology
Mayo Clinic
Scottsdale, AZ, USA

Videos can also be accessed at
http://link.springer.com/book/10.1007/978-3-319-14415-3

ISBN 978-3-319-14414-6   ISBN 978-3-319-14415-3   (eBook)
DOI 10.1007/978-3-319-14415-3

Library of Congress Control Number: 2015934005

Springer Cham Heidelberg New York Dordrecht London

Printed on acid-free paper

Springer International Publishing AG Switzerland is part of Springer Science+Business Media (www.springer.com)

Preface

Historically, small bowel disorders remained a diagnostic dilemma at a time that endoscopy and colonoscopy were routinely applied not only to the diagnosis but also to the treatment of acid peptic, neoplastic, and inflammatory gastrointestinal disorders. The midgut remained an endoscopic mystery. With the exception of surgically facilitated scope passage through a jejunal enterotomy, endoscopists nibbled at the edge of the small bowel, reaching the proximal jejunum with per os colonoscopes or overtube-assisted enteroscopes and the terminal ileum at time of colonoscopy. Other imaging wasn't much better: upper gastrointestinal and small bowel barium studies, Meckel's scan, and, only later, computed tomography enterography (CTE) scan looking for mass lesions, evidence of obstruction, or small bowel wall thickening.

The past several decades have seen an explosion in small bowel imaging leading to improved diagnosis and directed therapy. Although this is an endoscopic text, the editors would do the readers a disservice without putting endoscopy into perspective. As such, we direct your attention to the excellent chapters on conventional barium studies as well as the computed tomography enterography and magnetic resonance enterography.

This text describes the major advances in small bowel enteroscopy (capsule endoscopy, overtube-facilitated, and balloon-assisted) and their application for both common (gastrointestinal bleeding, malabsorptive disorders, Crohn's, etc.) and uncommon (small bowel tumors, Meckel's diverticulum, etc.) midgut disorders. The beauty of being able to visualize virtually the entire GI tract, of course, is improved diagnosis and treatment of our patients. The latter may be to direct appropriate medical or surgical therapy or to apply direct endoscopic therapy: removal of small bowel polyps and the dilation of midgut strictures whether they are the consequence of Crohn's disease, non-steroidal anti-inflammatory drugs (NSAIDs), or a previous surgical anastomosis. Small bowel enteroscopy may also allow access to the pancreaticobiliary tree in patients with surgically altered anatomy, performance of a direct percutaneous endoscopic jejunostomy (PEJ), and the evaluation and treatment of occult or actively bleeding GI lesions.

This text reviews not only the history and state of the art of small bowel endoscopy but also the near and potential future scenarios: improved capsule software, steerable capsules, and enteroscopes with improved optics and channel size to facilitate and enlarge our therapeutic capabilities.

The editors proffer this text to GI practitioners of all disciplines as well as those currently in training. It is our hope that it will aid you in the management of your patients with suspected or documented small bowel disorders.

Seattle, WA, USA   Richard Kozarek, M.D.
Scottsdale, AZ, USA   Jonathan A. Leighton, M.D.

Acknowledgements

We acknowledge Diane E. Lee, Virginia Mason Medical Center, and Maureen Pierce, Springer, for their invaluable assistance in manuscript preparation, editing, and collation and our families and staff for their support during the editing of this text.

Contents

Contributors

Brunella Barbaro, M.D. Department of Bioimaging and Radiological Sciences, Universita Cattolica del Sacro Cuore, Rome, Italy

Todd H. Baron, M.D., F.A.S.G.E. Division of Gastroenterology and Hepatology, University of North Carolina, Chapel Hill, Chapel Hill, NC, USA

Maximilien Barret, M.D., M.Sc. Sorbonne Paris Centre, Université Paris Descartes, Paris, France

Department of Gastroenterology and Digestive Endoscopy, Georges Pompidou European Hospital, Paris, France

Alessandra Bizzotto, M.D. Digestive Endoscopy Unit, Universita Cattolica del Sacro Cuore, Rome, Italy

David H. Bruining, M.D. Division of Gastroenterology and Hepatology, Mayo Clinic, Rochester, MN, USA

Emanuele Casciani, M.D., Ph.D. Department of Radiology, Emergency Department, "Umberto I" University Hospital, "Sapienza" University, Rome, Italy

Christophe Cellier, M.D., Ph.D. Sorbonne Paris Centre, Université Paris Descartes, Paris, France

Department of Gastroenterology and Digestive Endoscopy, Georges Pompidou European Hospital, Paris, France

Paola Cerro, M.D. Department of Radiology, Nuovo Regina Margherita Hospital, Rome, Italy

Michael V. Chiorean, M.D. Inflammatory Bowel Disease Center of Excellence, Department of Gastroenterology, Digestive Disease Institute, Virginia Mason Medical Center, Seattle, WA, USA

Manuel Berzosa Corella, M.D. Department of Gastroenterology, Mayo Clinic Florida, Jacksonville, FL, USA

Guido Costamagna, M.D., F.A.C.G. Digestive Endoscopy Unit, Universita Cattolica del Sacro Cuore, Rome, Italy

Salvatore Cucchiara, M.D., Ph.D. Pediatric Gastroenterology and Liver Unit, Department of Pediatrics and Childhood Neuropsychiatry, "Umberto I" University Hospital, Sapienza University of Rome, Rome, Italy

Edward J. Despott, M.R.C.P (Gastro), F.E.B.G.H, M.D. (Res) Royal Free Unit for Endoscopy, Royal Free Hospital, University College London, Institute for Liver and Digestive Health, London, UK

Joel G. Fletcher, M.D. Department of Radiology, Mayo Clinic, Rochester, MN, USA

Chris Fraser, M.B., Ch.B., M.D., F.R.C.P. Centre for Liver and Digestive Disorders, Royal Infirmary of Edinburgh, Edinburgh, UK

Wolfson Unit for Endoscopy, St. Mark's Hospital and Academic Institute, Harrow, Middlesex, UK

Lucia Fry, M.D., Ph.D., F.A.S.G.E. Division of Gastroenterology, Hepatology and Infectious Diseases, Otto-von-Guericke University, Magdeburg, Germany

Gianfranco Gualdi, M.D. Department of Radiology, Emergency Department, "Umberto I" University Hospital, Sapienza University of Rome, Rome, Italy

Amy B. Kolbe, M.D. Department of Radiology, Mayo Clinic, Rochester, MN, USA

Rosario Landi, Digestive Endoscopy Unit, Universita Cattolica del Sacro Cuore, Rome, Italy

Jonathan A. Leighton, M.D. Division of Gastroenterology and Hepatology, Mayo Clinic, Scottsdale, AZ, USA

Blair S. Lewis, M.D. Division of Gastroenterology, Mount Sinai School of Medicine, New York, NY, USA

Otto S. Lin, M.D., M.Sc. Digestive Disease Institute, Virginia Mason Medical Center, Seattle, WA, USA

Frank Lukens, M.D. Department of Gastroenterology, Mayo Clinic Florida, Jacksonville, FL, USA

Georgia Malamut, M.D., Ph.D. Sorbonne Paris Centre, Université Paris Descartes, Paris, France

Department of Gastroenterology and Digestive Endoscopy, Georges Pompidou European Hospital, Paris, France

Clelia Marmo, M.S. Digestive Endoscopy Unit, Universita Cattolica del Sacro Cuore, Rome, Italy

Klaus Mönkemüller, M.D., Ph.D., F.A.S.G.E. Division of Gastroenterology, University of Alabama at Birmingham, Birmingham, AL, USA

Giovanni Di Nardo, M.D., Ph.D. Pediatric Gastroenterology and Liver Unit, Department of Pediatrics, Sapienza University of Rome, Rome, Italy

John Ospina Nieto, M.D., M.S.C.C., M.S.C.H., M.A.S.G.E. Unidad de Estudios Digestivos, UNESDI, Bogotá, Colombia

Jessica Noelting, M.D. Department of Gastroenterology and Hepatology, Mayo Clinic Arizona, Scottsdale, AZ, USA

Salvatore Oliva, M.D. Paediatric Gastroenterology and Liver Unit, Department of Paediatrics, "Umberto I" University Hospital, Sapienza University of Rome, Rome, Italy

Fouad A. Otaki, M.D. Department of Gastroenterology, Weill Cornell/New York Presbyterian Hospital, New York, NY, USA

Gabriel Rahmi, M.D. Department of Gastroenterology and Digestive Endoscopy, Georges Pompidou European Hospital, Paris Cedex, France

Jean-Francois Rey, M.D. Department of Hepatology and Gastroenterology, Institut Arnault Tzanck, St. Laurent du Var, France

Maria Elena Riccioni, M.D. Digestive Endoscopy Unit, Universita Cattolica del Sacro Cuore, Rome, Italy

Andrew Ross, M.D. Digestive Disease Institute, Virginia Mason Medical Center, Seattle, WA, USA

Elia Samaha, M.D. Department of Gastroenterology and Digestive Endoscopy, Georges Pompidou European Hospital, Paris Cedex, France

Shabnam Sarker, M.D. Department of Internal Medicine, University of Alabama at Birmingham, Birmingham, AL, USA

Felice Schnoll-Sussman, M.D. Department of Medicine, Gastroenterology, New York Presbyterian Hospital/Weill Cornell Medical College, New York, NY, USA

Rakesh Sinha, F.R.C.R., M.D., M.B.B.S. Department of Clinical Radiology, Warwick Hospital, South Warwickshire NHS Foundation Trust, Warwick, Warwickshire, UK

Adam Templeton, M.D. Section of Gastroenterology, University of Washington Medical Center, Seattle, WA, USA

Christopher Teshima, M.D., M.Sc., Ph.D., F.R.C.P.C. Division of Gastroenterology, St. Michael's Hospital, University of Toronto, Toronto, ON, Canada

Hironori Yamamoto, M.D., Ph.D. Department of Medicine, Division of Gastroenterology, Jichi Medical University, Shimotsuke, Tochigi, Japan

Tomonori Yano, M.D. Department of Medicine, Division of Gastro-enterology, Jichi Medical University, Shimotsuke, Tochigi, Japan

Part I

Indications for Small Bowel Disorder Imaging

Indications for Imaging the Small Bowel

Jessica Noelting and Jonathan A. Leighton

Background

In recent years, science and technology have come a long way in imaging the small bowel. These new modalities have reinvigorated our interest and understanding of small bowel diseases. The small bowel has traditionally been difficult to evaluate because of the fact that it is approximately 600 cm in length and extremely tortuous. Throughout this book, you will learn about traditional methods of evaluating the small bowel, as well as the newer techniques that have revolutionized the way we approach the small bowel today.

Traditional imaging methods, such as the barium small bowel follow through, have been limited in their ability to detect small or subtle abnormalities. Enteroclysis provided more detail but was difficult to perform and associated with significant patient discomfort. Whereas small bowel follow through or enteroclysis is relatively

J. Noelting, M.D.
Department of Gastroenterology and Hepatology,
Mayo Clinic Arizona, 13400 East Shea Blvd.,
Scottsdale, AZ 85259, USA
e-mail: Noelting.jessica@mayo.edu

J.A. Leighton, M.D. (✉)
Division of Gastroenterology and Hepatology,
Mayo Clinic, 13400 E. Shea Blvd., Scottsdale,
AZ 85259, USA
e-mail: Leighton.jonathan@mayo.edu

safe and noninvasive, the yield is low [1, 2], especially for mucosal lesions such as angioectasias. Endoscopy is useful for the most proximal and distal aspects of the small bowel but failed to investigate the majority of this organ. Although the yield of intraoperative endoscopy is very good, this test is very invasive and carries significant risks including serosal tears, perforation, mortality, and postoperative complications.

In the "olden days," circa 2000, the evaluation of suspected small bowel disease, particularly obscure gastrointestinal bleeding, was therefore inefficient and not cost effective. Patients would often require multiple hospitalizations, extensive diagnostic testing, and repeated blood transfusions without identifying a source. Patients would undergo repeat upper and lower endoscopy, push enteroscopy, small bowel follow through, or enteroclysis followed by angiography or intraoperative endoscopy. The historical challenges related to these tests included a high miss rate for small bowel lesions, limited availability, and accuracy of these older diagnostic tests, and thus the need for more invasive intraoperative enteroscopy and exploratory laparotomy to adequately examine the small bowel.

We are now in a "new age" with regard to imaging the small bowel. With the introduction of capsule endoscopy (CE) in 2001 and balloon-assisted enteroscopy in 2004, there was a true paradigm shift in the approach to suspected small bowel disease. This was followed by the development of more sophisticated software for

R. Kozarek and J.A. Leighton (eds.), *Endoscopy in Small Bowel Disorders*,
DOI 10.1007/978-3-319-14415-3_1, © Springer International Publishing Switzerland 2015

cross-sectional imaging and the introduction of CT enterography and MR enterography. Together, these new modalities are seen as "disruptive technology" in that they led to a complete change in how we view the small bowel. Prior to these new techniques, the gastrointestinal tract was viewed as the upper tract, proximal to the ligament of Treitz, and the lower tract, distal to the ligament of Treitz. With the advent of these technologies, we can now view not only the upper and lower tract, but also the middle tract, i.e., the small bowel. Obscure gastrointestinal bleeding is no longer so obscure. The small bowel is no longer the "black box" of the gastrointestinal tract thanks, in particular, to capsule endoscopy and deep enteroscopy.

Capsule Endoscopy

In the following chapters, you will become more familiar with CE and its indications. Capsule endoscopy is truly an archetypical example of "disruptive" technology. It allows for a direct, noninvasive visual examination of the small bowel mucosa without discomfort or the need for sedation. Capsule endoscopy is an elegant solution in that the camera is not tethered to an apparatus, and thus is able to travel the entire length of the small bowel. The capsule measures from 24 mm to 31 mm × 11 mm to 13 mm, and is propelled through the small bowel by peristalsis. It is ingested orally or delivered into the small bowel by endoscopic assistance. It can visualize the entire small intestine in 79–90 % of cases [3]. As such, CE has become the gold standard in the evaluation of suspected small bowel disease.

Studies have shown that its diagnostic yield for small bowel lesions is superior to most other modalities [4, 5]. Its main utility lies in its high positive and negative predictive value as well as its ability to direct further therapeutic intervention and/or surgery [6]. While CE has had a huge impact in gastroenterology, we must recognize its limitations. These include a lack of therapeutic capabilities, inability to control movement, a high rate of incidental findings, and difficulty in localizing lesions. Finally, there is a potential to

miss single-mass lesions and for capsule retention in high-risk individuals. In most situations, the benefits of CE outweigh these limitations.

Deep Enteroscopy

In addition to the development of CE, deep enteroscopy techniques have also added to our armamentarium for evaluating the small bowel. These new devices include double-balloon and single-balloon enteroscopy, as well as spiral enteroscopy. The main concept of all three techniques is to plicate the intestine over the endoscope, using a series of push-and-pull maneuvers. Unlike CE, therapeutic interventions such as biopsy, cauterization, and polypectomy can be performed and are undertaken in approximately 33 % of deep enteroscopies [7]. The major drawback of deep enteroscopy is the high resource utilization, with procedures lasting upwards of 60 min, and the need for anesthesia, assistants, and fluoroscopy. Its overall diagnostic yield is comparable to CE [8], but deep enteroscopy is more invasive, requires sedation or anesthesia, and is associated with higher resource utilization. The new device-assisted enteroscopy techniques can achieve a total enteroscopy by combined oral and anal approach in 8–63 % of cases, depending on the experience of the endoscopist [5]. As you will learn in the following chapters, all forms of deep enteroscopy are comparable in terms of yield, safety, and learning curve. The advent of this new technology has indeed brought the small bowel within the reach of the endoscopist.

Indications for Evaluating the Small Bowel

Although gastroenterologists most often are called to evaluate the stomach and colon, there are many reasons to image the small bowel (Table 1.1). The main ones can be divided into vascular, inflammatory, and neoplastic disorders. Overall, the single most common reason to evaluate the small bowel is for obscure gastrointestinal bleeding. Other indications include suspected

Table 1.1 Reasons to image the small bowel

Vascular	Inflammatory	Neoplastic	Other
• Angioectasia	• Peptic ulcer disease	• Carcinoid	• Abnormal imaging study
• Arteriovenous malformation	• Inflammatory bowel disease	• GIST	• Symptom evaluation
• Dieulafoy lesion	• NSAID enteropathy	• Adenocarcinoma	
• Varices	• Celiac disease	• Lymphoma	
• Hemorrhoids		• Ampullary carcinoma	
• Radiation enteritis		• Metastases	

Adapted from Leighton, JA. (2012, May 20). Archival appraisal defined. Powerpoint lecture presented at the AGA Postgraduate Course, San Diego Convention Center

small bowel disease, tumors and polyposis syndromes, Crohn's disease, and malabsorptive disorders. As you will see throughout this book, the approach to these different disorders may vary depending on the individual scenario and there is, to date, very little evidence-based medicine to determine specific practice guidelines. Imaging of the small bowel is done for obscure gastrointestinal bleeding, tumors and/or polyps, inflammatory bowel disease (IBD), malabsorptive syndromes, as well as symptomatology.

Obscure Gastrointestinal Bleeding

The most common indication for CE and deep enteroscopy is the evaluation of suspected small bowel bleeding. Obscure gastrointestinal bleeding (OGIB) is persistent bleeding from the gastrointestinal tract after negative esophagogastroduodenoscopy, colonoscopy, and small bowel radiologic test. It can be either overt (visible bleeding) or occult (iron-deficiency anemia without visible bleeding) [9]. The differential diagnosis is quite extensive and includes vascular, inflammatory, and neoplastic lesions, as well as hemobilia, hemosuccus pancreaticus, and vasculitis.

The diagnosis may be straightforward, as in the patient with multiple, bleeding, arteriovenous malformations or an ulcerated mass seen on capsule endoscopy. However, of all indications for evaluating the small bowel, obscure gastrointestinal bleeding can also be the most challenging because lesions can be located anywhere throughout the small bowel and, in the case of certain vascular lesions, may be difficult to identify

when they are not bleeding. Lesions may be missed due to patient conditions (e.g., hypotension), the fleeting nature of the lesion (e.g., Dieulafoy), or human error. Lesions include, in order of decreasing prevalence, angiodysplasia, ulcer, varices, bleeding polyp, tumor, and other rare causes [10].

While many lesions are ultimately found in the distal small bowel, a significant amount can be located in regions accessible with standard endoscopes [11]. As such, this bleeding can be caused by lesions proximal to the ligament of Treitz or in the colon that were missed on initial endoscopic evaluation. Thus, second-look endoscopy is recommended prior to embarking on an extensive small bowel evaluation. It is also important to rule out other causes of anemia such as bone marrow diseases and malabsorption, before concluding that the cause is gastrointestinal bleeding. Once gastrointestinal bleeding has been documented or iron-deficiency anemia confirmed and malabsorption and hematologic causes have been excluded, and second-look endoscopy is negative, then one can proceed with a small bowel evaluation.

In most cases, Capsule endoscopy will be the next best test. Depending on results, deep enteroscopy may be indicated to follow up on suspicious lesions. Deep enteroscopy complements CE. One study showed that there is excellent concordance between deep enteroscopy and CE [12]. The results of CE can be used to identify a lesion and guide further management. Generally, if the lesion is present within the first 75 % of small bowel transit time, we use an antegrade approach, and otherwise use a retrograde approach. Cost-effectiveness models suggest that DBE is the most cost-effective approach for obscure overt gastrointestinal bleeding; however, CE-guided DBE may be associated with better long-term outcomes due to decreased risk for complications and appropriate resource utilization [13]. Cross-sectional imaging techniques including CT angiography and CT enterography can also be used to localize a source of bleeding with a diagnostic yield of 10–40 % [12, 13], which is lower than CE and deep enteroscopy. However, in difficult cases of OGIB, cross-sectional imaging, capsule endoscopy, and deep enteroscopy can be complementary. That is, complex cases will require all three modalities for diagnosis and treatment of the condition.

Tumors and Polyposis Syndromes

Tumors of the small bowel often present with OGIB. In the USA in 2014, cancers of the small intestine represented 0.5 % of total cancer cases and 0.2 % of cancer deaths [14]. Primary small bowel tumors comprise approximately 2–5 % of all primary gastrointestinal neoplasms [15, 16]. The most common malignant small intestine malignant neoplasms, in decreasing order of incidence, are carcinoid, adenocarcinoma, lymphoma, and stromal tumors [17].

Capsule endoscopy now plays an important role in the diagnosis and management of small bowel tumors. A meta-analysis found CE to be superior to push enteroscopy and small bowel follow through, in the setting of OGIB [4]. CE can provide initial diagnosis, estimated location, characteristics (size, shape, ulceration, etc.), and extent/number of mass lesions present. It can also be used for surveillance after polypectomy. However, CE can miss single-mass lesions in the small intestine at a rate approximating 19 % [18]. Factors that can affect the visualization in CE include rapid transit and poor/lack of preparation. In one study, most (74 %) missed lesions were located in the proximal small bowel [19]. Thus, CE and push enteroscopy may be complementary studies in this setting. CE is superior to MRE for evaluation of tumors in patients with Peutz-Jeghers syndrome (PJS) and

familial adenomatous polyposis (FAP) [20, 21]. However, one study did suggest that MRE may be better at estimating the size of large polyps [22].

Deep enteroscopy also plays a role in the evaluation of small bowel tumors, particularly because of the ability to attain a tissue diagnosis. DBE has a diagnostic yield between 94 and 100 % for all small bowel tumors. Thus, this test may be helpful in cases where CE is negative but suspicion for a tumor remains high. It also has the advantage of being able to obtain a histopathologic diagnosis and, potentially, treat with polypectomy. However, DBE is more invasive and has a risk of perforation (1.3 %) and pancreatitis (0.6 %) [19].

At this time, there are limited evidence-based guidelines for small bowel imaging for suspected tumors. We suggest capsule endoscopy, in most cases, as the initial test of choice. It is suggested to perform CE prior to deep enteroscopy due to increased patient tolerance, ability to visualize the entire small intestine, and less invasive nature of the test. If a tumor is identified on CE, it can help direct the approach to deep enteroscopy. Thus these two tests work well together in the diagnosis and management of small bowel tumors.

Two polyposis syndromes with increased risk of small intestinal malignancy are PJS and FAP. In patients with PJS the risk ratio of small intestinal tumors is 520 [23], and thus some have recommended capsule endoscopy every 3 years starting at age 8 [24]. Most patients with FAP will have duodenal adenomas and it is estimated that they occur in 54–74 %. By age 75, >95 % of patients with FAP will have duodenal adenomas [25].

Regarding polyposis syndromes, there are limited studies on the benefits of CE, either for diagnosis or surveillance. Research in this area is limited mostly by the rarity of each condition. It has been suggested to screen patients with Peutz-Jeghers syndrome and others [26, 27], and can be justified in patients presenting with gastrointestinal bleeding. The role of deep enteroscopy in these patients is to sample and/or remove polyps. Deep enteroscopy can also be combined with surgery when very large polyps are identified.

Inflammatory Bowel Disease

Small bowel imaging can play an important role in the evaluation of patients with IBD with also have small bowel involvement. The diagnosis of IBD, particularly Crohn's disease, can be challenging because there is no single gold standard test. The disease involves the small bowel in approximately 70 % of patients and up to 30 % of patients have disease confined to the small bowel, usually the distal ileum [28]. Furthermore, even when the disease is not confined to the small intestine, involvement of this part of the GI tract can confer a worst prognosis and higher likelihood of recurrence [29]. In a subgroup of patients, identification of small bowel inflammation proximal to the terminal ileum can be difficult. Cross-sectional imaging has become popular for evaluation and monitoring of Crohn's disease due to its noninvasive nature and relative ease of use (especially when compared to deep enteroscopy). The role of CE and deep enteroscopy in this area remains controversial and has yet to be determined. Notably, cross-sectional imaging is helpful in assessing transmural inflammation and fistulae; however, it probably does not assess mucosal disease as well as CE and deep enteroscopy.

Capsule endoscopy can be used to evaluate the small bowel, particularly when colonoscopy with ileoscopy is negative. The advent of capsule technology has facilitated the evaluation of suspected CD, allowing for a more thorough assessment of the mucosa. The technology appears to have additional diagnostic yield of up to 70 % for CD isolated to the small bowel following a negative ileocolonoscopy. CE has the potential to be used not only in the diagnosis of IBD, but also in assessing the severity and extent of disease, post-surgical recurrence, and, perhaps, response to therapy. Findings of aphthous ulcers, fissuring ulcers, granularity, loss of vascular patter, and mucosal edema are similar on CE as on traditional endoscopy.

Capsule endoscopy may also be of benefit in patients with established CD. It may be complementary to ileocolonoscopy and upper endoscopy and has been shown to affect medical and surgical decision making [30]. In particular, CE may be useful in assessing the extent and severity of small bowel inflammation, particularly in patients with unexplained symptoms. In addition, CE may be useful for assessing mucosal healing once therapy has been initiated. There are studies to suggest that it may play a role in the evaluation of postoperative recurrence when ileocolonoscopy is not successful or needs to be avoided [29]. Finally, CE may be of value in assessing indeterminate colitis and reclassifying a subgroup as CD.

There are definite concerns and unanswered issues with CE in CD. The risk of capsule retention, due to stricturing disease, is higher in patients with known Crohn's disease, and in one study was reported to be 13 % [31]. Although CE has a high sensitivity (83–93 %), it has a low specificity (53–84 %) for diagnosing small bowel Crohn's disease [32, 33]. Furthermore, it remains to be seen whether or not CE is cost effective in the diagnosis of Crohn's disease [34].

The role of deep enteroscopy in IBD is less clear due to limited randomized controlled trials assessing the utility of this modality for CD. Deep enteroscopy has the advantage of obtaining tissue samples and being able to perform therapeutic interventions such as stricture dilatation. Histological evaluation can be particularly helpful in confirming active IBD, both for initial diagnosis and monitoring of IBD. Regarding the diagnostic yield, a meta-analysis of 11 studies comparing CE and DBE showed that they were comparable for small bowel disease, including inflammatory lesions [12]. However, DBE is more invasive and should be reserved for cases where CE is contraindicated, to obtain a tissue diagnosis after a positive study, to perform endotherapy, or to retrieve a retained capsule.

In contrast to obscure gastrointestinal bleeding, radiologic imaging can be particularly useful in the assessment of patients with CD. On cross-sectional imaging, transmural inflammation manifests as bowel wall thickening and enhancement. Both magnetic resonance enterography (MRE) and computed tomography enterography (CTE) have a good accuracy (0.86–0.93) compared to endoscopic evaluation with a sensitivity (0.81–0.90) and specificity (0.88–1.0) for assessing disease activity by bowel wall thickening and enhancement [35]. However, both CTE and MRE lack the ability to visualize the mucosa and false-positive results can be seen if the bowel is under-distended.

In the majority of cases, ileocolonoscopy is the first test of choice in the assessment of patients with CD. However, it is reasonable to evaluate the small bowel, with either cross-sectional imaging or CE when suspicion of CD is high despite negative ileocolonoscopy. These new methods for evaluating the small bowel disease can assist clinicians in making a more timely and accurate diagnosis in patients with IBD, and can assist in determining prognosis and likelihood of recurrence. Armed with this information, the clinician can make better recommendations for treatment. Then, these methods can be used for monitoring response to treatment or disease recurrence.

Celiac Disease and Other Autoimmune Enteropathies

The exact role of small bowel imaging in celiac disease is evolving. Celiac disease is an immune reaction to eating gluten manifesting as inflammation of the small intestine that affects 1 % of the white American population [36]. Other enteropathies include autoimmune, hypogammaglobulinemic sprue and drug-induced (e.g., olmesartan). Typically, patients present with chronic diarrhea, postprandial abdominal pain, bloating, and weight loss. For diagnosis of celiac disease, initial testing with serology (i.e., tissue transglutaminase antibodies) is followed by duodenal biopsies. Macroscopically, enteropathy appears as villous atrophy, nodularity, fissures, scalloping, layered or stacked folds, and a mosaic appearance of the mucosa [37, 38]. Duodenal biopsies show intraepithelial lymphocytes, crypt hyperplasia, and/or villous atrophy.

Although histology is the gold standard for diagnosing celiac disease, CE may play a role in evaluating those patients with positive serology and negative histology, for patients unwilling or unable to undergo upper endoscopy, and for complicated or refractory celiac disease. In patients who are symptomatic despite a gluten-free diet, especially if they have alarm symptoms such as weight loss, fever, and pain, up to 60 % may have evidence of ongoing villous atrophy, ulcers or erosions, or cancer [39–41]. Capsule endoscopy has a sensitivity of 89 % and specificity of 95 % for detecting enteropathy [42].

Deep enteroscopy techniques may also be useful in patients with refractory or complicated celiac disease. In one study of 21 patients who were symptomatic and had villous flattening on duodenal biopsies despite maintaining a strict gluten-free diet, referred for double-balloon enteroscopy, 5 patients were diagnosed with enteropathy-associated T cell lymphoma (EATL) and 2 with ulcerative jejunitis. CT scan of these patients only detected EATL in four patients and did not detect ulcerative jejunitis in any. The authors conclude that deep enteroscopy should be reserved for patients with refractory celiac disease or those with a history of EATL [43]. In another study of 12 patients with unexplained malabsorption, double-balloon enteroscopy with small bowel biopsies yielded a diagnosis in 8 patients (including amyloidosis and Crohn's disease) even though duodenal biopsies were normal [44].

The role of radiologic evaluation is limited. Small bowel barium studies may show decreased jejunal folds, jejunal dilation, increased ileal fold thickness, and intussusceptions; however, this cannot reliably differentiate celiac disease or malabsorption from irritable bowel syndrome [45]. MRE, enteroclysis, and CTE, in contrast, can be useful in evaluating complicated celiac disease (malignancy, ulceration) [46].

Although upper endoscopy is usually sufficient for diagnosis and evaluation of celiac disease, small bowel imaging can be useful in complicated or refractory cases or when lymphoma is suspected. Capsule endoscopy can also be used for patients who cannot tolerate upper endoscopy. There is little role for cross-sectional imaging in this disease, other than to look for complications.

Symptom Evaluation and Abnormal Imaging Studies

The role of CE and deep enteroscopy in the evaluation of nonspecific symptoms is not clear. Small bowel imaging in patients with gastrointestinal symptoms is most useful when "alarm" features are present. Such "alarm" symptoms include weight loss, elevated erythrocyte sedimentation rate or C-reactive protein, thrombocytosis, anemia, and/or fevers. In patients with abdominal pain and diarrhea alone without these "alarm" symptoms, the yield tends to be quite low.

In a study of 165 nonbleeding patients referred for CE, the most common indications were diarrhea and abdominal pain. Among the 30 patients with diarrhea alone, only 8 (27 %) had positive findings [47]. In a study of 72 patients with chronic abdominal pain, with or without diarrhea, the diagnostic yield of CE was poor (21 and 0 %) in patients with normal inflammatory markers but was 67 and 90 % in patients with positive inflammatory markers. Diagnoses included IBD, small bowel tumors, enteritis, and NSAID enteropathy [48]. Similarly, in another group of 50 patients with chronic abdominal pain, the only additional sign that was associated with positive findings on CE was evidence of inflammation [49].

Conclusion

New endoscopic techniques, including CE and deep enteroscopy, in conjunction with cross-sectional imaging, have revolutionized our approach to the evaluation of small bowel disorders. Physicians are now armed with several methods of investigating the small intestine. These advances in technology have also improved patients' tolerance to testing and may reduce their exposure to radiation and complications by using less invasive methods.

These new techniques have transformed our approach to patients with OGIB. In many ways, OGIB is no longer "obscure" because of our ability to adequately image the small bowel. With the arrival of these new methods, patients previously labeled "OGIB" may be further subdivided into missed lesions (within reach of the upper endoscope or colonoscope), small bowel bleeding, and truly "obscure" gastrointestinal bleeding. With this ease of access, we may increase the diagnosis of small bowel tumors and enteropathy, and more accurately assess for disease activity in IBD.

In the twentieth century, no one would have imagined being able to reach the entire length of the small intestine endoscopically. What will come next? Research is currently under way with remote-controlled capsules using magnets, which could quickly be guided to a point of interest for more detailed inspection, and capsules that release gas to distend the lumen for better visualization. The logical next step would be to have that capsule take samples of the mucosa or deliver drugs to a specific lesion as well. Research in this area is also under way. The future is bright for imaging of the small bowel and evaluating small bowel diseases.

References

1. Rondonotti E, Villa F, Mulder CJ, Jacobs MA, de Franchis R. Small bowel capsule endoscopy in 2007: indications, risks and limitations. World J Gastroenterol. 2007;13(46):6140–9 [Review].
2. Delvaux M, Fassler I, Gay G. Clinical usefulness of the endoscopic video capsule as the initial intestinal investigation in patients with obscure digestive bleeding: validation of a diagnostic strategy based on the patient outcome after 12 months. Endoscopy. 2004;36(12):1067–73 [Validation Studies].
3. Gerson LB, Batenic MA, Newsom SL, Ross A, Semrad CE. Long-term outcomes after double-balloon enteroscopy for obscure gastrointestinal bleeding. Clin Gastroenterol Hepatol. 2009;7(6): 664–9.
4. Triester SL, Leighton JA, Leontiadis GI, Fleischer DE, Hara AK, Heigh RI, et al. A meta-analysis of the yield of capsule endoscopy compared to other diagnostic modalities in patients with obscure gastrointestinal bleeding. Am J Gastroenterol. 2005;100(11):2407–18 [Comparative Study Meta-Analysis].
5. Pennazio M, Santucci R, Rondonotti E, Abbiati C, Beccari G, Rossini FP, et al. Outcome of patients with obscure gastrointestinal bleeding after capsule endoscopy: report of 100 consecutive cases. Gastroenterology. 2004;126(3):643–53 [Clinical Trial Multicenter Study Research Support, Non-U.S. Gov't].
6. Nakamura M, Niwa Y, Ohmiya N, Miyahara R, Ohashi A, Itoh A, et al. Preliminary comparison of capsule endoscopy and double-balloon enteroscopy in

patients with suspected small-bowel bleeding. Endoscopy. 2006;38(1):59–66 [Comparative Study].

7. Gross SA, Stark ME. Initial experience with double-balloon enteroscopy at a U.S. Center. Gastrointest Endosc. 2008;67(6):890–7 [Comparative Study].

8. Raju GS, Gerson L, Das A, Lewis B. American Gastroenterological A. American gastroenterological association (aga) institute technical review on obscure gastrointestinal bleeding. Gastroenterology. 2007;133(5):1697–717 [Review].

9. Zaman A, Katon RM. Push enteroscopy for obscure gastrointestinal bleeding yields a high incidence of proximal lesions within reach of a standard endoscope. Gastrointest Endosc. 1998;47(5):372–6 [Clinical Trial].

10. Marmo R, Rotondano G, Casetti T, Manes G, Chilovi F, Sprujevnik T, et al. Degree of concordance between double-balloon enteroscopy and capsule endoscopy in obscure gastrointestinal bleeding: a multicenter study. Endoscopy. 2009;41(7):587–92 [Clinical Trial Comparative Study Multicenter Study].

11. Somsouk M, Gralnek IM, Inadomi JM. Management of obscure occult gastrointestinal bleeding: a cost-minimization analysis. Clin Gastroenterol Hepatol. 2008;6(6):661–70.

12. Pasha SF, Leighton JA, Das A, Harrison ME, Decker GA, Fleischer DE, et al. Double-balloon enteroscopy and capsule endoscopy have comparable diagnostic yield in small-bowel disease: a meta-analysis. Clin Gastroenterol Hepatol. 2008;6(6):671–6 [Comparative Study Meta-Analysis Research Support, Non-U.S. Gov't].

13. Gerson L, Kamal A. Cost-effectiveness analysis of management strategies for obscure GI bleeding. Gastrointest Endosc. 2008;68(5):920–36.

14. Siegel R, Ma J, Zou Z, Jemal A. Cancer statistics, 2014. CA Cancer J Clin. 2014;64(1):9–29.

15. Giuliani A, Caporale A, Teneriello F, Alessi G, Serpieri S, Sammartino P. Primary tumors of the small intestine. Int Surg. 1985;70(4):331–4.

16. Schottenfeld D, Beebe-Dimmer JL, Vigneau FD. The epidemiology and pathogenesis of neoplasia in the small intestine. Ann Epidemiol. 2009;19(1): 58–69 [Research Support, N.I.H., Extramural Review].

17. Bilimoria KY, Bentrem DJ, Wayne JD, Ko CY, Bennett CL, Talamonti MS. Small bowel cancer in the united states: changes in epidemiology, treatment, and survival over the last 20 years. Ann Surg. 2009;249(1): 63–71 [Research Support, Non-U.S. Gov't].

18. Lewis BS, Eisen GM, Friedman S. A pooled analysis to evaluate results of capsule endoscopy trials. Endoscopy. 2005;37(10):960–5 [Comparative Study Evaluation Studies].

19. Honda W, Ohmiya N, Hirooka Y, Nakamura M, Miyahara R, Ohno E, et al. Enteroscopic and radiologic diagnoses, treatment, and prognoses of small-bowel tumors. Gastrointest Endosc. 2012;76(2):344–54 [Comparative Study Evaluation Studies Research Support, Non-U.S. Gov't].

20. Urquhart P, Grimpen F, Lim GJ, Pizzey C, Stella DL, Tesar PA, et al. Capsule endoscopy versus magnetic resonance enterography for the detection of small bowel polyps in Peutz-Jeghers syndrome. Fam Cancer. 2014;13:249–55.

21. Akin E, Demirezer Bolat A, Buyukasik S, Algin O, Selvi E, Ersoy O. Comparison between capsule endoscopy and magnetic resonance enterography for the detection of polyps of the small intestine in patients with familial adenomatous polyposis. Gastroenterol Res Pract. 2012;2012:215028.

22. Gupta A, Postgate AJ, Burling D, Ilangovan R, Marshall M, Phillips RK, et al. A prospective study of MR enterography versus capsule endoscopy for the surveillance of adult patients with Peutz-Jeghers syndrome. AJR Am J Roentgenol. 2010;195(1):108–16 [Comparative Study Research Support, Non-U.S. Gov't].

23. Giardiello FM, Brensinger JD, Tersmette AC, Goodman SN, Petersen GM, Booker SV, et al. Very high risk of cancer in familial Peutz-Jeghers syndrome. Gastroenterology. 2000;119(6):1447–53 [Meta-Analysis Research Support, Non-U.S. Gov't Research Support, U.S. Gov't, P.H.S.].

24. Beggs AD, Latchford AR, Vasen HF, Moslein G, Alonso A, Aretz S, et al. Peutz-Jeghers syndrome: a systematic review and recommendations for management. Gut. 2010;59(7):975–86 [Consensus Development Conference].

25. Groves CJ, Saunders BP, Spigelman AD, Phillips RK. Duodenal cancer in patients with familial adenomatous polyposis (fap): results of a 10 year prospective study. Gut. 2002;50(5):636–41.

26. Giardiello FM, Trimbath JD. Peutz-Jeghers syndrome and management recommendations. Clin Gastroenterol Hepatol. 2006;4(4):408–15 [Research Support, N.I.H., Extramural Research Support, Non-U.S. Gov't Review].

27. Dunlop MG. Guidance on gastrointestinal surveillance for hereditary non-polyposis colorectal cancer, familial adenomatous polypolis, juvenile polyposis, and Peutz-Jeghers syndrome. Gut. 2002;51 Suppl 5:V21–7 [Guideline Practice Guideline].

28. Farmer RG, Hawk WA, Turnbull Jr RB. Clinical patterns in Crohn's disease: a statistical study of 615 cases. Gastroenterology. 1975;68(4 Pt 1):627–35.

29. Pons Beltran V, Nos P, Bastida G, Beltran B, Arguello L, Aguas M, et al. Evaluation of postsurgical recurrence in Crohn's disease: a new indication for capsule endoscopy? Gastrointest Endosc. 2007;66(3):533–40 [Comparative Study].

30. Cotter J, Dias de Castro F, Moreira MJ, Rosa B. Tailoring Crohn's disease treatment: the impact of small bowel capsule endoscopy. J Crohn's Colitis. 2014;8:1610–5.

31. Cheifetz AS, Kornbluth AA, Legnani P, Schmelkin I, Brown A, Lichtiger S, et al. The risk of retention of the capsule endoscope in patients with known or suspected Crohn's disease. Am J Gastroenterol. 2006;101(10):2218–22.

32. Solem CA, Loftus Jr EV, Fletcher JG, Baron TH, Gostout CJ, Petersen BT, et al. Small-bowel imaging

in Crohn's disease: a prospective, blinded, 4-way comparison trial. Gastrointest Endosc. 2008;68(2): 255–66 [Clinical Trial Comparative Study Research Support, Non-U.S. Gov't].

33. Girelli CM, Porta P, Malacrida V, Barzaghi F, Rocca F. Clinical outcome of patients examined by capsule endoscopy for suspected small bowel Crohn's disease. Dig Liver Dis. 2007;39(2):148–54 [Clinical Trial].

34. Levesque BG, Cipriano LE, Chang SL, Lee KK, Owens DK, Garber AM. Cost effectiveness of alternative imaging strategies for the diagnosis of small-bowel Crohn's disease. Clin Gastroenterol Hepatol. 2010;8(3):261–7. 267 e261–264 [Research Support, Non-U.S. Gov't Research Support, U.S. Gov't, P.H.S.].

35. Fiorino G, Bonifacio C, Peyrin-Biroulet L, Minuti F, Repici A, Spinelli A, et al. Prospective comparison of computed tomography enterography and magnetic resonance enterography for assessment of disease activity and complications in ileocolonic Crohn's disease. Inflamm Bowel Dis. 2011;17(5):1073–80 [Clinical Trial Comparative Study Validation Studies].

36. Fasano A, Berti I, Gerarduzzi T, Not T, Colletti RB, Drago S, et al. Prevalence of celiac disease in at-risk and not-at-risk groups in the United States: a large multicenter study. Arch Intern Med. 2003;163(3):286–92 [Multicenter Study Research Support, Non-U.S. Gov't].

37. Cellier C, Green PH, Collin P, Murray J. Icce consensus for celiac disease. Endoscopy. 2005;37(10):1055–9 [Consensus Development Conference Research Support, Non-U.S. Gov't].

38. Green PH, Rubin M. Capsule endoscopy in celiac disease. Gastrointest Endosc. 2005;62(5):797–9 [Comment Editorial].

39. Culliford A, Daly J, Diamond B, Rubin M, Green PH. The value of wireless capsule endoscopy in patients with complicated celiac disease. Gastrointest Endosc. 2005;62(1):55–61 [Comparative Study Research Support, Non-U.S. Gov't].

40. Joyce AM, Burns DL, Marcello PW, Tronic B, Scholz FJ. Capsule endoscopy findings in celiac disease associated enteropathy-type intestinal t-cell lymphoma. Endoscopy. 2005;37(6):594–6 [Case Reports].

41. Apostolopoulos P, Alexandrakis G, Giannakoulopoulou E, Kalantzis C, Papanikolaou IS, Markoglou C, et al. M2a wireless capsule endoscopy for diagnosing ulcerative jejunoileitis complicating celiac disease. Endoscopy. 2004;36(3):247 [Case Reports].

42. Rokkas T, Niv Y. The role of video capsule endoscopy in the diagnosis of celiac disease: a meta-analysis. Eur J Gastroenterol Hepatol. 2012;24(3):303–8 [Evaluation Studies Meta-Analysis].

43. Hadithi M, Al-toma A, Oudejans J, van Bodegraven AA, Mulder CJ, Jacobs M. The value of double-balloon enteroscopy in patients with refractory celiac disease. Am J Gastroenterol. 2007;102(5):987–96.

44. Fry LC, Bellutti M, Neumann H, Malfertheiner P, Monkemuller K. Utility of double-balloon enteroscopy for the evaluation of malabsorption. Dig Dis. 2008;26(2):134–9 [Clinical Trial].

45. Kumar P, Bartram CI. Relevance of the barium follow-through examination in the diagnosis of adult celiac disease. Gastrointest Radiol. 1979;4(3):285–9 [Comparative Study].

46. Tennyson CA, Semrad CE. Small bowel imaging in celiac disease. Gastrointest Endosc Clin N Am. 2012;22(4):735–46 [Review].

47. Katsinelos P, Tziomalos K, Fasoulas K, Paroutoglou G, Koufokotsios A, Mimidis K, Terzoudis S, Maris T, Beltsis A, Geros C, Chatzimavroudis G. Can capsule endoscopy be used as a diagnostic tool in the evaluation of nonbleeding indication in daily clinical practice? A prospective study. Med Princ Pract. 2011;20:362–7.

48. Katsinelos P, Fasoulas K, Beltsis A, Chatzimavroudis G, Paroutoglou G, Maris T, et al. Diagnostic yield and clinical impact of wireless capsule endoscopy in patients with chronic abdominal pain with or without diarrhea: a Greek multicenter study. Eur J Intern Med. 2011;22(5):e63–6.

49. May A, Manner H, Schneider M, Ipsen A, Ell C. Prospective multicenter trial of capsule endoscopy in patients with chronic abdominal pain, diarrhea and other signs and symptoms (cedap-plus study). Endoscopy. 2007;39(7):606–12.

Part II

History of Small Bowel Imaging

Barium Studies

2

Emanuele Casciani, Paola Cerro, Giovanni Di Nardo,
Salvatore Oliva, Gianfranco Gualdi,
and Salvatore Cucchiara

E. Casciani, M.D., Ph.D.
Department of Radiology, Emergency Department,
"Umberto I" University Hospital, Sapienza
University, Viale del Policlinico 155, Rome
00161, Italy
e-mail: emanuelecasciani@gmail.com

P. Cerro, M.D.
Department of Radiology, Nuovo Regina Margherita
Hospital, Via Morosini 30, Rome 00153, Italy
e-mail: pcerro@hotmail.it; paolo.cerro@aslroma.it

G. Di Nardo, M.D., Ph.D.
Pediatric Gastroenterology and Liver Unit,
Department of Pediatrics, Sapienza University
of Rome, Viale Regina Elena 324, Rome 00161, Italy
e-mail: giovanni.dinardo3@olice.it;
giovanni.dinardo@uniroma1.it

S. Oliva, M.D.
Paediatric Gastroenterology and Liver Unit,
Department of Paediatrics, "Umberto I" University
Hospital, Sapienza University of Rome,
Rome 00161, Italy

G. Gualdi, M.D.
Department of Radiology, Emergency Department,
"Umberto I" University Hospital, Sapienza University
of Rome, Viale del Policlinico 155,
Rome 00165, Italy
e-mail: gianfrancogualdi@tiscali.it

S. Cucchiara, M.D., Ph.D. (✉)
Pediatric Gastroenterology and Liver Unit,
Department of Pediatrics and Childhood
Neuropsychiatry, "Umberto I" University Hospital,
Sapienza University of Rome, Viale Regina Elena
324, Viale del Policlinico 155, Rome 00161, Italy
e-mail: salvatore.cucchiara@uniroma1.it

Introduction

For many years, the small bowel follow-through (SBFT) has been the most widely used radiologic modality to evaluate small bowel (SB) diseases. This method has been partly replaced by enteroclysis, which was rejuvenated in the 1970s and has now become a primary tool of gastrointestinal (GI) radiologists [1].

During the last two decades, we have witnessed a slow but steady reduction in the number of barium studies performed both in Europe and in the USA [2].

However, DiSantis observed a large decrease approximating 47 % and 46 % in the number of upper GI studies and of barium enemas, respectively, in a period of only 8 years—from 1998 to 2006 [3]. From 2001 to 2006, the nationwide volume fell by 37 % (from 533,650 to 337,882 examinations) [3]. These numbers include both upper GI procedures alone and those which included SB studies. The barium SB examination, in turn, had a dip of just 7 % (from 117,790 to 109,039 examinations) [3].

Barium can take several hours to opacify all the SB loops, a consequence of their considerable length and transit time. In addition, study duration is influenced by gastric emptying time and the possible presence of lesions. The deterioration of barium, from a mere flaky appearance of the suspension to a fully developed flocculation, which inevitably occurs in long examinations, can produce different grades of non-adherence to

R. Kozarek and J.A. Leighton (eds.), *Endoscopy in Small Bowel Disorders*,
DOI 10.1007/978-3-319-14415-3_2, © Springer International Publishing Switzerland 2015

the mucosa with consequent difficulties in morphological evaluation of the loops. For this reason, the SBFT is not reliable in highlighting early or small lesions.

The proper distension of the bowel loops necessary for their optimal visualization can be achieved by the placement of a feeding tube through the esophagus, stomach, and duodenum to the ligament of Treitz (enteroclysis).

The use of enteroclysis has increased the diagnostic accuracy in small bowel disorders because improved distension of the lumen allows direct visualization of the mucosal surface and a clear and simultaneous evaluation of all the dilated bowel loops. This technique also avoids overlapping artifacts.

Enteroclysis can be performed with single or double contrast (barium with methylcellulose or barium with air) and requires an optimal intestinal preparation [4, 5]. The double-contrast method has allowed the first extra-operative assessment in vivo of an anatomic parameter: the length of the intestine. The latter is important for the prognosis and prediction of chronic intestinal insufficiency, particularly in short bowel syndromes [6].

In 1973, the first monoslice computed tomography (CT) commercial scanner was introduced. This changed the diagnostic evaluation and the clinical management of multiple GI diseases, to include diverticulitis, appendicitis, intestinal obstruction, inflammatory bowel diseases, and tumors.

The monoslice CT was subsequently improved with the helical (1989) and multidetector-row techniques (MDCT) allowing faster acquisitions and thinner collimations. This resulted in a better visualization of bowel loops and mesentery, as well as the possibility of reformatting the images in different planes.

Another important step in the evaluation of the intestines and anorectum has been the introduction of magnetic resonance (MR) imaging, particularly for its high soft tissue contrast. Accuracy may also be enhanced by the use of different enteral contrast agents and of multiple ultrafast sequences.

Moreover, MR enterography provides the same information as CT enterography without the use of ionizing radiation, which makes this method particularly suitable for the study of the SB in pediatric patients and for the follow-up of chronic diseases [7, 8] (Fig. 2.1).

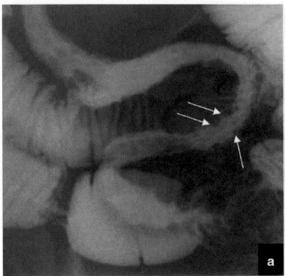 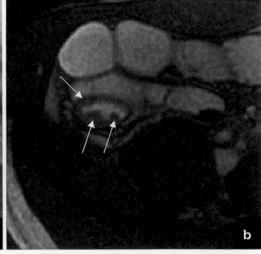

Fig. 2.1 Conventional enteroclysis versus MR enterography. Conventional enteroclysis (**a**) shows small nodular defects (*arrows*) corresponding to pseudopolyps shown by transverse steady-state MR enterography sequence (*arrows* in **b**) in a patient with Crohn's disease

Video capsule endoscopy (CE), introduced in 2000, has further contributed to the reduction in the use of barium examinations allowing the direct evaluation of the SB wall with a higher accuracy in the detection of early and superficial lesions [9–11].

The availability of these new radiological methods with a resulting reduction in the demand for barium studies has also made radiologists progressively less interested and able to perform these types of examinations [2].

Moreover, although these new imaging methods are less accurate than traditional radiology in the assessment of mural lesions, they allow evaluation of the bowel wall, its relationship with the parenchymal organs, peritoneal recesses, and the surrounding tissues. Recent literature shows a gradual replacement of the barium studies with new radiological methods (CE or CT or MR enterography) in most clinical situations.

Currently, a cross-sectional imaging study is the examination of choice for the evaluation of an SB neoplasm as it allows, with a single study, detection of a mass, its extraparietal extension, and the presence of pathologic lymph nodes or distant metastases [12].

Currently, according to new guidelines, CE and/or MR enterography have also supplanted barium studies in the screening of patients with familial adenomatous polyposis [13] and in other important clinical situations, such as suspected high small bowel obstruction (SBO) [14] and active obscure GI bleeding [15] in which MDCT, endoscopy, and CE are considered more accurate. In fact, a noninvasive MDCT scan allows evaluation of the obstruction or bleeding in terms of location, cause, and severity, with the application of multiplanar reconstruction images [14, 15].

Finally, the clinical and diagnostic approach to the patient with abdominal pain has significantly changed with ultrasound (US)—almost always the initial examination in a wide range of situations.

However, barium examinations, such as SBFT, are still the most common and accessible radiological methods for studying the small bowel [10], and their application is important especially in situations where other new techniques are limited.

As such, these procedures can provide the correct diagnosis at a lower cost and with fewer complications (e.g., those due to sedation required for endoscopy) [2]. Moreover, they are often used as a second-line test to confirm CT, MR, or US findings and are considered the diagnostic study of choice to exclude the presence of a bowel stenosis before performing a CE.

Barium Imaging in Intestinal Malrotation

Intestinal malrotation, which is defined as a congenital abnormal position of the gut within the peritoneal cavity, may lead to potentially fatal sequelae, such as midgut volvulus. The midgut rotation process can be divided into three stages. In stage I, from the 5th to the 10th week of gestation, the midgut elongates forming the primary intestinal loop, which undergoes a physiological herniation into the umbilical coelom where it grows and rotates 90° counterclockwise around the axis of the superior mesenteric artery (SMA). Failure to return to the abdomen during stage I results in the development of an omphalocele. In stage II, during the 10th to the 12th week of gestation, the midgut retracts into the abdominal cavity. The small intestine returns first completing its final 90-degree counterclockwise rotation and thereby passing posterior to the SMA. The large intestine enters later making an additional 180-degree counterclockwise rotation resulting in the normal configuration of the colon. In conclusion, the normal whole rotation of the intestine is 270° in a counterclockwise direction. Rotational defects during this process can result in a number of abnormal conditions. Nonrotation of the midgut, also called left-sided colon, is the most common rotation anomaly that occurs if the primary intestinal loop fails to undergo the second rotation of 180°. The result is an aberrant positioning of the colon and cecum on the left side of the abdominal cavity with the small intestinal loops situated in the right side. The duodenum has its first and second parts normally situated but the third and fourth parts slope down to the right of the SMA. This condition can lead to midgut volvulus and duodenal obstruction. The reversed rotation, instead, arises when the primary intestinal loop undergoes an incorrect 180-degree clockwise rotation after the first 90-degree counterclockwise rotation resulting in a total 90-degree clockwise rotation with an abnormal position of the transverse colon in the retroperitoneal space, posterior to the duodenum and the SMA. Finally, mixed rotations of the midgut (also called malrotations) can occur, due to an uncoordinated rotation of the duodenum and the colon with one malrotated segment and the other partially or nonrotated [16]. The most frequent type of malrotation arises when the cephalic limb and the caudal limb of the primary intestinal loop undergo only the initial 90-degree rotation and the later 180-degree rotation, respectively. The result is a correct positioning of the distal end of the duodenum and a cecal position just inferior to the gastric pylorus, near the midline in a subhepatic or central position. This causes an increased risk of intestinal obstruction as a consequence of SB compression, especially the duodenum.

In stage III, from the 12th week up until the term of gestation, the mesentery of some intestinal segments becomes fixed to the posterior abdominal wall, whereas some others disappear. Initially, following rotation, the duodenum and pancreas are situated in the right upper quadrant. There, due to the pressure of the colon, they are compressed against the posterior abdominal wall with which their peritoneums fuse, disappearing, and the resulting retroperitoneal position of most of the duodenum and head of the pancreas. In addition, the mesentery of the ascending and descending colon fuses with the peritoneum of the posterior abdominal wall with both the ascending, except for about 3 cm of its caudal portion, and descending colon becoming retroperitoneal.

The mesenteries of the appendix, lower end of the cecum, and sigmoid colon remain free.

What undergoes major changes is the mesentery of the primary intestinal loop, also called the mesentery proper, which, at the end of the process, in case of normal rotation and fixation, extends from the duodenojejunal junction (ligament of Treitz) in the left upper quadrant to the ileocecal junction in the right iliac fossa.

Also in this stage, some different abnormalities may occur due to altered fixation processes.

Firstly an incomplete or, in extreme cases, a total lack of fixation of the ascending colon to the posterior abdominal wall can lead to an abnormal motility of the cecum alone (mobile cecum) or of both the cecum and other colonic segments, respectively, with an increased risk of volvulus. A malfixation of the mesentery proper may result in a reduced distance between the ligament of Treitz and the ileocecal junction, resulting in loose loops of bowel hanging on an unsteady and narrow pedicle that is prone to twisting, volvulus, and strangulation.

Furthermore, an incomplete fusion of the mesentery with the posterior wall of the colon can lead to the formation of retrocolic recesses, most frequently posterior to the ascending colon, with the risk of herniation and entrapment of SB loops.

Finally, if the cecum fails to descend to its normal position in the right iliac fossa, it can develop an abnormal fixation in the right upper quadrant with dense fibrous bands (Ladd's bands) extending from the cecum to the retroperitoneum across the duodenum (Fig. 2.2) or, less frequently, between the colon and the duodenum (Fig. 2.3). The major risk is a variable degree of compression until complete obstruction of the duodenal loop.

Of all cases of malrotation, 60–80 % present in the first month of life, mostly in the first week. The most common symptoms of midgut volvulus are a generalized discomfort of the infant and bilious vomiting that needs an immediate investigation even in the absence of acute abdominal pain [17]. Similarly, a malrotation/volvulus must be suspected in any case of acute abdomen, even if bilious vomiting is absent.

However, the clinical presentation can be very variable and ambiguous, including both acute symptoms such as diarrhea, non-bilious vomiting, suspected infection or sepsis, shock or GI bleeding, and long-standing conditions of malabsorption and growth defects.

In the diagnosis of malrotation, the plain X-ray is rarely sufficient, except in cases of obvious complete duodenal occlusion, and an upper GI imaging is the preferred diagnostic modality, especially with the use of water-soluble contrast medium. Ionic hypertonic solutions, such as

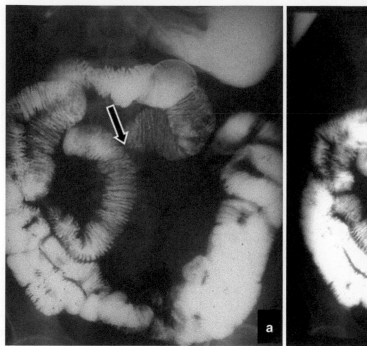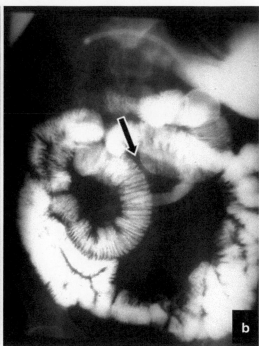

Fig. 2.2 Malrotation with duodenal bands. Radiographs show an abnormal location of the duodenojejunal junction (*arrow*) and the proximal part of the jejunum in the right upper abdominal quadrant and the ileum in the left abdominal quadrants. In (**b**) the *small black arrow* shows narrowing of a jejunal loop due to adhesion (Ladd's bands)

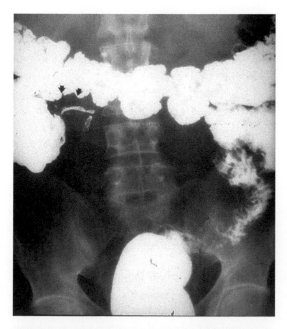

Fig. 2.3 Ladd's bands. Radiograph shows the cecum fixed in the right upper quadrant due to adhesions (Ladd's bands), histologically confirmed

gastrografin, are to be avoided as aspiration causes pulmonary edema that may be fatal. A nasogastric tube is required to administrate oral contrast medium, because the duodenum may be obscured by a contrast-filled and distended stomach. Upper GI malrotation can present with some pathognomonic signs that include an abnormally positioned duodenojejunal junction (Fig. 2.4), a spiral, "corkscrew" or Z-shaped configuration of the distal duodenum and proximal jejunum, and a right located proximal jejunum (Fig. 2.5). The duodenojejunal junction is usually situated in the retroperitoneal cavity and to the left of the spine at the same level or higher than the duodenal bulb. In an anatomical variant, the junction can be displaced inferiorly due to the relative mobility of the ligament of Treitz, and can mimic a malrotation [18]. There are some other conditions that can mimic malrotations on upper GI exams, especially for the duodenum (a mobile, wandering, or inversum duodenum) and peritoneal ligaments. In case of acute intestinal

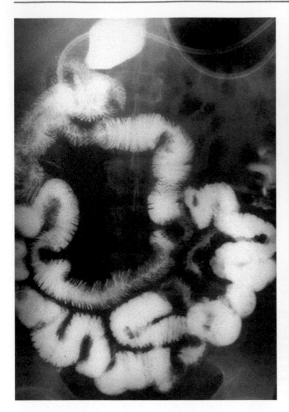

Fig. 2.4 Intestinal malrotation. Enteroclysis shows that the duodenum and jejunum are to the right of the spine

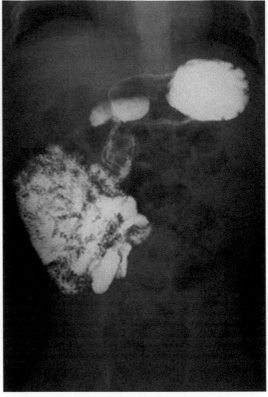

Fig. 2.5 Intestinal malrotation. Delayed radiograph shows the location of jejunal loops in the upper right side of the abdomen

obstruction, especially in children, upper GI images can show some pathognomonic findings such as a narrowed bowel, partially or completely occluded, with consequent dilatation of the proximal duodenum and a characteristic spiral or "corkscrew configuration" of the twisted distal duodenum.

When the obstruction is complete, the typical "corkscrew" image may not be seen because contrast medium may not enter the volvulized loops.

If the obstruction is caused by peritoneal bands, the duodenum can assume also a Z-shaped configuration [18].

The sensitivity of the upper GI series for the diagnosis of malrotation approximates 93 % [19] to 100 % [20]. However, in a retrospective study of 72 patients a significant number of false-positive upper GI diagnoses, supported by subsequent negative laparotomy, were observed. Particularly, 13 patients (18 %) were incorrectly diagnosed. In fact, after laparotomy, 6 (8.3 %)

had normal anatomy, 3 (4.2 %) did not have a volvulus, and 4 (5.5 %) had a malrotation without a volvulus [21].

The diagnostic accuracy of upper GI in diagnosing malrotation may be improved by various maneuvers [18]. First of all, the correct position of the duodenojejunal junction should be detected at the beginning of the exam with the first bolus and studied in both the frontal and lateral projections. In fact, the duodenum may be later displaced or obscured by contrast-filled jejunal loops or by the stomach so that it is important not to overfill the proximal gut initially.

Once it has been established that the duodenojejunal junction is normally positioned, manual epigastric compression can help in the differential diagnosis between malrotation and normal duodenal motility [22]. Sometimes, an immediate contrast enema or delayed abdominal films may be necessary to identify the correct position

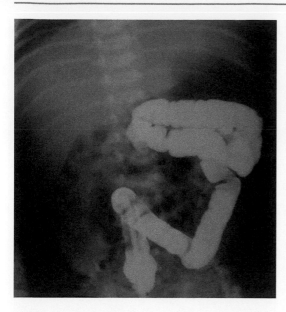

Fig. 2.6 Nonrotation of the colon. Radiograph shows that the entire colon is on the *left*

of the cecum. While the position of the colon may be normal in a child with malrotation, 80 % of individuals with malrotation have an abnormal cecal position (Fig. 2.6). Generally, the shorter the distance between the duodenojejunal junction and the cecal apex, the shorter the length of the SB mesentery and the greater the risk of volvulus. Finally, an inversion of the normal relationship of the SMA and vein seen on US or CT has been described as suggestive of malrotation. Unfortunately, however, this is neither highly specific nor highly sensitive, but when noted should warrant further evaluation for malrotation with an upper GI exam [23].

Barium Imaging of the Small Bowel in Crohn's Disease

Crohn's disease (CD) is a lifelong disease characterized by patchy, transmural inflammation, which may affect any part of the GI tract. The highest annual incidence of CD is 12.7 per 100,000 person-years in Europe, 5.0 person-years in Asia and the Middle East, and 20.2 per 100,000 person-years in North America [24]. The highest prevalence values for inflammatory bowel disease (IBD) are reported in Europe (ulcerative colitis [UC], 505 per 100,000 persons; CD, 322 per 100,000 persons) and North America (UC, 249 per 100,000 persons; CD, 319 per 100,000 persons). In time-trend analyses, 75 % of CD studies and 60 % of UC studies had a statistically significant increased incidence over time ($P < 0.05$) [24].

Establishing the diagnosis and exact distribution of the disease pattern with available local resources is crucial for planning the treatment strategy. A single gold standard for the diagnosis of CD is not available [25, 26]. For suspected CD, ileocolonoscopy and biopsies of both the terminal ileum and each colonic segment are the first-line procedures to establish the diagnosis, for they can verify microscopic evidence of CD. Irrespective of the findings at ileocolonoscopy, further investigation is recommended to examine the location and extent of the disease [25]. CD may affect a part of the ileum not reachable by the endoscope or may involve more of the proximal SB (10 % of patients). Additionally, at the time of diagnosis 15.5–36 % of patients have stricturing or penetrating disease (fistulas, phlegmons, or abscesses) [27, 28]. Endoscopy and radiology are complementary techniques to define the site and extent of the disease, which is important for the treatment plan [25].

Barium contrast examinations have long been the only imaging method providing morphological information of the SB, and have proven valuable in the diagnosis and management of CD. In the last decade, a progressive improvement of cross-sectional imaging has significantly changed the diagnostic and therapeutic work-up of patients [8, 29]. Indeed, these tools can reveal mucosal alterations as well as transmural and perienteric inflammation, leading to a new disease staging, detecting asymptomatic disease and assessing response to therapy [30]. For these reasons, on several systematic reviews and guidelines, modern cross-sectional imaging has replaced the barium studies for visualization of the SB in adult and pediatric populations [25, 26, 31]. In fact, there are definite advantages for the patient using the newer cross-sectional imaging modalities, particularly MR imaging, with the lack of

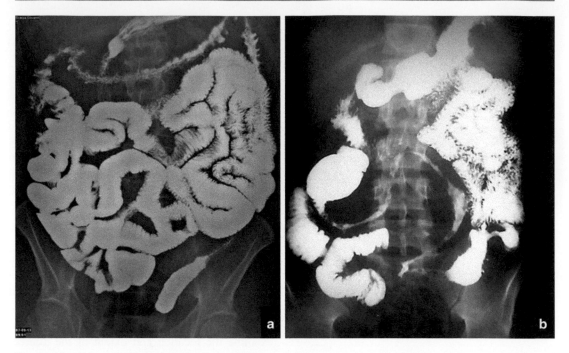

Fig. 2.7 Small bowel follow-through showing the normal filling pattern of the jejunum and ileum loops (**a**), and marked narrowing and mucosal irregularity of several loops of the jejunum in a patient with Crohn's disease (**b**)

ionizing radiation and increased accuracy in the detection of disease. There is, however, limited access to MR in most hospitals and the use of US depends on local expertise. For these and other reasons, to include cost, and the fact that they are noninvasive and easy to read and to perform, barium examinations are still the most available methods for investigating the SB in the majority of radiology departments [32]. Barium studies are a well-established method to investigate the SB in suspected or recurrent CD. In particular, SBFT remains the most commonly performed method for the investigation of SB diseases because of its ease of performance. SBFT can effectively depict transmural CD, but it may be imprecise in cases of mild disease, such as aphthous ulcers or other subtle mucosal abnormalities (Fig. 2.7). This disadvantage can be avoided with the use of enteroclysis, considered in the literature as the most accurate radiologic method in the diagnosis of CD [33]. In fact, it allows a careful estimate of disease extent, the identification of discrete lesions, characterization of strictures, and measurement of the length of unaffected bowel. Moreover, enteroclysis can depict early mucosal alterations, such as

lymphoid nodular hyperplasia, aphthous ulcers, and valvulae conniventes swelling, particularly when double-contrast enteroclysis is performed with air instead of methylcellulose (Fig. 2.8) [34]. Finally, enteroclysis may help in the differential diagnosis between CD and granulomatous enteritis as well as ulcerative colitis. A newer application of barium studies is to exclude an SB stricture in patients with suspicious or known CD before performing CE.

Characteristic findings of CD on barium studies include irregular thickening and alteration of the circular folds and narrowing of the bowel lumen with the presence of different kinds of ulcers, aphthous, larger, linear, and anastomotic. These signs are more often seen in the terminal ileum (Fig. 2.9) and in the first part of the colon, but they may affect any part of the GI tract, from the mouth to the anus. CD has a marked predilection for the terminal ileum with its high concentration of lymphoid tissue; however, additional "skip" lesions can be seen in the proximal SB (Fig. 2.10).

As more severe CD develops, small ulcers become enlarged and deeper and may connect to one another forming stellate, serpiginous, and

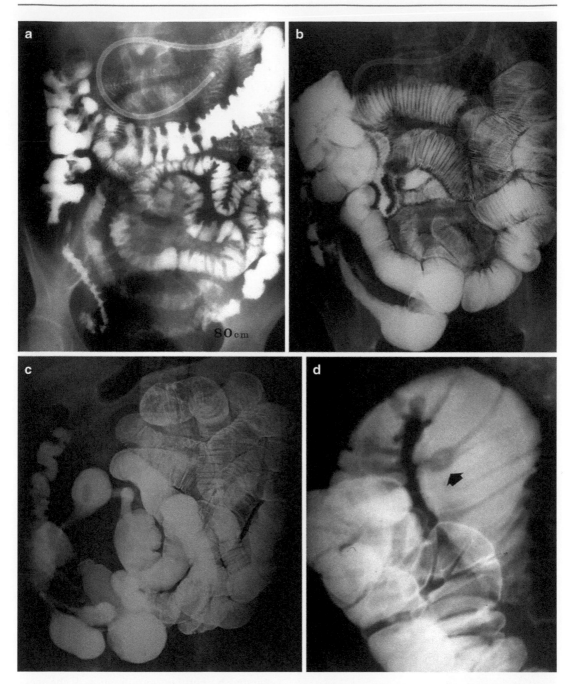

Fig. 2.8 Crohn's disease. (**a**) Enteroclysis shows focally thickened irregular folds and ulcerations of terminal ileum starting from the ileocecal valve extended to 80 cm. (**b**) Enteroclysis shows distal ileum stricturing with fistula. (**c**) Enteroclysis shows multiple stricturing of the distal ileum ("skip" lesions). (**d**) Frontal spot image from enteroclysis shows aphthoid ulcer in a jejunal loop as punctate collections of barium surrounded by radiolucent mounds of edema (*arrow*)

linear ulcers (Fig. 2.11). On SB series or enteroclysis, a mesenteric border ulcer appears as a long 1- to 2-mm barium collection parallel to a short and straight mesenteric border. A radiolucent collar can be usually seen at the margin of the ulcer, parallel to the linear barium collection.

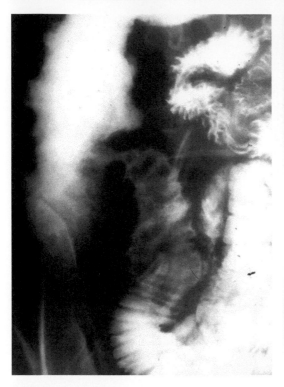

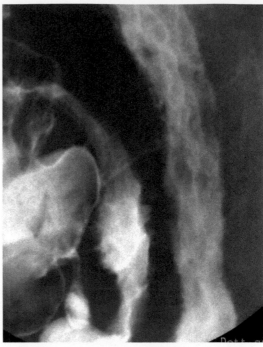

Fig. 2.9 Crohn's disease. Enteroclysis shows thickened irregular valvulae conniventes and mucosal nodularity of the terminal ileum

Fig. 2.11 Crohn's disease. Frontal spot image from enteroclysis demonstrates linear longitudinal and transverse ulcerations that create a cobblestone appearance in the distal ileum

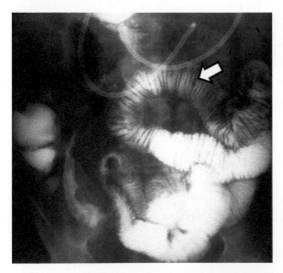

Fig. 2.10 Crohn's disease. Enteroclysis shows mucosal changes of Crohn's disease in the distal ileum, and focally thickened irregular folds in the jejunal loop (*arrow*)

The antimesenteric border of the bowel is usually uninvolved and pulled into the ulcer collar, creating radiating folds. As inflammation penetrates

the submucosa and muscularis layers, deep knife-like linear clefts form the basis of "cobblestoning" that can lead to fissure or fistula formation. They appear as a barium-filled reticular network of grooves that surround round or ovoid radiolucent islands of mucosa. Eventually, transmural inflammation causes a decrease in luminal diameter and a limited wall distensibility, which lead to a radiographic aspect called "string sign," due to a combination of severe edema and spasm or fibrosis. Other radiological signs include antimesenteric border sacculations, focally thickened irregular folds, loop adhesions, and ileal loops separated by fibrofatty proliferation of the mesentery [35] (Figs. 2.12 and 2.13).

Conventional enteroclysis has been shown to be highly accurate, with a sensitivity of 95 % and a specificity of 96.5 % in diagnosing SB diseases. It also permits detection of partially or nonobstructive lesions that may not be demonstrated with cross-sectional imaging techniques [36].

Some investigators have compared SBFT with SBE studies and reported comparable results

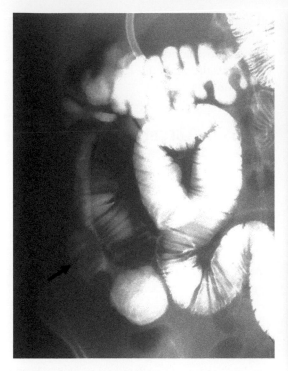

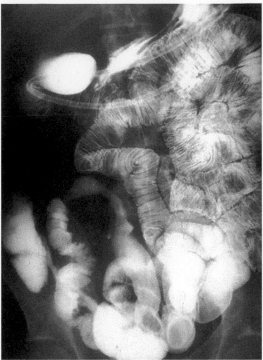

Fig. 2.12 Crohn's disease. Enteroclysis shows pseudodi-verticula (*arrow*) of the antimesenteric wall of the narrowed distal ileum

Fig. 2.13 Crohn's disease. Enteroclysis shows the relatively greater involvement of the mesenteric side of the terminal ileum and the displacement of the involved loop away from the normal small bowel secondary to mesenteric inflammation and fibrofatty proliferation

[37, 38]. However, the per-oral study is preferable as a screening examination because of its noninvasiveness, its safety, the short time required, the lower radiation exposure, and its higher accuracy in detecting gastroduodenal disease compared to SBE. A normal SBFT obviates the need to perform SBE.

Air double-contrast enteroclysis allows detection of subtle surface changes such as mucosal granularity and aphthae better than other radiological methods, but consistently reliable images may be more difficult to obtain [39].

SBFT and SBE show a low, albeit significant, correlation with surgical findings in the assessment of stenotic lesions in terms of number, localization, and extension (Fig. 2.14). These examinations may identify SB obstructions but cannot depict the cause and have a low sensitivity in the detection of extraluminal complications. For these reasons, it is often necessary to perform additional diagnostic exams such as CT or MRI (Fig. 2.15).

In general, the principal disadvantage of barium studies is the limited accuracy in evaluating the state of the bowel wall and the extramural extension of CD, especially in case of overlapping bowel loops.

Moreover, the high radiation dose is another important disadvantage, particularly in young patients and if fluoroscopy time is not kept to a minimum [40]. Gaca et al. [40] studied a total of 176 children with CD who underwent an average of 1.2 SBFTs with an average duration of 5.1 min and about 3.3 abdominal radiographs. The effective doses (mSv) for a 5-min fluoroscopy were 0.15 for the central abdomen, 0.35 for the right lower quadrant, and 0.56 for the pelvis, yielding an average effective dose for SBFT (5-min fluoroscopy, 3.3-min abdominal radiographs) of 1.8–2.2 mSv. Although 5 min of fluoroscopy time for an SBFT might seem excessive, this was calculated based on the average of

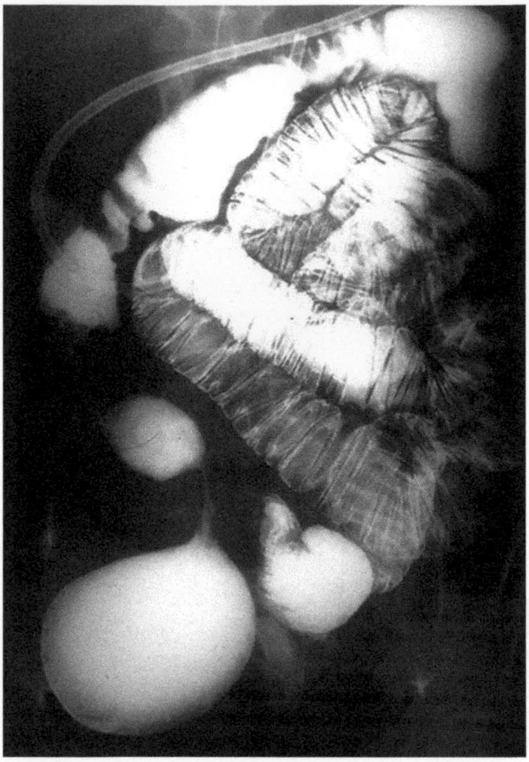

Fig. 2.14 Crohn's disease. Enteroclysis shows multiple narrowed distal ileal segments unchanged during the exam, indicative of fibrotic narrowing

30 examinations performed by five experienced pediatric radiologists. In a young population of CD patients, the ionizing radiation required for SBE limits the use of this technique for follow-up of disease.

Comparison of SBE, SBFT, CE, US, CT, MRI, and Scintigraphy

In a recent study SBFT, CT, and MRI were compared and appeared to be equally accurate in the identification of SB active inflammation. Although the sensitivity values of CT (89 %) and MRI (83 %) were slightly higher than those of SBFT (67–72 %) with regard to active terminal ileitis, these differences were not significant [41].

A prospective blinded trial [42] to assess the sensitivity and specificity of CE, CT enterography (CTE), ileocolonoscopy, and SBFT in the diagnosis of SB CD showed a sensitivity of CE for detecting active inflammation of 83 %, not significantly higher than CTE (83 %), ileocolonoscopy (74 %), or SBFT (65 %). Moreover, its specificity (53 %) was significantly lower than that of the other tests ($P<0.05$). These findings,

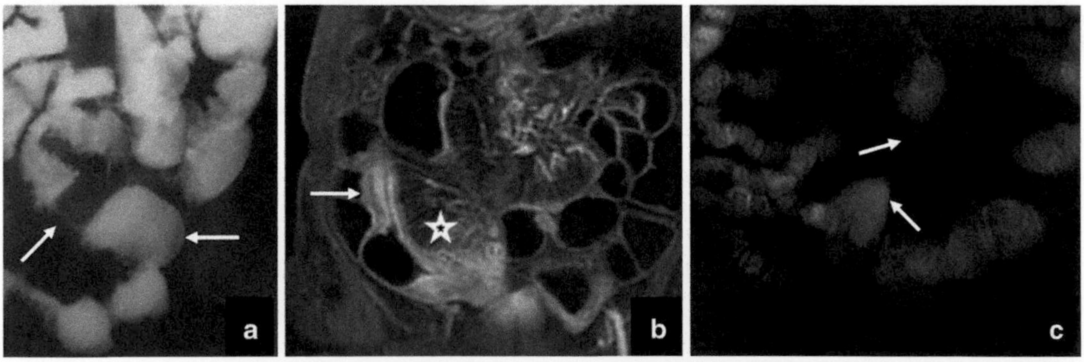

Fig. 2.15 Crohn's disease. Enteroclysis (**a**) shows the presence of marked narrowing of the lumen of the terminal ileum (*arrow*) with dilatation of the proximal bowel loop (*thick arrows*). In the same patient, coronal enhanced T1 GRE MR enteroclysis image (**b**) shows segmental wall thickening with layered enhancement of the wall (mural stratification) causing marked narrowing of the lumen of the terminal ileum (*arrow*), and increased vascularity (*asterisks*), named "comb sign," adjacent to a hyperenhancing thickened segment of ileum. These MR findings are typical of "active" Crohn's disease. MR fluoroscopy sequence (**c**) shows, also, the high-grade stenosis (*arrow*) with dilatation of the bowel loop proximally (*thick arrow*)

in addition to the need to perform an SB radiography to exclude asymptomatic partial SB obstruction that could cause capsule retention, may limit the utility of CE as a first-line test in the diagnosis of CD unless a patency capsule is initially used. A meta-analysis including 33 out of 1,406 studies compared the accuracies of US, MRI, scintigraphy, CT, and positron emission tomography (PET) for diagnosis in patients with suspected or known IBD, mainly CD [29]. The study showed that mean sensitivities for the diagnosis of IBD on a per-patient basis were high and not significantly different among the imaging modalities (90 %, 93 %, 88 %, and 84 % for US, MRI, white blood cell [WBC] scintigraphy, and CT, respectively). The only significant difference in values was found between scintigraphy and US ($P = 0.009$). Mean per-bowel-segment sensitivities were lower: 74 % for US, 70 % for MRI, 77 % for WBC scintigraphy, and 67 % for CT. Mean per-bowel-segment specificities were of 93 % for US, 94 % for MRI, 90 % for WBC scintigraphy, and 90 % for CT. CT proved to be significantly less sensitive and less specific compared to WBC scintigraphy ($P = 0.006$) and MRI ($P = 0.037$). There have been no studies published that have defined the accuracy of PET in the diagnosis of IBD. The authors concluded that no significant differences in diagnostic accuracy among US, CT, MRI, and WBC scintigraphy were observed, and that, because patients with IBD often need frequent reevaluation, the use of a diagnostic modality not involving ionizing radiation is preferable. Conventional enteroclysis is superior to MR enteroclysis in visualizing early and superficial mucosal lesions [8], but CE will probably become the best method for assessing mucosal changes. However, since the inflammatory process in CD does not stop at the mucosa, MR enteroclysis, because of its superb soft tissue contrast, functional information, direct multiplanar capabilities, and lack of radiation exposure, can answer all major clinical questions relevant to patients' treatment and has the potential to become a real one stop shop in the evaluation of CD.

References

1. Maglinte DDT, Rubesin S. Advances in intestinal imaging. Radiol Clin N Am. 2003;41:xi–xii.
2. Levine MS, Rubesin SE, Laufer I. Barium studies in modern radiology: do they have a role? Radiology. 2009;250:18–22.
3. DiSantis DJ. Gastrointestinal fluoroscopy: what are we still doing? AJR. 2008;191:1480–2.
4. Maglinte DDT, Herlinger H. Single contrast and biphasic enteroclysis. In: Herlinger H, Maglinte DDT, editors. Clinical radiology of the small intestine. Philadelphia: WB Sauders; 1989. p. 107–19.
5. Di Mizio R. Morbo di Crohn del tenue. Atlante di Radiologia. Rome: Verduci Editore; 2002.
6. Fanucci A, Cerro P, Fraracci L, Ietto F. Small bowel length measured by radiography. Gastrointest Radiol. 1984;9:349–51.
7. Casciani E, Masselli G, Di Nardio G. MR enterography versus capsule endoscopy in paediatric patients with suspected Crohn's disease. Eur Radiol. 2011;21:823–31.
8. Masselli G, Casciani E, Polettini E, et al. Assessment of Crohn's disease in the small bowel prospective comparison of magnetic resonance enteroclysis with conventional enteroclysis. Eur Radiol. 2006;16:2817–27.
9. Liangpunsakul S, Maglinte DD, Rex DK. Comparison of wireless capsule endoscopy and conventional radiologic methods in the diagnosis of small bowel disease. Gastrointest Endosc Clin N Am. 2004;14:43–50.
10. Hara AK, Leighton JA, Sharma VK, Fleischer DE. Small bowel: preliminary comparison of capsule endoscopy with barium study and CT. Radiology. 2004;230:260–5.
11. Costamagna G, Shah SK, Riccioni ME, et al. A prospective trial comparing small bowel radiographs and video capsule endoscopy for suspected small bowel disease. Gastroenterology. 2002;123:999–1005.
12. Pappalardo G, Gualdi G, Nunziale A, et al. Impact of magnetic resonance in the preoperative staging and the surgical planning for treating small bowel neoplasms. Surg Today. 2013;43:613–9.
13. Beggs AD, Latchford AR, Vasen HFA, et al. Peutze Jeghers syndrome: a systematic review and recommendations for management. Gut. 2010;59:975–86.
14. Ros PR, Huprich JE. ACR Appropriateness Criteria on suspected small-bowel obstruction. J Am Coll Radiol. 2006;3:838–41.
15. Artigas JM, Martì M, Soto J, et al. Multidetector CT angiography for acute gastrointestinal bleeding: technique and findings. Radiographics. 2013;33:1453–70.
16. Long FR, Kramer SS, Markowitz RI, Taylor GE. Radiographic patterns of intestinal malrotation in children. Radiographics. 1996;16:547–56.
17. Millar AJ, Rode H, Cywes S. Malrotation and volvulus in infancy and childhood. Semin Pediatr Surg. 2003;12:229–36.

18. Applegate KJ, Anderson JM, Klatte EC. Intestinal malrotation in children: a problem-solving approach to the upper gastrointestinal series. Radiographics. 2006;26:1485–500.
19. Lin JN, Lou CC, Wang KL. Intestinal malrotation and midgut volvulus: a 15-year review. J Formos Med Assoc. 1995;94(4):178–81.
20. Seashore JH, Touloukian RJ. Midgut volvulus: an ever-present threat. Arch Pediatr Adolesc Med. 1994;148:43–6.
21. Stephens LR, Donoghue V, Gillick J. Radiological versus clinical evidence of malrotation, a tortuous tale—10-year review. Eur J Pediatr Surg. 2012;22:238–42.
22. Lim-Dunham JE, Ben-Ami T, Yousefzadeh DK. Manual epigastric compression during upper gastrointestinal examination of neonates: value in diagnosis of intestinal malrotation and volvulus. AJR. 1999;173:979–83.
23. Strouse PJ. Disorders of intestinal rotation and fixation ("malrotation"). Pediatric Radiol. 2004;34: 837–51.
24. Molodecky NA, Soon IS, Rabi DM, et al. Increasing incidence and prevalence of the inflammatory bowel diseases with time, based on systematic review. Gastroenterology. 2012;142:46–54.
25. Van Assche G, Dignass A, Panes J, et al. The second European evidence-based consensus on the diagnosis and management of Crohn's disease: definitions and diagnosis. J Crohn's Colitis. 2010;4: 7–27.
26. Panes J, Bouhnik Y, Reinisch W, et al. Imaging techniques for assessment of inflammatory bowel disease: joint ECCO and ESGAR evidence-based consensus guidelines. J Crohn's Colitis. 2013;7: 556–85.
27. Mylonaki M, Langmead L, Pantes A, et al. Enteric infection in relapse of inflammatory bowel disease: importance of microbiological examination of stool. Eur J Gastroenterol Hepatol. 2004;16:775–8.
28. Aloi M, Viola F, D'Arcangelo G, et al. Disease course and efficacy of medical therapy in structuring paediatric Crohn's disease. Dig Liver Dis 2013;45: 464–8.
29. Horsthuis K, Bipat S, Bennink RJ, Stoker J. Inflammatory bowel disease diagnosed with US, MR, scintigraphy, and CT: meta-analysis of prospective studies. Radiology. 2008;247:64–79.
30. Mackalski BA, Bernstein CN. New diagnostic imaging tools for inflammatory bowel disease. Gut. 2006;55:733–41.
31. Huprich JE, Rosen MP, Fidler JL, et al. ACR Appropriateness Criteria® on Crohn's disease. J Am Coll Radiol. 2010;7:94–102.
32. Hafeez R, Greenhalgh R, Rajan J, et al. Use of small bowel imaging for the diagnosis and staging of Crohn's disease—a survey of current UK practice. Br J Radiol. 2011;84:508–17.
33. Maglinte DD, Kohli MD, Romano S, Lappas JC. Air (CO_2) double-contrast barium enteroclysis. Radiology. 2009;252(3):633–41.
34. Levine MS, Rubesin SE, Laufer I. Pattern approach for diseases of mesenteric small bowel on barium studies. Radiology. 2008;249:445–60.
35. Makò EK, Mester AR, Tarjan Z, et al. Enteroclysis and spiral CT examination in diagnosis and evaluation of small bowel Crohn's disease. Eur J Radiol. 2000;35:168–75.
36. Ott DJ, Chen YM, Gelfand DW, et al. Detailed per-oral small bowel examination vs. enteroclysis. Part I: expenditures and radiation exposure. Radiology. 1985;155:29–31.
37. Thoeni RF, Gould RG. Enteroclysis and small bowel series: comparison of radiation dose and examination time. Radiology. 1991;178:659–62.
38. Maglinte DDT, Gourtsoyiannis N, Rex D, et al. Classification of small bowel Crohn's subtypes based on multimodality imaging. Radiol Clin N Am. 2003;41:285–303.
39. Patel DR, Levine MS, Rubesin S. Comparison of small bowel follow through and abdominal CT for detecting recurrent Crohn's disease in neoterminal ileum. Eur J Radiol. 2013;82:464–71.
40. Gaca AM, Jaffe TA, Delaney S, et al. Radiation doses from small-bowel follow-through and abdomen/pelvis MDCT in pediatric Crohn disease. Pediatr Radiol. 2008;38:285–91.
41. Solem CE, Loftus Jr EV, Fletcher JG, et al. Small-bowel imaging in Crohn's disease: a prospective, blinded, 4-way comparison trial. Gastrointest Endosc. 2008;68:255–66.
42. Triester SL, Leighton JA, Leontiadis GI, et al. A meta-analysis of the yield of capsule endoscopy compared to other diagnostic modalities in patients with non-stricturing small bowel Crohn's disease. Am J Gastroenterol. 2006;101:954–64.

Endoscopy

3

Blair S. Lewis

Introduction

To look back at the history of endoscopy is to see the driving force and vision of individuals challenging the accepted knowledge of the time. Gastroenterologists are no different from most people and they do not embrace change easily. Early on, conventional wisdom resisted the need for gastroscopy let alone upper endoscopy including the duodenum at the technique's inception. Even the addition of biopsy capability to endoscopes was felt unnecessary by many in the beginning.

The evolution of enteroscopy has been largely the same and did not gain widespread acceptance until recently. Indeed, even the use of capsule endoscopy was a slow evolution. I fully realize that this chapter is not the most practical one in this volume, but a perspective on the development of small bowel imaging is still important. I have been involved in the field of enteroscopy since 1985 and this summary illustrates the work of many others in the field and their commitment to expanding the field of endoscopy despite criticism and resistance from colleagues. Swain referred to enteroscopists as "a tiny band of enthusiasts in showy endoscopy units" performing "an esoteric and rather terrifying procedure" [1]. He was correct, except for the part

B.S. Lewis, M.D. (✉)
Division of Gastroenterology,
Mount Sinai School of Medicine,
1067 Fifth Avenue, New York, NY 10128, USA
e-mail: Blairlewismd@me.com

about "showy endoscopy units." Indeed, when you look through the references you will see a handful of names who carried the torch for a while. But enteroscopy has now come of age and is a rather routine examination revolutionized by capsule endoscopy and overtube assisted devices (e.g., double balloon, single balloon, and spiral enteroscopy). But that is not how it all started.

Flexible upper endoscopy with the ability to view the duodenum began with the development of the Hirschowitz ACMI 4990 fiberscope in October of 1960 [2]. Previous gastroscopes typically only viewed the esophagus and stomach and only rarely could be directed through the pylorus [3]. Previous biopsy forceps were passed alongside the gastroscope and thus directed biopsies were not possible and often the specimens were poor. Although flexible endoscopy was a huge advance over previous rigid and semirigid instruments, many doctors felt that the fiberscope had no future and, indeed, it was difficult to enter the duodenum. Norman Cohen reported 1,000 fiberscope exams in 1966, but stated it was unclear if the duodenum was entered in any examination [4]. Despite lack of acceptance and its own limitations based on size and maneuverability, many new instruments were developed and Olympus began producing a longer, 105 cm, model GIF in 1971. This endoscope became the workhorse of upper endoscopy until the development of video instruments in the 1990s.

Enteroscopy was initially a technology with little application, which slowed its acceptance.

R. Kozarek and J.A. Leighton (eds.), *Endoscopy in Small Bowel Disorders*,
DOI 10.1007/978-3-319-14415-3_3, © Springer International Publishing Switzerland 2015

The small intestine was thought to be a rare site for any pathology and the ability to look at the most proximal and distal ends, during upper endoscopy and colonoscopy, was all that was needed in the evaluation of most patients. Some physicians doubted enteroscopy's clinical usefulness and thus expressed skepticism at the field's development. It was even stated that the development of sonde enteroscopy was unnecessary and most likely too expensive. Incredibly, similar opinions were voiced following the development of capsule endoscopy. But it is now clear that the power to peer into the small bowel changed medical practice and the technology has revolutionized the field.

This is especially true when dealing with a patient with unexplained gastrointestinal bleeding. Prior to the development of these technologies, patients with obscure bleeding were simply transfused. Small bowel cancers were diagnosed late and thus carried a very poor prognosis. Mortalities associated with obscure gastrointestinal bleeding were high. In 1980, Herbsman reported that survival of more than 6 months for adenocarcinoma of the small bowel was rare [5]. In 2006, there were 5,420 new cases of small bowel cancer reported along with 1,070 deaths [6]. It has been shown that early diagnosis improves survival. Early enteroscopy helped determine the etiology of bleeding in such cases and helped determine the most appropriate treatment algorithms. Of 71 patients treated for obscure gastrointestinal bleeding, Szold reported 19 patients with tumors detected early by enteroscopy [7]. In this series, 13 patients were long-term survivors and six died of metastatic disease. In a 2006 retrospective review of 144 patients with primary cancer of the small intestine, the overall 5-year survival was 57 % and the median survival was 52 months [8]. Not surprisingly, survival was best for early-stage tumors and those that could be completely resected. With the development of newer and more effective technologies, the relatively primitive and challenging techniques of rope-way and sonde enteroscopy have been abandoned and forgotten. In addition, there is less of a role for surgery guided by intraoperative enteroscopy. Yet it is important to recognize

that they were instrumental in paving the way forward to where we are today.

Endoscopy of the small bowel was considered to be the last frontier of flexible endoscopy [9]. The usual diagnostic techniques applied to the small bowel were confounded by the small intestine's length and tortuosity, its free intraperitoneal location, and vigorous contractility. These characteristics, in turn, limited the diagnostic ability of barium small bowel studies and limited the identification of specific sites by special imaging techniques such as nuclear medicine scans and angiography. The yield of a barium small bowel series for diagnosing tumors of the small intestine remains quite low as does enteroclysis and even CT enterography.

There was clearly a need to improve the evaluation of the small bowel. Push enteroscopy was one of the early attempts to visualize the small bowel endoscopically. During push enteroscopy, an endoscope is pushed beyond the ligament of Treitz into the proximal jejunum. Push enteroscopy was termed deep upper endoscopy, extended upper endoscopy or simply enteroscopy. Though there is tremendous experience using orally passed colonoscopes as push enteroscopes, the first report of push enteroscopy was in 1973 using an instrument specifically designed for that purpose. Physicians and staff were concerned about the cleanliness of a colonoscope. Though we now accept that a clean instrument is a "clean" instrument, this was not true in the 1970s. Ogoshi reported in 1973 using an Olympus SIF-B to evaluate the proximal small bowel [10]. The instrument was 162 cm in length and had a 1 cm tip diameter. Fluoroscopy was used during intubation and it was estimated that 30 cm of jejunum were visualized. Several more reports followed using this instrument.

Push enteroscopy changed in 1983 when Parker and Agayoff reported that a colonoscope could be safely used instead of a designated instrument [11]. They gas sterilized the instrument prior to its use. This advancement made enteroscopy available to all endoscopists. The other major advance was the acceptance of push enteroscopy as the preferred method to obtain small bowel biopsies. The idea of visually

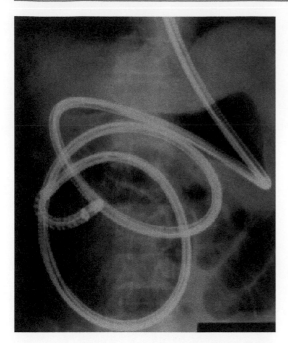

Fig. 3.1 X-ray of push enteroscopy using a 2 m long instrument

directed biopsies was attractive and Parker and Agayoff confirmed that the tissue samples obtained allowed for an adequate diagnosis when compared with suction tube biopsies—the standard at that time. Several studies confirmed the value of obtaining small bowel biopsies with an endoscope. The advantage of endoscopy over the Rubin tube was twofold. First, the endoscopist could visually inspect the mucosa and second, repeated biopsies were possible without removing the instrument.

Push enteroscopy took its next step when longer instruments were developed, measuring 200–225 cm in working length (Fig. 3.1). Stiffening overtubes were also created to allow even deeper small bowel intubation. By 1984, push enteroscopy had become mainstream. Several indications were proffered including evaluation of patients with obscure gastrointestinal bleeding and for the placement of jejunal feeding tubes. Messer, using a pediatric colonoscope, reported finding the bleeding site in 20 of 52 patients with obscure gastrointestinal bleeding [12]. Findings included angiodysplasias in 9 and small bowel tumors in 11. Foutch used an orally

passed adult colonoscope and reported a yield of 38 % in 39 patients [13]. Chong reported finding a possible cause of bleeding in 64 % of 55 patients using the newer push enteroscope in combination with an overtube [14]. Push enteroscopy was therapeutic as well. Using bipolar cautery, Foutch was able to fulgurate angiodysplasias in 11 of 12 patients [13] and control of bleeding was attained in 8 of 11 treated patients. Askin and Lewis followed 55 patients who had cauterization of jejunal angiodysplasias for an average of 3 years [15]. This group required significantly fewer total transfusions when compared with their precauterization status as well as when compared to a cohort of patients who were not cauterized. Morris confirmed the effectiveness of cauterization at push enteroscopy in a group of 11 transfusion dependent patients [16].

It was 1982 when the first report demonstrated the use of enteroscopy in the diagnosis of a small bowel tumor. Shinya reported on the initial use of both sonde and push enteroscopy and described finding a duodenal adenocarcinoma and a jejunal hemangiolymphangioma [17]. The role of enteroscopy in the diagnosis of small bowel tumors has developed since that time. Often, small bowel tumors were diagnosed by other means and were confirmed by enteroscopy. Parker reported finding a large neurofibroma within the proximal jejunum [11]. Hashmi reported a 22-year-old woman presenting with melena [18]. The jejunal leiomyoma was diagnosed initially by angiography and was subsequently confirmed by push enteroscopy and enteroclysis. Shigematsu reported three patients with lymphangiomas of the small bowel diagnosed on small bowel series and subsequently confirmed on push enteroscopy [19]. Watatani reported, in 1989, a 73-year-old woman with nausea and vomiting in whom a small bowel series showed a distal duodenal lesion [20]. Push enteroscopy not only confirmed this lesion, but a biopsy was performed that revealed this to be adenocarcinoma preoperatively.

Push enteroscopy was also used to place jejunal feeding tubes. The initial idea was to carry a transgastric jejunal tube through a previous gastrostomy into the jejunum. Direct percutaneous jejunostomies were the next to be described.

Nasojejunal feeding tubes were also placed. The enteroscope was advanced to the jejunum, a guidewire was advanced through the instrument and the instrument was removed leaving the guidewire. The wire was transferred through the nasal passage and then using the Seldinger technique, the nasojejunal tube was positioned. This was used for feeding as well as to place catheters for enteroclysis and to obtain cholangiograms in patients after Roux-en-Y hepatic jejunostomies. Polypectomies were described as well as surveillance of patient with polyposis syndromes.

The rope-way method of enteroscopy was the oldest method to totally intubate the small intestine [21, 22]. It was in 1972, 4 years after the first description of colonoscopy, that Classen reported this procedure. The technique involved having a patient swallow a guide string and allowing it to pass through the rectum. The string was then exchanged for a somewhat stiffer Teflon tube over which an endoscope was passed. A complete endoscopic examination was obtained with this method. The instruments were fully therapeutic including cauterization and polypectomy. Unfortunately, the exam was painful due to tightening of the guide-tube and often-required general anesthesia. Due to patient discomfort, length of time necessary for string passage and development of better-tolerated techniques, the rope-way method was abandoned. Classen abandoned the technique shortly after his first report and described it as a "rigorous procedure" that was "traumatic to the patient." Video rope-way enteroscopes were also developed but these had the same limitations of the non-video versions [23].

Another development was endostomy, a procedure that involved creating an enterocutaneous fistula that could then allow a thin endoscope to intubate the small bowel [24]. Frimberger reported this technique in one patient. The fistulae were created using standard Ponsky gastrostomy techniques in the jejunum and in the cecum. After the tracts matured in 8–10 days, thin (4 mm diameter) prototype endoscopes were inserted through the jejunostomy and cecostomy to evaluate the intestine. Although innovative, this procedure was never accepted.

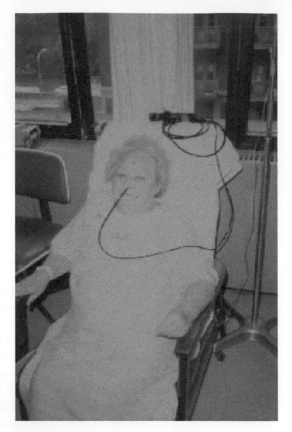

Fig. 3.2 Patient undergoing sonde enteroscopy while the instrument was carried into the small bowel by peristalsis

The last of the historical procedures is sonde enteroscopy. This was termed small bowel enteroscopy or long tube enteroscopy. The term sonde came from the French word for probe. In essence, it was an endoscopic Cantor tube, used for small bowel obstruction. A thin transnasal endoscope had a hood or balloon on its tip that allowed peristalsis to drag the instrument distally (Fig. 3.2). The endoscopic exam was performed during withdrawal of the scope. Development of sonde enteroscopy spanned nearly 13 years [25]. Prototype SSIF (sonde small intestinal fiberscope) I thru IV had narrow fields of vision (60°) and a large diameter (11 mm). Initially, a metal hood was placed at the instrument tip and used to induce distal passage. Subsequent prototypes had utilized a balloon at the tip that was inflated upon placement in the small bowel. Early enteroscopes were fitted with magnifying lenses to evaluate villi shape and were used in the diagnosis of

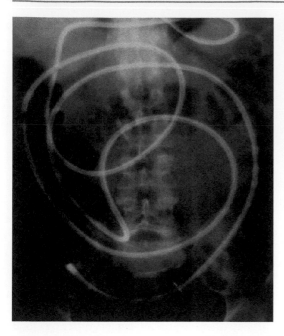

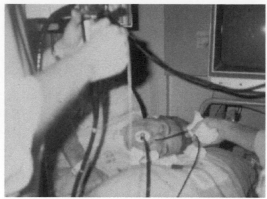

Fig. 3.4 Insertion of sonde enteroscope with orally passed colonoscope

Fig. 3.3 X-ray of sonde enteroscopy with total small bowel intubation

tuberculosis and malabsorption states [26]. Attempts to introduce tip deflection capability in the fifth prototype made the instrument too stiff for distal intubation [27, 28]. Oral passage, which was required with these thick instruments, was associated with patient salivation, gagging, and considerable discomfort [29]. A thin, flexible, transnasal enteroscope was developed in 1986 [30] with a tip diameter of 5 mm and a length of 2,560 mm. The instrument's forward angle of view was initially 90°, but was subsequently increased to 120°. This instrument, in contrast to a push enteroscope, had no biopsy or therapeutic capability and no tip deflection. An attempt to add biopsy capability to this instrument in the tenth prototype was successful, but targeting the biopsy remained a problem since there was no tip deflection [31]. The major standard sonde enteroscope, the SIF-SW (small intestinal fiberscope—sonde, wide) did not have this biopsy channel, but remained transnasally passed with a fisheye lens (Fig. 3.3). Video technology was also applied to sonde enteroscopy. Dabezies reported on a video sonde enteroscope used in seven patients [32]. The instrument's tip measured 11 mm, due to the presence of the video chip, necessitating

oral passage. The instrument did not use a balloon, and depth of intubation was limited.

The original technique to position a sonde enteroscope within the jejunum was to pass the instrument transnasally, lay the patient on their right side and follow the patient with sequential fluoroscopy. My first exposure to sonde enteroscopy was watching a videotape of Dr. Tada performing the examination on himself! A technique to rapidly place the enteroscope into the jejunum was developed to shorten the examination time. This rapid technique used a push enteroscope to grasp a suture affixed to the sonde instrument tip and actually "push" the scope into the jejunum (Fig. 3.4). The advantage of this technique was that it permitted total or near total small bowel intubation within 8 h and thus allowed the procedure to be performed on an ambulatory basis. The original technique averaged 24 h.

Sonde enteroscopy proved itself useful in the evaluation of the patient with presumed small intestinal bleeding. Initially, Lewis and Waye reported results of the technique in 60 patients with obscure gastrointestinal bleeding. In this report, a small bowel site of blood loss was detected in 33 % [33]. A later report by Lewis detailed results in 504 patients [34]. In patients with obscure gastrointestinal bleeding, combined push and sonde enteroscopy documented findings in 42 % of patients. Eighteen percent of the lesions were found in the region covered by push enteroscopy but distal to the area examined by standard upper endoscopy. Twenty-six percent of the lesions were found in the remaining bowel examined by sonde enteroscopy. Vascular ectasias constituted 80 % of the findings overall and small bowel tumors accounted for 10 %. Several of the tumors discovered occurred in patients after a falsely negative enteroclysis [35]. Similar experience using sonde enteroscopy was reported by Barthel with a yield of 27.8 % in 18 patients [36], by Gostout with a yield of 26 % in 35 patients [37], and by Morris with a yield of 38 % in 65 patients [38].

Significantly, the nature of vascular lesions was better understood from these studies. Lewis reported an average age of 69 years in 102 patients with small intestinal angiodysplasias, without a sex predilection [33]. Angiodysplasias of the small bowel presented with either brisk or occult bleeding. Patients usually had only fecal occult blood test positivity or melena. Red or maroon blood per rectum was uncommon. Lewis reported that melena was the presenting sign in 64 % of 102 patients with bleeding small bowel angiodysplasias, while 36 % had occult blood in the stool. His findings also confirmed autopsy data by Meyer [39] who reviewed 218 angiodysplasias and found 2.3 % in the duodenum, 10.5 % in the jejunum, and 8.5 % in the ileum. Lewis also found that most patients had only a few vascular lesions that were countable, and all could be found within the same segment of small bowel. Diffuse lesions were much less common and were seen in less than 3 % of all patients with small bowel vascular lesions.

Despite numerous advances in sonde enteroscopy, it became clear that sonde enteroscopy had distinct disadvantages. The time required made it tedious for both patient and physician. Adhesions, strictures, and motility disturbances limited passive passage of the instrument. Even when complete small bowel intubation was achieved, total mucosal inspection was never complete. The lack of tip deflection and the inability to readvance the instrument once withdrawal had begun limited the mucosal view. Instruments also proved to be fragile and only one patient could be examined per day using the one instrument. Although this technology was a major advance and helped

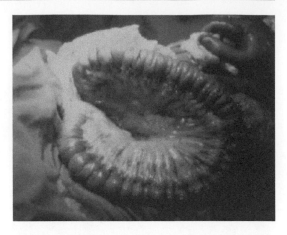

Fig. 3.5 The entire small bowel pleated onto a sterile colonoscope during intraoperative enteroscopy

define obscure gastrointestinal bleeding, sonde enteroscopy was found to be inefficient. At its heyday there were 29 centers offering sonde enteroscopy, but by 1999 there were only 10, and today it is totally forgotten.

Intraoperative enteroscopy remains the fallback procedure to allow total small bowel endoscopic examination when other procedures are unsuccessful. Colonoscopes are routinely employed for this examination, though a push enteroscope may also be used (Fig. 3.5). The instrument does not need to be sterile, since the recommended technique involves peroral intubation of the small intestine. The proximal jejunum is intubated prior to the performance of the laparotomy, since once the abdomen is open, it may be difficult to advance the instrument around the ligament of Treitz due to excessive, and unopposed, bowing of the endoscope shaft along the greater curvature of the stomach. With oral intubation of an adult colonoscope, the endotracheal tube cuff may need to be deflated to permit passage of the wide caliber endoscope. Once the colonoscope is placed within the proximal jejunum, laparotomy is performed. A non-crushing clamp is placed across the ileocecal valve to prevent distention of the colon with insufflated air. Colonic distention can lead to difficulties with subsequent abdominal closure.

The endoscopic exam is performed by having the surgeon grasp the endoscope tip and hold a short segment of bowel straight to allow endoscopic

Fig. 3.6 Intraoperative enteroscopy with instrument placed in sterile sleeve and then advanced into the small bowel

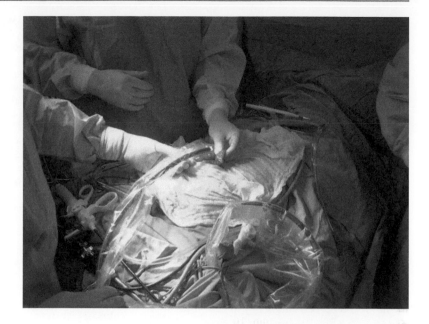

inspection. The view is best seen by dimming the overhead lights, which also allows the surgeon to visualize the transilluminated bowel. Once examined both internally and externally, the small bowel is pleated onto the shaft of the endoscope and the next section of bowel is examined. Active bleeding within the small bowel may limit the effectiveness of this examination. Generally, examination is performed only during intubation since mucosal trauma occurs with the pleating and may be confused with the appearance of angioectasia on withdrawal [40]. Lesions identified with intraoperative enteroscopy are marked by the surgeon with a suture placed on the serosal surface of the small intestine. At the end of the examination, the endoscope is withdrawn and sites of resection are identified by the sutures. There are other techniques of intraoperative enteroscopy. This author performs an enterotomy through which an enteroscope covered by a sterile plastic sheath is placed (Fig. 3.6).

Intraoperative endoscopy has been used for several reasons. It is presently the endoscopic method most widely used in identifying small intestinal sites of bleeding (Fig. 3.7). This most typically involves a bleeding site identified on capsule endoscopy and not approachable by other endoscopic means. Intraoperative enteroscopy is also used in cases where surgical guidance is

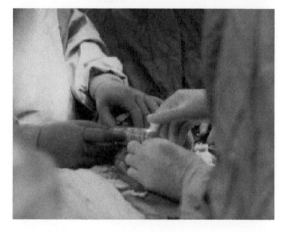

Fig. 3.7 Surgeons pleat the small bowel onto a colonoscope at intraoperative enteroscopy

needed to limit small bowel resection. This is especially true in patients with hereditary hemorrhagic telangiectasia (HHT) syndrome where there are often diffuse lesions that are limited to the jejunum. The diffuse nature often limits enteroscopic management, and the surgeon needs to know where these lesions are located. Intraoperative enteroscopy is also used in patients with small bowel polyposis such as Peutz–Jeghers. Multiple polypectomies can be performed, and the specimens can be removed through enterotomy, limiting resection. Finally, intraoperative enteroscopy has been used to identify and guide resection of diaphragm disease of the small bowel caused by nonsteroidal anti-inflammatory drugs. These stenotic diaphragms of the small bowel are not palpable, and endoscopic guidance is often necessary intraoperatively.

Conclusion

Enteroscopy has changed dramatically since these early days, and no longer is the small bowel considered the rare site of pathology nor considered an area not accessible by endoscopic means. Yet the development of present-day capsule endoscopy or balloon or overtube assisted enteroscopy came from the steady work of individuals who did not accept the norm and pushed endoscopy to new vistas.

References

1. Appleyard M, Fireman Z, Glukhovsky A, Jacob H, Shreiver R, Kadirkamanathan S, Lavy A, Lewkowicz S, Scapa E, Shofti R, Swain P, Zaretsky A. A randomized trial comparing wireless capsule endoscopy with push enteroscopy for the detection of small-bowel lesions. Gastroenterology. 2000;119:1431–8.
2. Hirschowitz B. Endoscopic examination of the stomach and duodenal cap with the fiberscope. Lancet. 1961;1:1074–78.
3. Modlin I. Brief history of endoscopy. Milano, Italy: MultiMed; 2000.
4. Cohen N, Hughes R, Manfredo H. Experience with 1000 fibergastroscope examinations of the stomach. Am J Dig Dis. 1966;11:943–50.
5. Herbsman H, Wetstein L, Rosen Y, et al. Tumors of the small intestine. Curr Probl Surg. 1980;17:121.
6. American Cancer Society; Cancer facts and figures 2005. p. 4; http://www.cancer.org/acs/groups/content/@nho/documents/document/caff2005f4pwsecuredpdf.pdf.
7. Szold A, Katz LB, Lewis BS. Surgical approach to occult gastrointestinal bleeding. Am J Surg. 1992;163(1):90–2.
8. North JH, Pack MS. Malignant tumors of the small intestine: a review of 144 cases. Am Surg. 2000;66(1):46–51.
9. Lewis B, Waye J. Small bowel enteroscopy in 1988: pros and cons. Am J Gastroenterol. 1988;83:799–802.
10. Ogoshi K, Hara Y, Ashizawa S. New technic for small intestinal fiberoscopy. Gastrointest Endosc. 1973;20:64–5.
11. Parker H, Agayoff J. Enteroscopy and small bowel biopsy utilizing a peroral colonoscope. Gastrointest Endosc. 1983;29:139–40.
12. Messer J, Romeu J, Waye J, Dave P. The value of proximal jejunoscopy in unexplained gastrointestinal bleeding. Gastrointest Endosc. 1984;30:151.
13. Foutch PG, Sawyer R, Sanowski R. Push-enteroscopy for diagnosis of patients with gastrointestinal bleeding of obscure origin. Gastrointest Endosc. 1990;36:337–41.
14. Chong J, Tagle M, Barkin JS, Reiner DK. Small bowel push-type fiberoptic enteroscopy for patients with occult gastrointestinal bleeding or suspected small bowel pathology. Am J Gastroenterol. 1994;89:2143–6.
15. Askin MP, Lewis BS. Push enteroscopic cauterization: long-term follow-up of 83 patients with bleeding small intestinal angiodysplasia. Gastrointest Endosc. 1996;43(6):580–3.
16. Morris AJ, Mokhashi M, Straiton M, Murray L, Mackenzie JF. Push enteroscopy and heater probe therapy for small bowel bleeding. Gastrointest Endosc. 1996;44:394–7.
17. Shinya H, McSherry C. Endoscopy of the small bowel. Surg Clin North Am. 1982;62:821–4.
18. Hashmi M, Sorokin J, Levine S. Jejunal leiomyoma: an endoscopic diagnosis. Gastrointest Endosc. 1985;31:81–3.
19. Shigematsu A, Iida M, Hatanaka M, et al. Endoscopic diagnosis of lymphangioma of the small intestine. Am J Gastroenterol. 1988;83:1289–93.
20. Watatani M, Yasuda N, Imamoto H, et al. Primary small intestinal adenocarcinoma diagnosed by endoscopic examination prior to operation. Gastroenterol Jpn. 1989;24:402–6.
21. Deyhle P, Jenny S, Fumagalli J. Endoscopy of the whole small intestine. Endoscopy. 1972;4:155–7.
22. Classen M, Fruhmergen P, Koch H. Peroral enteroscopy of the small and large intestine. Endoscopy. 1972;4:157–62.
23. Sato N, Tamegai Y, Yamakawa T, Hiratsuka H. Clinical applications of the small intestinal videoendoscope. Endoscopy. 1992;24:631 (abstr).
24. Frimberger E, Hagenmuller F, Classen M. Endostomy: a new approach to small-bowel endoscopy. Endoscopy. 1989;21:86–8.
25. Tada M, Kawai K. Small bowel endoscopy. Scand J Gastroenterol. 1984;19 Suppl 102:39–52.
26. Tada M, Misaki F, Kawai K. Endoscopic observation of villi with magnifying enterocolonoscopes. Gastrointest Endosc. 1982;28:17–9.
27. Tada M, Akasaka Y, Misaki F, et al. Clinical evaluation of a sonde-type small intestinal fiberscope. Endoscopy. 1977;9:33–8.
28. Tada M, Misaki F, Kawai K. Pediatric enteroscopy with a sonde-type small intestinal fiberscope (SSIF VI). Gastrointest Endosc. 1983;29:44–7.
29. Lewis B, Waye J. A comparison of 2 sonde-type small bowel enteroscopes in 100 patients: the SSIF VII and the SSIF VI KAI. Gastroenterology. 1988;94:A261.
30. Tada M, Shimizu S, Kawai K. A new transnasal sonde-type fiberscope (SSIF VII) as a pan-enteroscope. Endoscopy. 1986;18:121–4.
31. Tada M, Shimizu S, Kawai K. Small bowel endoscopy with a new transnasal sonde-type fiberscope (SSIF-Type 10). Endoscopy. 1992;24:631 (abstr).

32. Dabezies M, Fisher R, Krevsky B. Video small bowel enteroscopy: early experience with a prototype instrument. Gastrointest Endosc. 1991;37:60–2.

33. Lewis B, Waye J. Gastrointestinal bleeding of obscure origin: the role of small bowel enteroscopy. Gastroenterology. 1988;94:1117–20.

34. Berner J, Mauer K, Lewis B. Push and sonde enteroscopy for obscure GI bleeding. Am J Gastroenterol. 1994;89:2139–42.

35. Lewis B, Kornbluth A, Waye J. Small bowel tumors: the yield of enteroscopy. Gut. 1991;32:763–5.

36. Barthel J, Vargo J, Sivak M. Assisted passive enteroscopy and gastrointestinal tract bleeding of obscure origin. Gastrointest Endosc. 1990;36:222.

37. Gostout CJ. Sonde enteroscopy. Technique, depth of insertion, and yield of lesions. Gastrointest Endosc Clin N Am. 1996;6:777–92.

38. Morris A, Wasson L, MacKenzie J. Small bowel enteroscopy in undiagnosed gastrointestinal blood loss. Gut. 1992;33:887–9.

39. Meyer C, Troncale F, Galloway S, Sheahan D. Arteriovenous malformations of the bowel: an analysis of 22 cases and a review of the literature. Medicine. 1981;60:36–48.

40. Frank M, Brandt L, Boley S. Iatric submucosal hemorrhage: a pitfall of intraoperative endoscopy. Am J Gastroenterol. 1981;75:209–10.

Part III

Recent Noninvasive Imaging Modalities

CT Enterography

4

Joel G. Fletcher, Amy B. Kolbe,
and David H. Bruining

Overview

CT enterography (CTE) has become a key component for the diagnosis and management of small intestinal diseases and lesions. As a radiologic modality designed to optimize visualization of the small bowel and surrounding structures, it can be utilized for an extremely diverse set of indications. CTE in adult and pediatric Crohn's disease patients can detect active inflammation, stricturing disease, and penetrating complications, and assess response to medical therapy. It can also demonstrate extraintestinal inflammatory bowel disease manifestations and alternate etiologies for a patient's symptoms of abdominal pain or diarrhea. Additional CTE applications include the diagnosis of small bowel tumors and vascular lesions in patients with obscure gastrointestinal bleeding. These features have made CTE a vital tool in the clinician's small bowel imaging armamentarium.

4

J.G. Fletcher, M.D. (✉) • A.B. Kolbe, M.D.
Department of Radiology, Mayo Clinic,
200 First Street SW, Rochester, MN 55905, USA
e-mail: fletcher.joel@mayo.edu

D.H. Bruining, M.D.
Division of Gastroenterology and Hepatology,
Mayo Clinic, 200 First Street SW, Rochester,
MN 55905, USA
e-mail: bruining.david@mayo.edu

Introduction

CTE has gained widespread acceptance in abdominal imaging and gastroenterology as a powerful technique to visualize small bowel inflammation and masses and to guide therapeutic decision making. Its adoption was initially aided by recognition that small bowel fluoroscopy is limited in its visualization of mucosal detail compared to modern endoscopic techniques [1, 2]. The past decade has provided evidence for the complementarity and uniqueness of CTE findings compared to capsule and balloon-assisted endoscopy, e.g., intramural and perienteric findings that provide important adjunctive information not provided by direct luminal visualization [3–5]. For example, many small bowel tumors can arise within the small bowel wall with intact, overlying mucosa, and many complications of Crohn's disease (such as perienteric fistula or mesenteric venous thromboses) can directly affect management of care and are usually not that visualized at endoscopy. While vascular lesions are directly visualized with endoscopic techniques, CTE can provide important information relating to size and arteriovenous shunting that may influence treatment [6]. In this chapter, we highlight the imaging findings at CTE, with an emphasis on differential diagnosis, summarize indications and evidence for use of CTE, as well as review technical adaptations that maximize patient benefit while minimizing risk. Finally, we suggest a perspective for incorporating CTE into multimodality adult and pediatric GI practices.

General Principles and Patient Preparation

Prior to reviewing imaging findings, a basic understanding of CTE patient preparation is necessary. CTE is an abdominopelvic CT in which patient preparation and image acquisition and reconstruction methods have been adapted to maximize visualization of the small bowel lumen, wall, and perienteric mesentery. Patient preparation requires ingestion of a relatively large volume of enteric contrast (900–1,800 cc) administered over 45–60 min prior to CT examination to distend the small bowel lumen [7–9]. The enteric contrast agent is selected based on potential pathologies and the patient's ability to ingest different agents, but most small bowel pathologies are best visualized with the use of neutral enteric contrast, which possesses CT attenuation similar to water. Hyperenhancing masses and inflammation and vascular structures are conspicuous when juxtaposed against low-attenuation perienteric fat and a neutral enteric contrast agent [10, 11]. Most neutral contrast agents contain sugar alcohols or similar substances, which retard water absorption along the small bowel to result in better luminal distension [9]. Owing to the need for patient ingestion, CTE is generally performed as an outpatient procedure; when performed in the emergency room or hospital, it is often performed only with water. CTE is usually performed as a single acquisition, usually in the "enteric phase" of contrast enhancement, approximately 50 s after the start of intravenous injection, as this is the time period of maximal small bowel enhancement [12]. When synchronous imaging of other organs, such as the liver, is required, hepatic phase imaging can also be performed without demonstrable loss in performance for identification and staging of Crohn's disease [13]. For patients with potential pancreatic or small bowel pathology, the timing of the "pancreatic phase"

of enhancement is identical to the enteric phase. Multiphase CTE is reserved for detection and characterization of causes of obscure gastrointestinal bleeding, as multiphasic exams are required to confidently diagnose active bleeding (as demonstrated by extravasation of intravenous contrast into the bowel lumen) and vascular lesions [14]. Patient preparation, image acquisition, and reconstruction parameters are tailored to meet the individual needs of each patient and their indication for imaging, or diagnostic task (see later section: Adaptations).

Imaging Findings

Visual review of CTE findings can be classified according to the small bowel segment (i.e., duodenum, jejunum, or ileum); mural thickening and enhancement, symmetry, and location within the bowel wall (i.e., intramural, luminal, or related to diverticula); and perienteric findings. The distribution and enhancing nature of the lesions will further aid in differential diagnosis and guide subsequent imaging and treatment options.

The Normal Small Bowel

Radiologists and gastroenterologists should be familiar with the appearance of the normal bowel at CTE. The jejunum demonstrates numerous feathery folds, the valvulae conniventes. The jejunal and ileal wall thickness should be 3 mm or less when the small bowel is distended, but can be thicker when collapsed or in peristalsis. Owing to the feathery valvulae conniventes, the jejunum wall is often falsely interpreted as having mural thickening when the lumen is only collapsed and the folds are coapting with each other (Fig. 4.1). The duodenum has a similar appearance to the jejunum, with the transverse portion crossing underneath the SMA to enter the left upper quadrant. The proximal jejunum may be located in the left upper quadrant or may cross into the right lower quadrant. Both the duodenum and jejunum will enhance to a substantially greater degree than the ileum during the enteric phase, with

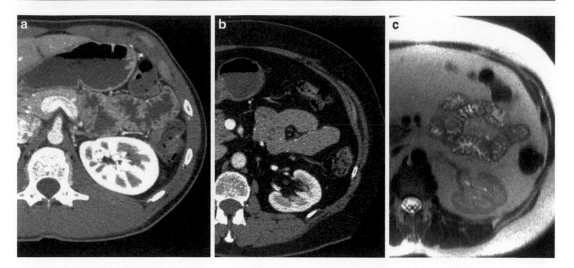

Fig. 4.1 Normal appearance of jejunum at CT enterography. Note thin and regularly spaced valvulae conniventes in distended jejunum (**a**). Collapsed jejunum in another patient at CT enterography (**b**) shows normal appearance as lumen collapses and jejunal folds coapt together. Forty minutes after CT in (**b**), patient underwent MR enterography showing normal jejunal loops and folds (**c**)

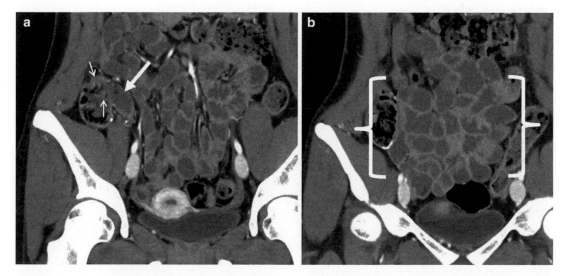

Fig. 4.2 Coronal CT enterography images showing normal appearance of terminal (**a**, *arrow*) and distal (**b**, *between brackets*) ileum. Note paucity of folds, thin wall, and slightly decreased mural enhancement. *Small arrows* (**a**) show ileocecal valve, which is located within a haustral fold in the cecum

enhancement becoming more similar across the length of the small bowel in later phases of enhancement [15]. The terminal ileum enters the cecum at the ileocecal valve, which has a "fish-mouth" shape and is located within a cecal fold (Fig. 4.2). It is normal for the terminal ileum to contain intramural fat, and this should not be regarded as a sign of chronic inflammation within the terminal ileum, as it is in other enteric locations [16]. The small bowel vasculature should be carefully evaluated along with the small bowel. The mesenteric arteries are best evaluated on the sagittal view; the mesenteric veins are best appreciated on coronal images.

Mural Findings

Mural hyperenhancement is generally seen in the presence of mural thickening, and it is a nonspecific sign of inflammation or altered perfusion. The combination of segmental mural hyperenhancement and mural thickening is specific for Crohn's disease when the enhancement and mural thickening are asymmetric with respect to the bowel lumen—for example, worse along the mesenteric border (Fig. 4.3). Similar to findings at small bowel follow-through where the mesenteric border linear ulcers are pathopneumonic for Crohn's disease, inflammation as represented by CT findings of hyperenhancement and mural thickening are seen most prominently along the mesenteric border, often with pseudosacculation along the anti-mesenteric border, with prominent vasa recta that supply the inflamed bowel segment. Jejunal Crohn's involvement occurs in about 15 % of Crohn's

patients, is associated with an increased incidence of stricturoplasty and hospitalizations [17], and is frequently overlooked by novice radiologists and gastroenterologists (Figs. 4.4 and 4.5). While there are a number of other causes of segmental jejunal hyperenhancement and mural thickening, including infection (often giardia), ulcerative jejunitis in sprue, vasculitis, and systemic infiltrating diseases, only Crohn's disease typically involves the bowel in an asymmetric fashion (whether proximal or distal). Segmental hyperenhancement without wall thickening can be seen in early Crohn's disease, as well as other causes of hyperenhancement, and generally reflects more mild degrees of inflammation. Radiation enteritis and NSAID-related diaphragm disease also demonstrate segmental hyperenhancement in conjunction with focal strictures in the mid to distal small bowel. Both types of strictures are short (often 1–2 cm) and symmetric with respect to the bowel lumen

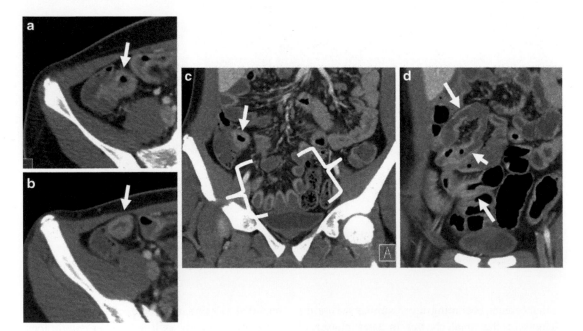

Fig. 4.3 Typical appearance of Crohn's ileitis at CT enterography in patient with erythematous mucosa at ileoscopy. Note mural thickening and hyperenhancement of terminal ileum on axial and coronal images (**a**–**c**, *arrows*). In distal ileal loops, inflammation as demonstrated by hyperenhancement and wall thickening is more prominent along the mesenteric border (**c**, *between brackets*), so is asymmetric with respect to bowel lumen. Multiple skip lesions (**d**, *arrow*) are present in the mid-ileum. Findings demonstrate the complementarity of CT enterography with endoscopic assessment. Biopsy at ileoscopy showed active and chronic ileitis

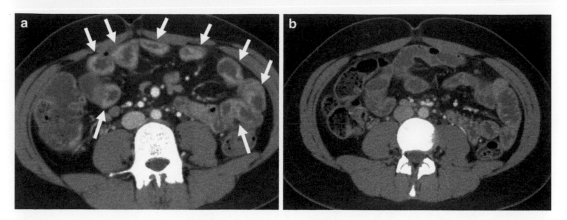

Fig. 4.4 Typical findings of jejunal Crohn's disease in 18-year-old Crohn's patient with asymmetric thickening and hyperenhancement of multiple loops (**a**, *arrows*). After combination therapy (infliximab combined with azathioprine), CT enterography 2 years later demonstrates normal appearance to the previously inflamed jejunal loops (**b**)

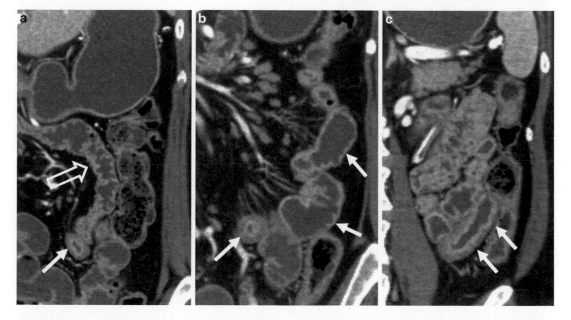

Fig. 4.5 CT enterography images from another patient with jejunal Crohn's disease show normal-appearing jejunum (*open arrow*, **a**) superior to inflamed jejunum (**a**, *solid white arrow*). Note prominent vasa recta along mesenteric border of other jejunal loops (**b**, *arrows*), in addition to disruption of fold pattern and asymmetric enhancement. Some inflamed loops have a layered or stratified appearance to the thickened bowel wall (**a–c**, *arrow*)

[18, 19]. Strictures in the setting of radiation enteritis occur in small bowel with abnormal enhancement, while those in diaphragm disease have variable (often mild) hyperenhancement with intervening regions of normal-appearing bowel. Celiac sprue typically manifests as normally enhancing jejunal loops that have lost valvulae conniventes due to villous atrophy, usually with fold reversal (or increased number of folds) in the ileum (Fig. 4.6). Hypoenhancing bowel can be a worrisome finding for ischemia, and when pneumatosis is present, infarction is often present. As ischemia generally frequently occurs in the setting of high-grade small bowel

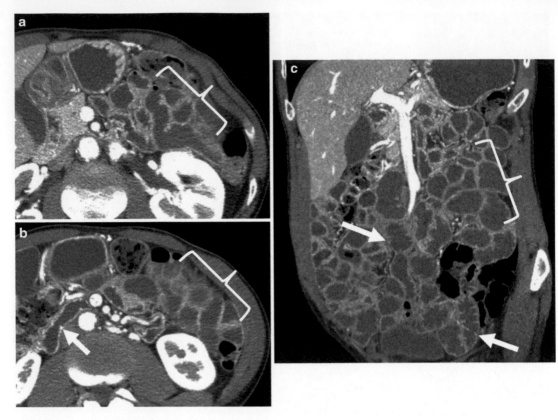

Fig. 4.6 CT enterography images demonstrating typical findings of celiac sprue, including normally enhancing jejunal loops with loss of folds (**a–c**, *brackets*). Note fea-tureless duodenum (**b**, *arrows*) and increased number of folds in the ileum (fold reversal; **c**, *arrows*)

obstruction or vascular occlusion, pneumato-sis cystoides coli and benign pneumatosis are not infrequently observed in outpatient CTE (Fig. 4.7). Focal regions of wall thickening with hypo- or isoenhancement may also represent intramural hemorrhage or lymphoma (described later) [20].

Mural thickening is generally considered to be present when greater than 3 mm in a distended bowel segment. When segmental mural thicken-ing is combined with segmental hyperenhance-ment, findings usually reflect inflammatory or infectious etiologies. Symmetrical involvement in the proximal small bowel can be seen in ulcer-ative jejunitis and/or infectious jejunitis, such as neutropenic enteritis or giardia. For ulcerative jejunitis, other findings such as relative loss of valvulae conniventes are helpful. Symmetrical

mural thickening combined with straightened and dilated bowel loop is often seen in ACE-related angioedema, venous compromise (such as from SMV thrombosis or carcinoid tumor), or pancreatitis. ACE-related angioedema is usually seen in women and may or may not be associated with first exposure to an ACE inhibitor. It is man-ifest by general bowel wall edema, and segmental luminal dilation, often with localized ascites and mesenteric edema [21]. Hyperenhancement of affected loops is normal or relatively mild with symmetric bowel wall edema present. SMV thrombosis, and segmental hemorrhage in antico-agulated patients, can also present with long segment mural thickening with or without hyper-enhancement, and correlative findings in the SMV or solid organs should be searched for. Infiltrating diseases such as systemic IgG-related

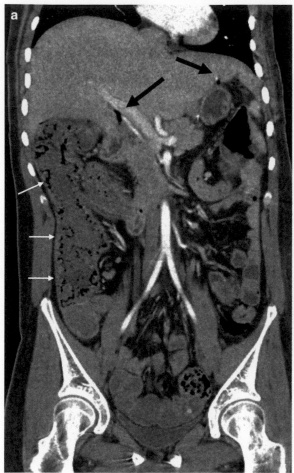

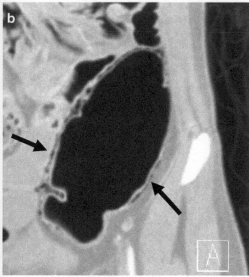

Fig. 4.7 Pneumatosis is observed throughout the ascending colon (**a**, *small white arrows*), with a small amount of free air underneath the liver (**a**, *black arrows*) on CT enterography performed for anemia. Coronal image of sigmoid colon also shows pneumato-sis (**b**, *black arrows*). Patient was observed in hospital without treatment without deterioration. Imaging findings felt to represent benign pneumatosis potentially due to pseudo-obstruction or multiple prior enteroenteric anastomoses

disease, mastocytosis, and amyloidosis are rarely seen, but they can also cause segmental bowel wall thickening (Fig. 4.8). In general, for inflammatory, vascular, and infiltrative diseases, the bowel wall thickening will be less than 1.5 cm in diameter; neoplasm should be considered for focal regions of bowel wall thickening of greater degree [22]. Diffuse small bowel thickening can be seen in cirrhosis, graft-versus-host disease, and shock bowel, where correlation with patient history and other imaging findings usually suggests the diagnosis. Diffuse hyperenhancement of the bowel with mild and symmetric wall thickening is seen in conjunction with CT signs of hypotension (e.g., flat IVC) in patients with trauma-induced shock bowel, but similar findings are seen in other conditions such as septic shock and cardiac arrest that cause hypotension [23].

Focal mural findings in the small bowel are generally neoplastic or vascular, whereas luminal findings include active bleeding and polyps or neoplasia. While adenocarcinoma is generally considered one of the more common small bowel neoplasms, carcinoid (neuroendocrine) tumors,

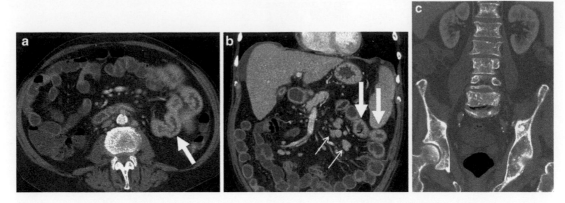

Fig. 4.8 Diffuse and continuous jejunal mural thickening and enhancement (**a** and **b**, *arrows*) due to mastocytosis. Note mesenteric adenopathy (*small white arrow*, **b**), small amount of ascites (**b**), and diffuse sclerotic lesions in the bones (**c**)

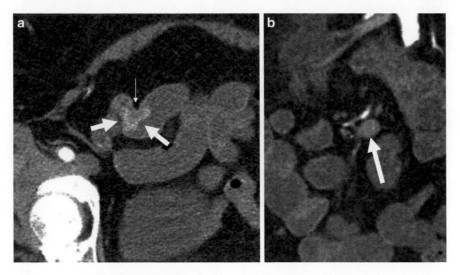

Fig. 4.9 Multiphase CT enterography performed for obscure GI bleeding demonstrates an enhancing ileal tumor (**a**, *arrows*). The mass demonstrates intense enhancement and serosal puckering (*small white arrow*), which is indicative of carcinoid tumors. Nodal metastases from carcinoid tumors typically occur close to mesenteric vessels (**b**, *arrows*)

gastrointestinal stromal tumors (GIST), and lymphoma are much more frequently seen at cross-sectional enterography. Now that multiphase CTE is often performed to evaluate for obscure GI bleeding, the unique morphologies of many of these tumors are being better appreciated.

Carcinoid tumors can appear as small hyperenhancing polyps, which grow within the bowel wall and over time will often become flat or plaque-like masses, often with luminal shouldering and serosal puckering or retraction (Figs. 4.9 and 4.10) [24]. Multifocal neuroendocrine tumors are frequently seen and are clustered within a small bowel (usually ileal) segment. As the tumor infiltrates through the vessel wall, typical patterns of metastatic lymphadenopathy are seen (Fig. 4.10). Neuroendocrine mesenteric and nodal metastases will often cluster along the regional mesenteric vessels and eventually cause vascular compromise. Eventually, liver metastases will develop.

GIST tumors are generally hyperenhancing tumors, often with an exoenteric component,

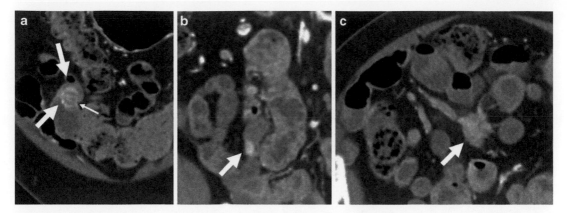

Fig. 4.10 CT enterography performed for abdominal pain shows multiple enhancing ileal masses (**a** and **b**, *arrows*), one with characteristic serosal puckering (**a**, *small arrow*), indicating multifocal ileal carcinoid tumors.

Mesenteric nodal metastasis (**c**, *arrow*) demonstrates typical findings of enhancing mesenteric mass with radiating strands of desmoplasia to nearby small bowel loops and engorged mesenteric veins (due to obstruction)

Fig. 4.11 Typical appearance of small bowel gastrointestinal stromal tumor (GIST; *arrow*) at CT enterography. Axial image shows 2 cm hypervascular mass with intraluminal and exoenteric components

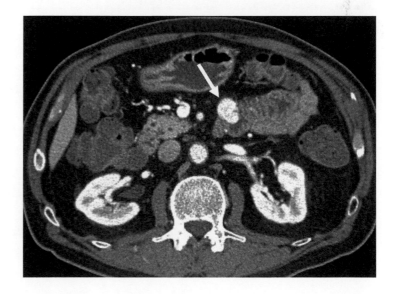

and may or may not show surface ulceration (Fig. 4.11). In contradistinction, some GIST tumors can be isoenhancing and intraluminal. Frequently, as the GISTs enlarge, they ulcerate and may lose typical hyperenhancement patterns. It may be useful to characterize the morphology of these masses with positive enteric contrast when needed. Occasionally, ectopic pancreas can mimic the appearance of GIST tumors in the proximal small bowel, as the ectopic tissue will also be exoenteric with respect to the bowel lumen.

Small bowel lymphomas occur as singular or multiple areas of focal bowel wall thickening. Unlike carcinoid or GIST tumors and Crohn's disease, lymphomas typically are iso- or hypoenhancing compared to the adjacent bowel wall. The classic pattern for lymphoma is that of "aneurysmal ulceration," meaning that the lumen of the small bowel tumor is markedly enlarged with thickening of the surrounding wall (Fig. 4.12) [25]. There will often be adjacent lymphadenopathy. Adenocarcinoma can be seen

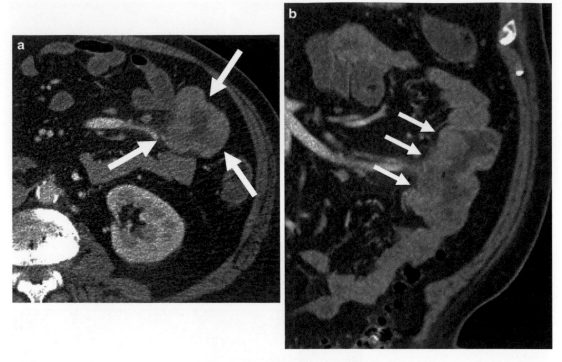

Fig. 4.12 Small bowel lymphoma (**a** and **b**, *arrows*) with marked wall thickening caused by iso- or hypo-attenuating tumor and enlargement of the bowel lumen (referred to as "aneurysmal ulceration")

Fig. 4.13 Adenocarcinoma (*arrows*) arising in setting Crohn's disease in a patient with multiple strictures. Note high-grade partial obstruction and nodularity to the extraluminal margin

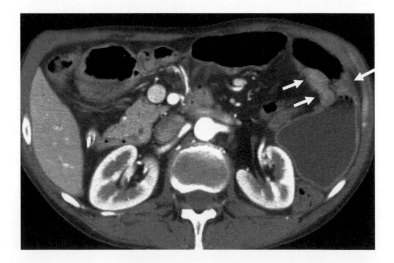

in isolation or in the setting of Crohn's disease, where it can appear as a focal stricture with mural nodularity (Fig. 4.13) [26]. Adenocarcinomas are infrequently detected at CTE and do not demonstrate a characteristic morphology.

Active bleeding at multiphase CTE is demonstrated by progressive accumulation of intraluminal contrast over subsequent phases of enhancement (Figs. 4.14 and 4.15). Active bleeding may be associated with a neoplasm or vascular etiology, but in the case of a Dieulafoy lesion or focal ulcer, no other abnormality will be appreciated. Several studies have shown that bleeding rates detectable at CT angiography and

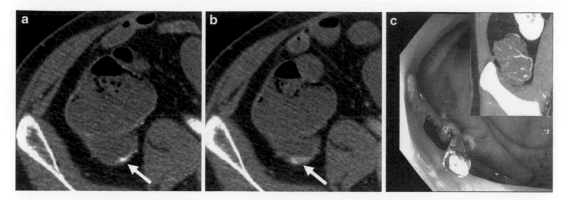

Fig. 4.14 Axial enteric and delayed-phase images (**a** and **b**, respectively) demonstrate progressive accumulation of intravenous contrast dependently within the cecum, indicating active bleeding (**a** and **b**, *arrows*). Coronal maxi- mum intensity projection images (**c**, *inset*) show nodular tufts of vessels in the wall of the cecum. Patient was treated with argon plasma coagulation and hemoclips

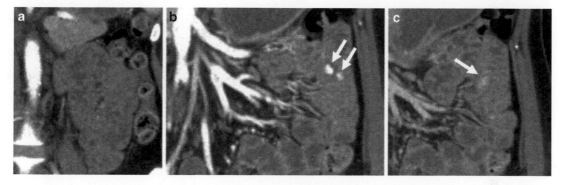

Fig. 4.15 Coronal arterial-, enteric-, and delayed-phase images (**a**, **b**, and **c**, respectively) from a multiphase CT enterography demonstrate progressive accumulation of intravenous contrast within the jejunal lumen between the arterial and enteric phases (**b**, *arrows*). Delayed-phase images show movement and dilution of intraluminal contrast (**c**, *arrow*). Findings indicate active jejunal bleeding. Small bowel enteroscopy identified a Dieulafoy lesion at this location, which was treated with argon plasma coagulation

multiphase CTE are comparable to catheter angiography [14]. Medication and radiopaque debris will also be bright at multiphase CTE, and will be unchanged in appearance between phases when slight movement of luminal contents due to peristalsis is taken into account.

Vascular lesions at CTE are generally classified according to the method of Huprich and Yano as angioectasias, arterial lesions, and venous lesions [6]. Angioectasias are frequently multiple and seen in elderly patients. They appear as small or round intramural lesions, usually best seen in the enteric phase of enhancement. They are frequently multiple and are generally underestimated by CT compared to endoscopy. They are thought to arise from mesenteric veins that lack an internal elastic layer, with arteriovenous communication developing as the precapillary sphincter becomes incompetent [6]. Angioectasias and arterial lesions are also seen in the cecum and ascending colon with some regularity at multiphase CTE exam, and in this location, they are generally associated with arterial shunting and an enlarged draining vein. Arterial lesions are best seen in the arterial phase and may or may not have an enlarged draining vein. Because of avid

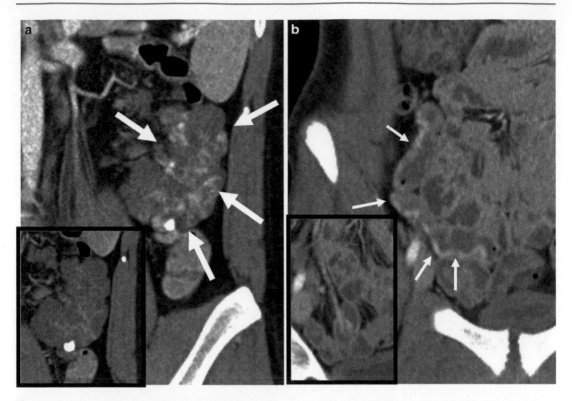

Fig. 4.16 Large jejunal vascular malformation with phleboliths on precontrast imaging (**a**, *inset*), and blood-filled spaces that enhanced slowly with time after contrast (**a**, *arrows*), in patient with presumed Klippel-Trenaunay- Weber. Another patient with an ileal vascular malformation with dilated intramural vessels (**b**, *arrows*) and a large draining vein (**b**, *inset*)

arterial enhancement, there is the potential for large amounts of bleeding. Arterial lesions include angioectasias with arterial shunting, Dieulafoy lesions, and arteriovenous fistulas. Venous lesions are a heterogeneous group of disorders, with varices frequently seen in patients with cirrhosis or chronic mesenteric venous thrombosis from Crohn's disease. Younger patients often have large congenital vascular malformations, often in conjunction with other known vascular lesions, e.g., Klippel-Trenaunay-Weber syndrome (Fig. 4.16).

CTE surveillance for polyps and masses can be performed in addition to magnetic resonance (MR) enterography or enteroclysis in patients with polyposis syndromes. In these patients, polyps and neoplasia occur within the lumen, so positive enteric contrast is often used. Because of the high attenuation differences between positive contrast and the filling defects of polyps, radiation doses can be markedly reduced to levels used for CT colonography (Fig. 4.17).

Morphologic abnormalities constitute a heterogeneous group of disorders, including malrotation, small bowel diverticulosis, Meckel's diverticulum, and postoperative anastomoses. Intestinal malrotation predisposes to midgut volvulus. Findings of small bowel nonrotation include ascending colon and cecum in the midline, redundant duodenum with ligament of Treitz in the right upper quadrant, and rounding of the uncinate process of the pancreas [27]. Patients with non-rotation and intermittent small bowel volvulus often present for outpatient imaging when the small bowel volvulus has resolved. They should be informed of findings so that they can present to the ER if acute, unrelenting pain occurs as prompt surgical treatment may be required.

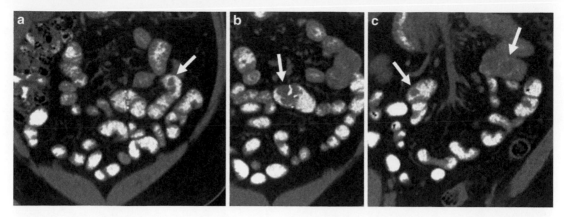

Fig. 4.17 Single-phase CT enterography with positive oral contrast demonstrates multiple polyps (**b–c**, *arrows*), including a recurrent polyp (**b**, *arrow*). Positive contrast enteroclysis or enterography can be performed at low radiation doses because suspected pathology is known to be located in the small bowel lumen, as opposed to the wall or perienteric tissues

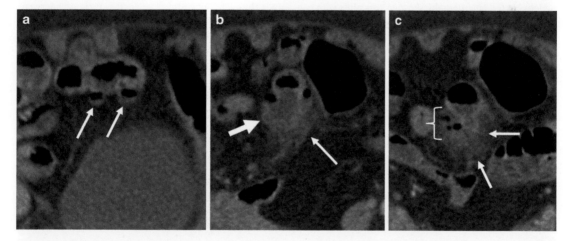

Fig. 4.18 Just superior to two ileal diverticula (**a**, *small arrows*), a large ileal diverticulum is seen (**b**, *arrow*) with stranding in the surrounding perienteric fat (**b** and **c**, *small arrows*) and localized perienteric air (**c**, *brackets*), indicating perforated ileal diverticulitis

Small bowel diverticula can be mistaken for a small bowel loop on a single cross-sectional image. In volumetric datasets from CT and MR enterography, the findings are unmistakable, but they are often overlooked. The lumen of the jejunum will have valvulae conniventes, whereas diverticula will not. Jejunal or ileal diverticulitis can occur when a diverticulum becomes inflamed or perforated (Fig. 4.18). Meckel's diverticulum is a frequent cause of obscure gastrointestinal bleeding in young and middle-aged patients. Bleeding from Meckel's can occur due to ulcer, inflammation, neoplasm, or ectopic gastric mucosa within the diverticulum. Often, the diverticulum will be large and may contain a focal area of hyperenhancement or luminal defect corresponding to one of these abnormalities.

Extraenteric Findings

Extraenteric findings can often be an important clue to inflammatory bowel disease or its complications (Fig. 4.19). Penetrating Crohn's

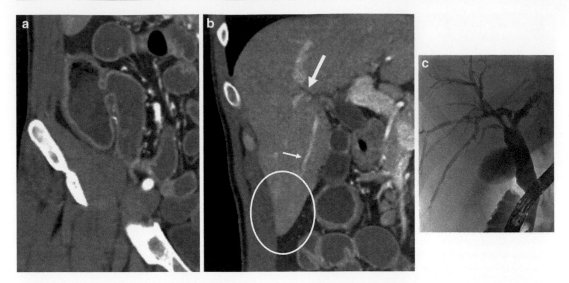

Fig. 4.19 Patient with history of indeterminate colitis underwent CT enterography showing pancolitis with patulous ileocecal valve (**a**), characteristic of ulcerative colitis. Coronal liver images show mild intrahepatic biliary dilation (**b**, *large arrow*) extending inferiorly into the right lobe (**b**, *small arrow*) with periductal perfusion abnormalities (**b**, *oval*), suggesting cholangitis. Patient underwent ERCP (**c**) demonstrating a localized stricture at the bifurcation of the intrahepatic ducts and mild changes of intrahepatic primary sclerosing cholangitis

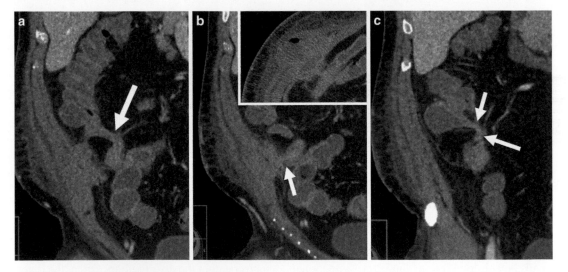

Fig. 4.20 CT enterography images from anterior to posterior demonstrate complex, penetrating ileocolic Crohn's disease. Fistulas appear as extraenteric tracts with tethering of affected bowel loops (enteroenteric fistula, **a**—*large arrow*; ileocecal fistula, **c**—*arrows*). *Middle image* shows fistula to abdominal wall (**b**, *arrow*) that has resulted in abdominal wall abscess (**b**, *inset*)

disease is manifest by sinus tracts, fistulae, inflammatory mass, and abscess. Small bowel fistulas (e.g., enterocolic fistula or entercutaneous fistulas) appear as enhancing, extraenteric tracts that arise from inflamed small bowel loops, and often distort or tether loops from which they arise [28]. Complex, branching fistulas will form asterisk-shaped fistulae complexes that will involve multiple small bowel loops (Figs. 4.20 and 4.21). Fistulas that extend to the retroperitoneum will often form abscesses along the iliopsoas muscle. Perianal fistulae

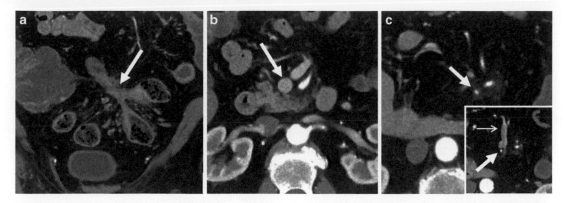

Fig. 4.21 Chronic superior mesenteric vein thrombosis in a patient with asterisk-shaped enteroenteric and enterocolic fistulae complex (**a**, *arrows*). Axial images demonstrate normal caliber superior mesenteric vein at the level of pancreatic head (**b**, *arrow*) that becomes diminutive inferiorly at the level of transverse duodenum (**c**, *arrow*). Even more inferiorly, enlarged peripheral mesenteric venous collaterals are seen (**c**, *inset*)

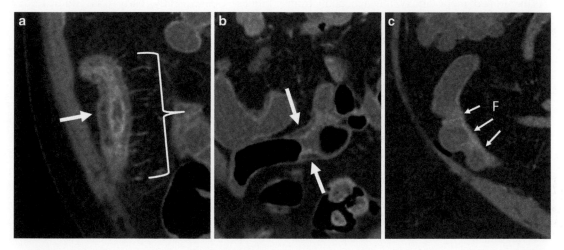

Fig. 4.22 Perienteric and acute and chronic Crohn's inflammation. Acute and chronic Crohn's inflammation is evidenced in small bowel loops with mural stratification with synchronous findings of submucosal fat (prior inflammation) and inner wall hyperenhancement (current inflammation; **a** and **b**, *arrows*). The "comb sign" (**a**, *brackets*) refers to engorged vasa that enter the small bowel or colon at a right angle (**a**, *bracket*). This imaging finding is associated with moderate to severe active inflammation. Mesenteric border inflammation (evidenced by mural hyperenhancement and wall thickening; *small arrows*, **c**) in a third patient is also indicative of Crohn's enteric inflammation, and is associated with antimesenteric sacculation and fibrofatty proliferation ("F")

suggest Crohn's disease as the etiology in patients with inflammatory colitis without small bowel involvement. While perianal fistulas and abscesses are often detected at CTE, they are poorly characterized in terms of their anatomic location compared to dedicated perineal MR imaging. Low-kV imaging techniques generally increase the conspicuity of perianal fistulas. Chronic perianal fistulas and anovaginal fistulas are often not seen at CTE.

Vascular and mesenteric findings are often associated with Crohn's disease. The "comb sign" represents engorged vasa recta that supply inflamed bowel segments (Fig. 4.22) and are associated with increased rates of hospitalization and TNF response [29]. Fibrofatty proliferation is often associated with mesenteric border inflammation, and displaces bowel loops (Fig. 4.22). Mesenteric venous thrombosis can be located centrally in the superior mesenteric vein and portal vein, or in smaller, peripheral mesenteric veins. Central mesenteric thromboses frequently completely recanalize, while peripheral ones often result in lasting venous narrowing (i.e., chronic peripheral mesenteric vein thrombosis), and result in collateral vessel formation, including the development of varices (Fig. 4.21) [30].

Reactive lymph nodes are a hallmark of Crohn's disease, where they are often numerous. For colorectal Crohn's disease, reactive lymph nodes are characteristically located in the pericolonic fat between the engorged vasa recta, whereas reactive mesenteric lymph nodes for small bowel Crohn's are usually located within the central mesentery. Lymph nodes greater than 1.5 cm are considered by some to be abnormal. As mentioned, metastatic lymphadenopathy from small bowel neuroendocrine tumors has a characteristic appearance. It clusters along lymph nodes, and owing to the serotonin release, often creates radiating strands of desmoplasia to adjacent small bowel loops, often with characteristic punctate calcification.

Indications and Evidence

Crohn's Disease

Natural History

The natural history of Crohn's disease in individual patients is varied. Different initial presentations of the disease, age at disease onset, and extent and location of disease involvement have been shown to suggest different phenotypes with different disease courses and complications. Therefore, the optimal imaging modality and timing will vary from patient to patient. Pigneur et al. showed that disease onset in childhood versus adulthood portends more active disease requiring more immunosuppressive therapy [31]. These patients require more frequent imaging specifically assessing for active inflammation and response to treatment changes. Cosnes et al. showed that the initial location of disease can predict the development of subsequent stricturing or penetrating complications [32]. Given the frequent asymptomatic nature of these complica-

tions in many patients [28, 33], cross-sectional radiologic surveillance to guide medical management is often helpful. And finally, Crohn's disease is a chronic disease process requiring ongoing imaging monitoring, with 70–80 % of patients requiring surgery at 20 years and many patients experiencing disease recurrence requiring reoperation within several years [34].

Mucosal Reference Versus Integrated Reference, and Endoscopic Skipping of the Terminal Ileum

Early studies of CTE compared CT findings to fluoroscopic small bowel follow-through, which is an inadequate reference standard for mucosal inflammation when compared to optical techniques. Consequently, early CTE studies compared results to endoscopy in the terminal ileum in patients that could be assessed at ileocolonoscopy [35]. Subsequent studies have suggested that the ileal mucosa can appear normal at ileocolonoscopy in the presence of synchronous intramural and proximal ileal inflammation [3, 36]. Indeed, in just over 50 % of Crohn's patients with normal findings in the terminal ileum at endoscopy [5], small bowel inflammation will be unequivocally present, either intramurally within terminal ileum or in the proximal small bowel. This phenomenon may occur in an even higher percentage of pediatric patients than adults [37, 38] and may herald aggressive disease. CTE is complementary to endoscopy in the assessment of small bowel involvement, as it readily shows disease involvement in segments of bowel not accessible by endoscope, as well as disease limited to the wall of the bowel and mesentery. Consequently, current reference standards for CTE studies usually include combined assessment using endoscopy or surgery, serum markers, and other confirmatory, cross-sectional imaging methods [3].

Clinical Benefit: Adult IBD

Several observational studies have demonstrated the benefit of CTE in making clinical decisions in the inpatient and outpatient settings. Higgins et al. showed that enterography imaging findings change the impression of steroid benefit in the majority of patients [39]. Bruining et al. prospectively assessed the clinical benefit of CTE in more than 250 patients with either established or suspected Crohn's disease [40]. After gastroenterologists examined the patient and obtained the clinical history, they were asked to detail their pre-imaging clinical management plan and level of confidence. After the CTE was performed, gastroenterologists were again asked for their management plan and level of confidence. Bruining et al. found that in approximately half of patients with either established or suspected Crohn's disease, CTE resulted in clinical management changes, and in 70 %, CTE findings substantially improved clinician level of confidence.

Two studies have examined the benefit of CT in the ER. Israeli et al. found that in a series of Crohn's patients presenting to the ER (80 % with abdominal pain), over 25 % had a small bowel obstruction and 8 % had penetrating disease, with management changes occurring on the basis of abdominal CT in over 80 % of patients (including 12 % of patients going to surgery) [41]. In a larger retrospective study of 648 Crohn's patients over an 8-year time frame, Kerner et al. found that the rate of penetrating disease, obstruction, or abscess was about 29 % and that about 35 % of patients had an abdominopelvic CT finding that necessitated treatment [42]. They concluded that "these numbers reflect the fact that patients with Crohn's disease are at high risk for complications given the nature of their disease and the risks of immunosuppression … Although radiation exposure in patients with Crohn's disease is a concern, clinicians must also weigh the risk of missing a potential urgent diagnosis when they forgo CT" [42].

Clinical Benefit: Pediatrics

Pediatric patients pose unique considerations for the imaging diagnosis and monitoring of inflammatory bowel disease and many factors need to be considered when determining the appropriate imaging modality to be used.

CTE is often used in conjunction with ileocolonoscopy as one of the first imaging studies to establish a diagnosis of inflammatory bowel disease and distinguish between ulcerative colitis

and Crohn's disease. CT offers superior spatial resolution and ability to assess all segments of bowel [43]. In addition, CT is often used in patients with known inflammatory bowel disease in the setting of acute abdominal pain with fever, leukocytosis, obstructive symptoms, or suspicion of penetrating complications or perforation, due to its wide availability, rapid performance, and good tolerability. In this scenario, positive oral contrast or water is often used in place of neutral enteric agents even though this may decrease sensitivity for identifying Crohn's small bowel inflammation. Finally, CTE is often used for procedure planning when invasive intervention, such as stricturoplasty, surgical resection, abscess drainage, or colectomy, is being considered. The most significant drawback of CTE is that because Crohn's disease has a chronic remitting course requiring lifelong imaging for acute complications often requiring medical and surgical intervention, the cumulative radiation dose of multiple CT exams can be substantial [44]. Therefore, in pediatric patients, medical justification rests on the perceived medical benefit for each exam (e.g., identification of abscess for antibiotic treatment, or obstruction evaluation for potential surgery).

MR enterography (MRE) is utilized most often for monitoring of disease activity and response to treatment, offering global assessment of the bowel wall and extraluminal disease manifestations like CTE. Because no ionizing radiation is utilized, MRE is the preferred imaging modality when evaluating asymptomatic patients [45]. MRE has been shown to be equally sensitive to CTE for the detection of bowel inflammation [36, 46], and is felt to be superior to CTE in the detection and characterization of perianal fistulizing disease and detection of fibrosis [47]. MRE can, however, suffer from various artifacts, such as air in the bowel lumen and motion. MRE also has the drawbacks of being a lengthy exam, which may not be well tolerated in very young patients, symptomatic patients, and claustrophobic patients, and is more costly compared to CTE. Some institutions routinely sedate younger patients for MRE to improve tolerance of the exam; others do not, citing potential risk of aspiration in anesthetized patients after oral contrast.

Both CTE and MRE require the ingestion of a large amount of enteric contrast, which can be poorly tolerated by pediatric patients. Ultrasound is emerging as a viable alternative for monitoring of Crohn's disease, with its application being particularly suitable to children and adolescents due to smaller body habitus and frequent lack of need for oral contrast. Ultrasound has the added benefit of interactive, real-time imaging, which allows the sonographer and radiologist to get feedback about symptom location and to assess for persistence of bowel wall thickening, narrowing, and dilatation. Real-time assessment can increase confidence that findings are not artifactual, e.g., by observing and distensibility in a potentially stenotic segment. Contrast-enhanced ultrasound using microbubbles has been shown to improve detection and confidence in active inflammation of the bowel wall over thickening alone [48]. Analysis of the bowel wall vascularity pattern after administration of microbubbles has also been shown to assist in the differentiation of inflammatory versus fibrotic strictures [49], and used to evaluate the response to treatment as manifested by wall enhancement and vascularity patterns [50–52]. Ultrasound may suffer from poor visualization of deeper bowel loops and decreased accuracy for global bowel assessment, particularly if enteric contrast is not utilized. Ultrasound is also heavily operator dependent, requiring experienced sonographers and radiologists for performance and interpretation.

Clinical Benefit: Obscure Gastrointestinal Bleeding (Adult)

Early capsule endoscopy studies showed that traditional radiologic imaging with small bowel follow-through and routine abdominal pelvic CT was ineffectual in detecting causes of obscure gastrointestinal bleeding [53]. Moreover, capsule endoscopy has a very high yield of positive findings in large series, particularly in patients with active bleeding [54–56]. However, as CTE and balloon-assisted endoscopy techniques have developed, it is also clear that capsule endoscopy fails to identify many small bowel tumors, owing largely to their

intermural or submucosal location. Compared to double-balloon endoscopy, capsule endoscopy may only identify about one-third of mass lesions [57]. In a retrospective study of 103 post-bulbar tumors, CTE found 91 % versus 30 % for capsule endoscopy, and in the subset of patients undergoing both studies, CTE found 2–3 times as many tumors [58]. Finally, Huprich et al. performed prospective and retrospective studies examining the role of multiphasic CTE in identification of small bowel bleeding sources in patients with obscure gastrointestinal bleeding [4, 59]. In a prospective study of 58 patients, capsule endoscopy demonstrated significant findings in 25 % of patients versus 44–48 % for CTE. In nine confirmed small bowel masses, CTE found 100 % versus 33 % for capsule endoscopy. The ASGE's 2011 practice guidelines recommend consideration of multiphase CTE after repeat endoscopy. Shin et al. additionally found that positive multiphase CTE findings occur more often in overt rather than occult obscure gastrointestinal bleeding, and that positive CTE findings are associated with specific treatments and diminished rates of rebleeding [60]. Additionally, multiphase CTE may be particularly helpful in patients with nondiagnostic capsule findings, such as nonspecific blood in the small intestine or lesions without bleeding [61, 62]. Based on these and other studies, multiphase CTE is considered complementary with capsule endoscopy in defining the site and cause of obscure gastrointestinal bleeding, particularly when nondiagnostic or questionable findings are seen at capsule endoscopy(e.g., due to stricture, motility, or dysphasia). Finally, multiphase CTE can be performed and interpreted on the same day to quickly guide diagnostic workup in these patients, and to select patients for surgery or therapeutic angiography in the case of small bowel tumors and active bleeding, or as an aid to visualization and treatment at subsequent balloon-assisted endoscopy.

Clinical Benefit: Obscure Gastrointestinal Bleeding (Pediatric)

Gastrointestinal bleeding in the pediatric population can be caused by a variety of conditions. Bleeding can be obscure and life threatening. Pediatric patients can experience obscure gastrointestinal bleeding secondary to the same etiologies as adults. In addition, some etiologies tend to present more commonly with gastrointestinal bleeding in children, such as Meckel's diverticulum, Crohn's disease, congenital vascular malformations, and polyps. After upper and lower endoscopy fail to reveal a cause, and capsule endoscopy is negative, radiologic workup is often initiated including nuclear medicine Meckel's scan, conventional CT and CTE, and catheter angiography.

The use of CTE for obscure gastrointestinal bleeding in the pediatric population has not been studied as extensively as in the adult population. In fact, only one case series was found in the literature reporting the use of CTE for this indication. Davis et al. reported a series of six patients with prior negative imaging studies such as ultrasound and Meckel's scan who underwent CTE [63]. In this cohort of patients, CTE was able to prospectively diagnose solitary polyps in two cases, multiple polyps in one case, a Meckel's diverticulum in two cases, and an inflamed duplication cyst in one case. No cases of vascular anomalies of the bowel wall were found in these patients. Diagnostic yield remains unknown as the cases with negative CTE were not reported.

Meckel's diverticulum in particular often poses a challenging clinical and radiologic diagnosis. Nuclear medicine Meckel's scan with Tc-99m pertechnetate is the first-line test ordered when a Meckel's diverticulum is suspected, with sensitivity and specificity reported to be 94 and 97 % in the literature [64]. However, false negatives do occur, and Meckel's without ectopic gastric mucosa are not diagnosed. CTE can potentially give the diagnosis in these cases.

The instance of vascular anomalies including hemangiomas and vascular malformations in the pediatric gastrointestinal tract is rare. These can be diffuse and associated with syndromes such as Klippel-Trenaunay, Osler-Weber-Rendu, and blue rubber bleb nevus syndrome. The most common symptom is gastrointestinal bleeding [65, 66]. The use of multiphase CTE exams in children has not been studied, and due to the concern of radiation exposure in young patients and the

need to adhere to the principles of ALARA in the pediatric population, until further dose reduction techniques and supportive data are established, use of these exams should be confined to pediatric patients with ongoing blood loss and negative endoscopic assessment.

Diarrhea and Abdominal Pain

Because CTE is often performed in patients with diarrhea, CTE may suggest noninflammatory bowel disease causes such as pancreatic insufficiency or mass, celiac disease, other causes of malabsorption, or bacterial overgrowth, due to motility disorder or small bowel diverticulosis. In these settings, CTE performed at routine abdominopelvic radiation dose settings can easily evaluate for pancreatic tumors and causes of diarrhea other than inflammatory bowel disease.

Adaptations of CTE Technique

CTE technique is adapted for patients of different sizes, ages, and clinical indications (called diagnostic tasks in the radiology literature). Obviously, single-phase CTE (in either the enteric/pancreatic or portal phase of enhancement) is performed for most indications. Multiphase examinations are performed for patients with obscure gastrointestinal bleeding, or patients with suspected pancreatic or neuroendocrine tumors. CTE is not performed for acute gastrointestinal bleeding, where enteric contrast is not needed [14]. Radiation dose is tailored to patient size and diagnostic task through use of the automatic exposure control on modern multidetector CT systems. Automatic exposure control modulates the X-ray tube current as the X-ray tube rotates around the patient as the patient passes through the CT gantry, and is designed to produce a constant level of image quality regardless of patient attenuation (e.g., with lower levels of tube current for projections going anterior to posterior in thin patients). It reduces radiation exposure by about 30 % over large numbers of patients. Newer CT systems also use tube energy (or kVp) to simultaneously minimize radiation exposure and increase iodine contrast to noise, which can increase conspicuity of inflamed bowel segments [67]. Lower tube energies and decreasing tube currents reduce radiation dose but increase CT image noise. Multiple studies have demonstrated that radiologists can perform quite well in diagnosing and staging Crohn's disease, even with lower dose CT images [68–70], but currently, multiple CT noise reduction methods exist, such as iterative reconstruction, and are available in most radiology departments [71, 72]. It is imperative that gastroenterologists and radiologists work together to make these lower dose technologies available to Crohn's patients who are young, who will incur greater lifetime radiation doses due to the recurrent nature of Crohn's complications [44]. In patients with renal insufficiency, contrast-enhanced CTE using half the routine amount of iodinated contrast can be performed by combining bolus-tracking, low kVp techniques, and iterative reconstruction. Positive enteric contrast can be used for polyposis patients, as mentioned earlier, and will permit exams to be performed without intravenous contrast at substantial dose reduction (Fig. 4.17).

CTE is often performed using a low-concentration barium solution containing sorbitol to promote gastric peristalsis and water retention within the bowel lumen. A variety of other commercially available products, as well as water, have been evaluated in a head-to-head comparison [9], but the low-concentration barium solution demonstrated the best lumen distension with fewer side effects. Studies have been performed looking for the optimal concentration, amount, and timing of enteric contrast [7, 9, 73]. Side effects are common, but are generally minor and time limited, including abdominal cramping, diarrhea, and nausea. Some patients have difficulty ingesting the required volume of enteric contrast, especially young patients or those with obstructive symptoms. In such cases the ingestion protocol is generally altered, such as giving less enteric contrast or having the patient switch to water ingestion. Administering the enteric contrast via enteric tube is an alternative available at some institutions due to patient preference.

Conclusion

CTE is an accepted cross-sectional imaging modality optimized for small bowel assessments, with CTE technique guided by both patient size and indication. Applications are numerous in patients with inflammatory bowel disease and obscure gastrointestinal bleeding as well as those with other gastrointestinal diseases. CTE can detect both intestinal and extraintestinal disease processes. Dose reduction techniques can be utilized to limit exposure, particularly in young patients.

References

1. American College of Radiology. Acr appropriateness criteria: Crohn's disease. http://wwwacrorg/Secondary MainMenuCategories/quality_safety/app_criteria/pdf/ ExpertPanelonGastrointestinalImaging/CrohnsDisease Doc5aspx (2008). Accessed 1 Nov 2010.
2. Fletcher JG, Huprich J, Loftus Jr EV, Bruining DH, Fidler JL. Computerized tomography enterography and its role in small-bowel imaging. Clin Gastroenterol Hepatol. 2008;6(3):283–9.
3. Faubion Jr WA, Fletcher JG, O'Byrne S, Feagan BG, de Villiers WJ, Salzberg B, et al. Emerging biomarkers in inflammatory bowel disease (embark) study identifies fecal calprotectin, serum mmp9, and serum il-22 as a novel combination of biomarkers for Crohn's disease activity: Role of cross-sectional imaging. Am J Gastroenterol. 2013;108:1891–900.
4. Huprich JE, Fletcher JG, Fidler JL, Alexander JA, Guimaraes LS, Siddiki HA, et al. Prospective blinded comparison of wireless capsule endoscopy and multiphase ct enterography in obscure gastrointestinal bleeding. Radiology. 2011;260(3):744–51.
5. Samuel S, Bruining DH, Loftus Jr EV, Becker B, Fletcher JG, Mandrekar JN, et al. Endoscopic skipping of the distal terminal ileum in Crohn's disease can lead to negative results from ileocolonoscopy. Clin Gastroenterol Hepatol. 2012;10(11):1253–9.
6. Huprich JE, Barlow JM, Hansel SL, Alexander JA, Fidler JL. Multiphase ct enterography evaluation of small-bowel vascular lesions. AJR Am J Roentgenol. 2013;201(1):65–72.
7. Ajaj W, Goehde SC, Schneemann H, Ruehm SG, Debatin JF, Lauenstein TC. Oral contrast agents for small bowel MRI: Comparison of different additives to optimize bowel distension. Eur Radiol. 2004;14(3):458–64.
8. Lauenstein T, Schneemann H, Vogt F, Herborn C, Ruhm S, Debatin J. Optimization of oral contrast agents for MR imaging of the small bowel. Radiology. 2003;228:279–83.

9. Young BM, Fletcher JG, Booya F, Paulsen S, Fidler J, Johnson CD, et al. Head-to-head comparison of oral contrast agents for cross-sectional enterography: Small bowel distention, timing, and side effects. J Comput Assist Tomogr. 2008;32(1):32–8.

10. Baker ME, Walter J, Obuchowski NA, Achkar JP, Einstein D, Veniero JC, et al. Mural attenuation in normal small bowel and active inflammatory Crohn's disease on ct enterography: location, absolute attenuation, relative attenuation, and the effect of wall thickness. AJR Am J Roentgenol. 2009;192(2):417–23.

11. Paulsen SR, Huprich JE, Fletcher JG, Booya F, Young BM, Fidler JL, et al. Ct enterography as a diagnostic tool in evaluating small bowel disorders: review of clinical experience with over 700 cases. Radiographics. 2006;26(3):641–57. discussion 657–662.

12. Schindera ST, Nelson RC, DeLong DM, Jaffe TA, Merkle EM, Paulson EK, et al. Multi-detector row ct of the small bowel: peak enhancement temporal window–initial experience. Radiology. 2007;243(2): 438–44.

13. Vandenbroucke F, Mortele KJ, Tatli S, Pelsser V, Erturk SM, de Mey J, et al. Noninvasive multidetector computed tomography enterography in patients with small-bowel Crohn's disease: is a 40-second delay better than 70 seconds? Acta Radiol. 2007;23:1–9.

14. Lee SS, Park SH. Computed tomography evaluation of gastrointestinal bleeding and acute mesenteric ischemia. Radiol Clin North Am. 2013;51(1):29–43.

15. Booya F, Fletcher JG, Huprich JE, Barlow JM, Johnson CD, Fidler JL, et al. Active Crohn's disease: Ct findings and interobserver agreement for enteric phase ct enterography. Radiology. 2006;241(3):787–95.

16. Harisinghani MG, Wittenberg J, Lee W, Chen S, Gutierrez AL, Mueller PR. Bowel wall fat halo sign in patients without intestinal disease. Am J Roentgenol. 2003;181(3):781–4.

17. Dave M. Crohn's disease with jejunal involvement: predictor of worse outcomes? J Clin Gastroenterol. 2013;47(5):379–80.

18. Flicek KT, Hara AK, De Petris G, Pasha SF, Yadav AD, Johnson CD. Diaphragm disease of the small bowel: a retrospective review of ct findings. AJR Am J Roentgenol. 2014;202(2):W140–5.

19. Macari M, Megibow AJ, Balthazar EJ. A pattern approach to the abnormal small bowel: observations at MDCT and CT enterography. AJR Am J Roentgenol. 2007;188(5):1344–55.

20. Altikaya N, Parlakgumus A, Demir S, Alkan O, Yildirim T. Small bowel obstruction caused by intramural hematoma secondary to warfarin therapy: a report of two cases. Turk J Gastroenterol. 2011;22(2):199–202.

21. Scheirey CD, Scholz FJ, Shortsleeve MJ, Katz DS. Angiotensin-converting enzyme inhibitor-induced small-bowel angioedema: clinical and imaging findings in 20 patients. AJR Am J Roentgenol. 2011;197(2):393–8.

22. James S, Balfe DM, Lee JK, Picus D. Small-bowel disease: categorization by ct examination. AJR Am J Roentgenol. 1987;148(5):863–8.

23. Ames JT, Federle MP. Ct hypotension complex (shock bowel) is not always due to traumatic hypovolemic shock. AJR Am J Roentgenol. 2009;192(5):W230–5.

24. Levy AD, Sobin LH. From the archives of the AFIP: gastrointestinal carcinoids: Imaging features with clinicopathologic comparison. Radiographics. 2007; 27(1):237–57.

25. Buckley JA, Fishman EK. Ct evaluation of small bowel neoplasms: spectrum of disease. Radiographics. 1998;18(2):379–92.

26. Weber NK, Fletcher JG, Fidler JL, Barlow JM, Pruthi S, Loftus EV, Jr., et al. Clinical characteristics and imaging features of small bowel adenocarcinomas in Crohn's disease. Abdom Imaging. 2014 [Epub ahead of print].

27. Pickhardt PJ, Bhalla S. Intestinal malrotation in adolescents and adults: spectrum of clinical and imaging features. AJR Am J Roentgenol. 2002;179(6): 1429–35.

28. Booya F, Akram S, Fletcher JG, Huprich JE, Johnson CD, Fidler JL, et al. Ct enterography and fistulizing Crohn's disease: clinical benefit and radiographic findings. Abdom Imaging. 2009;34(4):467–75.

29. Meyers MA, McGuire PV. Spiral ct demonstration of hypervascularity in Crohn's disease: "vascular jejunization of the ileum" or the "comb sign". Abdom Imaging. 1995;20:327–32.

30. Violi NV, Schoepfer AM, Fournier N, Guiu B, Bize P, Denys A. Prevalence and clinical importance of mesenteric venous thrombosis in the Swiss inflammatory bowel disease cohort. AJR Am J Roentgenol. 2014;203(1):62–9.

31. Pigneur B, Seksik P, Viola S, Viala J, Beaugerie L, Girardet JP, et al. Natural history of Crohn's disease: comparison between childhood- and adult-onset disease. Inflamm Bowel Dis. 2010;16(6):953–61.

32. Cosnes J, Gower-Rousseau C, Seksik P, Cortot A. Epidemiology and natural history of inflammatory bowel diseases. Gastroenterology. 2011;140(6):1785–94.

33. Solem CA, Loftus Jr EV, Fletcher JG, Baron TH, Gostout CJ, Petersen BT, et al. Small-bowel imaging in Crohn's disease: a prospective, blinded, 4-way comparison trial. Gastrointest Endosc. 2008;68(2):255–66.

34. Cosnes J, Cattan S, Blain A, Beaugerie L, Carbonnel F, Parc R, et al. Long-term evolution of disease behavior of Crohn's disease. Inflamm Bowel Dis. 2002;8(4):244–50.

35. Bodily KD, Fletcher JG, Solem CA, Johnson CD, Fidler JL, Barlow JM, et al. Crohn disease: mural attenuation and thickness at contrast-enhanced ct enterography–correlation with endoscopic and histologic findings of inflammation. Radiology. 2006; 238(2):505–16.

36. Siddiki HA, Fidler JL, Fletcher JG, Burton SS, Huprich JE, Hough DM, et al. Prospective comparison of state-of-the-art MR enterography and ct enterography in small-bowel Crohn's disease. AJR Am J Roentgenol. 2009;193(1):113–21.

37. Halligan S, Nicholls S, Bartram CI, Walker-Smith JA. The distribution of small bowel Crohn's disease in

children compared to adults. Clin Radiol. 1994;49(5): 314–6.

38. Lenaerts C, Roy CC, Vaillancourt M, Weber AM, Morin CL, Seidman E. High incidence of upper gastrointestinal tract involvement in children with Crohn disease. Pediatrics. 1989;83(5):777–81.

39. Higgins PD, Caoili E, Zimmermann M, Bhuket TP, Sonda LP, Manoogian B, et al. Computed tomographic enterography adds information to clinical management in small bowel Crohn's disease. Inflamm Bowel Dis. 2007;13(3):262–8.

40. Bruining DH, Siddiki HA, Fletcher JG, Sandborn WJ, Fidler JL, Huprich JE, et al. Benefit of computed tomography enterography in Crohn's disease: effects on patient management and physician level of confidence. Inflamm Bowel Dis. 2012;18(2):219–25.

41. Israeli E, Ying S, Henderson B, Mottola J, Strome T, Bernstein CN. The impact of abdominal computed tomography in a tertiary referral centre emergency department on the management of patients with inflammatory bowel disease. Aliment Pharmacol Ther. 2013;38(5):513–21.

42. Kerner C, Carey K, Mills AM, Yang W, Synnestvedt MB, Hilton S, et al. Use of abdominopelvic computed tomography in emergency departments and rates of urgent diagnoses in Crohn's disease. Clin Gastroenterol Hepatol. 2012;10(1):52–7.

43. Duigenan S, Gee MS. Imaging of pediatric patients with inflammatory bowel disease. AJR Am J Roentgenol. 2012;199(4):907–15.

44. Jaffe TA, Gaca AM, Delaney S, Yoshizumi TT, Toncheva G, Nguyen G, et al. Radiation doses from small-bowel follow-through and abdominopelvic MDCT in Crohn's disease. AJR Am J Roentgenol. 2007;189(5):1015–22.

45. Guimaraes LS, Fidler JL, Fletcher JG, Bruining DH, Huprich JE, Siddiki H, et al. Assessment of appropriateness of indications for ct enterography in younger patients. Inflamm Bowel Dis. 2010;16(2):226–32.

46. Lee SS, Kim AY, Yang SK, Chung JW, Kim SY, Park SH, et al. Crohn disease of the small bowel: Comparison of ct enterography, MR enterography, and small-bowel follow-through as diagnostic techniques. Radiology. 2009;251(3):751–61.

47. Quencer KB, Nimkin K, Mino-Kenudson M, Gee MS. Detecting active inflammation and fibrosis in pediatric Crohn's disease: prospective evaluation of MR-E and CT-E. Abdom Imaging. 2013;38(4):705–13.

48. Migaleddu V, Quaia E, Scanu D, Carla S, Bertolotto M, Campisi G, et al. Inflammatory activity in Crohn's disease: CE-US. Abdom Imaging. 2011;36(2):142–8.

49. Ripolles T, Rausell N, Paredes JM, Grau E, Martinez MJ, Vizuete J. Effectiveness of contrast-enhanced ultrasound for characterisation of intestinal inflammation in Crohn's disease: a comparison with surgical histopathology analysis. J Crohns Colitis. 2013;7(2): 120–8.

50. Guidi L, De Franco A, De Vitis I, Armuzzi A, Semeraro S, Roberto I, et al. Contrast-enhanced ultrasonography with sonovue after infliximab therapy in Crohn's disease. Eur Rev Med Pharmacol Sci. 2006;10(1):23–6.

51. Quaia E, Cabibbo B, De Paoli L, Toscano W, Poillucci G, Cova MA. The value of time-intensity curves obtained after microbubble contrast agent injection to discriminate responders from non-responders to anti-inflammatory medication among patients with Crohn's disease. Eur Radiol. 2013;23(6):1650–9.

52. Quaia E, Migaleddu V, Baratella E, Pizzolato R, Rossi A, Grotto M, et al. The diagnostic value of small bowel wall vascularity after sulfur hexafluoride-filled microbubble injection in patients with Crohn's disease. Correlation with the therapeutic effectiveness of specific anti-inflammatory treatment. Eur J Radiol. 2009;69(3):438–44.

53. Hara AK, Leighton JA, Sharma VK, Fleischer DE. Small bowel: preliminary comparison of capsule endoscopy with barium study and ct. Radiology. 2004;230(1):260–5.

54. Monkemuller K, Neumann H, Meyer F, Kuhn R, Malfertheiner P, Fry LC. A retrospective analysis of emergency double-balloon enteroscopy for small-bowel bleeding. Endoscopy. 2009;41(8):715–7.

55. Monkemuller K, Olano C, Fry LC, Ulbricht LJ. Small-bowel endoscopy. Endoscopy. 2009;41(10): 872–7.

56. Pennazio M. Bleeding update. Gastrointest Endosc Clin N Am. 2006;16(2):251–66.

57. Ross A, Mehdizadeh S, Tokar J, Leighton JA, Kamal A, Chen A, et al. Double balloon enteroscopy detects small bowel mass lesions missed by capsule endoscopy. Dig Dis Sci. 2008;53(8):2140–3.

58. Hakim FA, Alexander JA, Huprich JE, Grover M, Enders FT. Ct-enterography may identify small bowel tumors not detected by capsule endoscopy: eight years experience at Mayo Clinic Rochester. Dig Dis Sci. 2011;56(10):2914–9.

59. Huprich JE, Fletcher JG, Alexander JA, Fidler JL, Burton SS, McCullough CH. Obscure gastrointestinal bleeding: Evaluation with 64-section multiphase ct enterography—initial experience. Radiology. 2008; 246(2):562–71.

60. Shin JK, Cheon JH, Lim JS, Park JJ, Moon CM, Jeon SM, et al. Long-term outcomes of obscure gastrointestinal bleeding after ct enterography: does negative ct enterography predict lower long-term rebleeding rate? J Gastroenterol Hepatol. 2011;26(5):901–7.

61. Agrawal JR, Travis AC, Mortele KJ, Silverman SG, Maurer R, Reddy SI, et al. Diagnostic yield of dual-phase computed tomography enterography in patients with obscure gastrointestinal bleeding and a non-diagnostic capsule endoscopy. J Gastroenterol Hepatol. 2012;27(4):751–9.

62. Hara AK, Walker FB, Silva AC, Leighton JA. Preliminary estimate of triphasic ct enterography performance in hemodynamically stable patients with suspected gastrointestinal bleeding. AJR Am J Roentgenol. 2009;193(5):1252–60.

63. Davis JS, Ryan ML, Fields JM, Neville HL, Perez EA, Sola JE. Use of ct enterography for the diagnosis

of lower gastrointestinal bleeding in pediatric patients. J Pediatr Surg. 2013;48(3):681–4.

64. Sinha CK, Pallewatte A, Easty M, De Coppi P, Pierro A, Misra D, et al. Meckel's scan in children: a review of 183 cases referred to two paediatric surgery specialist centres over 18 years. Pediatr Surg Int. 2013;29(5):511–7.

65. Fishman SJ, Burrows PE, Leichtner AM, Mulliken JB. Gastrointestinal manifestations of vascular anomalies in childhood: varied etiologies require multiple therapeutic modalities. J Pediatr Surg. 1998;33(7): 1163–7.

66. Fremond B, Yazbeck S, Dubois J, Brochu P, Garel L, Ouimet A. Intestinal vascular anomalies in children. J Pediatr Surg. 1997;32(6):873–7.

67. Kaza RK, Platt JF, Al-Hawary MM, Wasnik A, Liu PS, Pandya A. Ct enterography at 80 kvp with adaptive statistical iterative reconstruction versus at 120 kvp with standard reconstruction: image quality, diagnostic adequacy, and dose reduction. AJR Am J Roentgenol. 2012;198(5):1084–92.

68. Allen BC, Baker ME, Einstein DM, Remer EM, Herts BR, Achkar JP, et al. Effect of altering automatic exposure control settings and quality reference mas on radiation dose, image quality, and diagnostic effi-cacy in MDCT enterography of active inflammatory Crohn's disease. AJR Am J Roentgenol. 2010;195(1): 89–100.

69. Kambadakone AR, Prakash P, Hahn PF, Sahani DV. Low-dose ct examinations in Crohn's disease: impact on image quality, diagnostic performance, and radiation dose. AJR Am J Roentgenol. 2010;195(1): 78–88.

70. Sagara Y, Hara AK, Pavlicek W, Silva AC, Paden RG, Wu Q. Abdominal ct: comparison of low-dose ct with adaptive statistical iterative reconstruction and routine-dose ct with filtered back projection in 53 patients. AJR Am J Roentgenol. 2010;195(3):713–9.

71. Del Gaizo AJ, Fletcher JG, Yu L, Paden RG, Spencer GC, Leng S, et al. Reducing radiation dose in ct enterography. Radiographics. 2013;33(4):1109–24.

72. Ehman EC, Yu L, Manduca A, Hara AK, Shiung MM, Jondal D, et al. Methods for clinical evaluation of noise reduction techniques in abdominopelvic ct. Radiographics. 2014;34(4):849–62.

73. Ajaj W, Goyen M, Schneemann H, Kuehle C, Nuefer M, Ruehm SG, et al. Oral contrast agents for small bowel distension in MRI: influence of the osmolarity for small bowel distention. Eur Radiol. 2005;15(7): 1400–6.

Magnetic Resonance Enterography

Rakesh Sinha

Introduction

Magnetic resonance enterography (MRE) examinations are carried out after ingestion of large volumes of oral contrast in order to distend the bowel lumen [1, 2]. MRE examinations allow concurrent assessment of the bowel lumen, bowel wall, surrounding mesentery, and other abdominal organs. A significant advantage is the lack of radiation associated with MR imaging. Real-time imaging for peristaltic activity and dynamic contrast studies are therefore possible with MRE without the associated radiation burden.

Recent advances in MRE techniques and faster imaging times are also proving useful for monitoring disease activity and severity in Crohn's disease in order to guide appropriate medical or surgical treatment. The emergence of diffusion-weighted MR imaging allows for detection of abnormalities at a cellular level. An MRE examination can provide comprehensive diagnostic information regarding anatomic, pathophysiological,

and cellular changes in the small bowel in a single, noninvasive procedure that is not possible with any other radiological modality.

Overview of MR Enterography in Small Intestinal Imaging

The main advantage of MRE examinations is that they allow simultaneous diagnostic assessment of the luminal, mural, and extramural structures. The alternative MR imaging technique of the small intestine is an MR enteroclysis examination that involves nasojejunal intubation. MR enteroclysis can provide excellent intestinal distension and by providing this volume challenge can be particularly useful in identifying subacute or partial strictures. However, nasojejunal intubation is usually uncomfortable for the patient and sedation or anxiolytics may be needed [1]. Furthermore, radiation is still involved during the placement of the nasojejunal catheter. It has been reported in several studies that patients prefer MRE to MR enteroclysis examinations [3, 4]. MRE examinations are also preferable in pediatric patients.

MR Imaging Versus Conventional Enteroclysis

Prospective comparative trials on MR enteroclysis as compared to conventional enteroclysis (CE) have reported sensitivity and specificity ranges of

Electronic supplementary material: The online version of this chapter (doi: 10.1007/978-3-319-14415-3_5) contains supplementary material, which is available to authorized users. Videos can also be accessed at http://link.springer.com/chapter/10.1007/978-3-319-14415-3_5.

R. Sinha, F.R.C.R., M.D., M.B.B.S. (✉)
Department of Clinical Radiology, Warwick Hospital, South Warwickshire NHS Foundation Trust, Lakin Road, Warwick, Warwickshire CV345BW, UK
e-mail: rakslide@gmail.com

82.5–89 % and 100 %, respectively, in the detection of bowel ulceration; 100 % and 88–92.9 % in the detection of stenosis; and 75–100 % and 97.8–100 % in the detection of fistulae in patients with Crohn's disease (CD) [4–9]. MR imaging detected a significantly higher number of extramural abnormalities such as abscesses, fibro-fatty proliferation, lymphadenopathy, and skip lesions as compared to CE [5–10]. In their study, Umschaden et al. [8] reported that MRI demonstrated abnormalities not seen at CE in up to a quarter of patients, whereas another study detected 70 % more abnormalities on MR imaging as compared to CE [9]. A critically appraised report concluded that MRE compares favorably with CE in terms of diagnostic yield but is inferior in detection of early mucosal abnormalities [9].

MRE Versus CT and Ultrasound

Studies have reported sensitivities of 80–86.3 % for computed tomography (CT) when compared with CE, and 80–88 % compared to ileocolonoscopy in the detection of Crohn's disease (CD) [10–12]. Maglinte et al. reported the overall sensitivity and specificity of CE in the diagnosis of CD to be 100 % and 99.3 %, respectively [13]. Other studies have also confirmed the high accuracy of CE in the detection of CD [14, 15]. Interestingly, one study has reported higher yield for state-of-the-art barium–carbon dioxide enteroclysis (as practiced in Japan) than even wireless capsule endoscopy (WCE) [14]. Ileocolonoscopy also has high accuracy in the detection of CD. Pera et al. reported an accuracy of 89 %, whereas Wilkins et al. reported sensitivity and specificity of 74 % and 100 % in the detection of CD [16, 17].

The major disadvantage of CT is the cumulative radiation dosage—especially since young patients with CD may undergo several imaging examinations during the disease process. Desmond et al. reported that CT accounted for up to 84.7 % of the cumulative dose imparted to patients with inflammatory bowel disease [18].

A comparative study of contrast-enhanced MRI with CT using oral contrast showed higher sensitivity and specificity for MR imaging in CD [19]. Another comparative study confirmed that MRE has the highest accuracy in the detection of terminal ileitis as compared to CT enterography and barium follow-through examinations [20]. Recent refinements in MRE technique have further enhanced its diagnostic accuracy as compared to surgical and histopathological standards (see later).

The advantages of ultrasonography are its noninvasiveness and widespread availability. However, ultrasonography is entirely dependent on operator expertise and it is not possible to view the gastrointestinal tract in its entirety. Ultrasonography has been shown to have high sensitivity in detection of CD, particularly disease involving the terminal ileum; a meta-analysis reported the sensitivity and specificity ranges of an ultrasound examination to range between 75–94 % and 67–100 %, respectively [21]. Both MR enterography and ultrasonography have the intrinsic advantage of being nonionizing, noninvasive, and patient-friendly examinations. The advantage of MRE over ultrasonography is that it allows multiplanar imaging and comprehensive assessment of the entire gastrointestinal tract. The ability to distinguish fibrotic from inflammatory strictures and higher sensitivity for detecting abscesses and fistulae are the other important advantages.

MRE vs Wireless Capsule Endoscopy

A prospective comparative study between MRE and WCE has shown WCE to be the more sensitive modality in the detection of CD [22]. MRE was less sensitive than WCE (83 % versus 100 %) although a statistically significant difference between the performance of WCE and MRE was not detected. Although several studies have reported higher diagnostic yield for WCE, they have also highlighted its limitations. Poor localization of bowel abnormalities, capsule retention, contraindications in obstructive disease, and false-positive results are some of the drawbacks of WCE. Furthermore as CD by nature has significant transmural or extraintestinal progression, radiological investigations that provide mural and extramural detail provide complementary information to the WCE examination [23, 24].

MRE Versus MR Enteroclysis

MR imaging of the small bowel can be performed after an enteroclysis examination. A meta-analysis reported that the sensitivity of MRE for diagnosing CD was lower than the sensitivity of MR entroclysis, whereas specificity values were comparable [7]. However, since that analysis, a prospective, randomized study showed a similar diagnostic sensitivity for MRE versus MR entero-clysis (88 % versus 88 %), and recommended enterographic examinations for follow-up of established CD [3]. Furthermore the MRE technique has been refined over the last few years and there is now greater experience amongst radiologists. Recent studies have reported that high-resolution MRE (HR-MRE) provided similar diagnostic results to invasive procedures such as MR enteroclysis in patients with CD [25, 26].

Current Clinical Role of MR Enterography

The major indication for MRE is in the diagnostic assessment and follow-up of CD. It can also be used as an alternative to endoscopy in the initial assessment of patients with symptoms of small bowel diseases. As mentioned previously, a nonionizing imaging modality such as MRE is preferable in younger patients and also in cases where repeated radiological imaging is anticipated during the course of the disease. MR imaging with its inherent superior tissue contrast resolution can help in categorizing disease status in CD and also guide treatment. As clinical symptoms may not accurately represent disease activity, MRE parameters may be used to grade disease activity in CD.

Other clinical uses of MRE are evolving and under research. There is documented evidence of its use in evaluation of celiac disease, benign and malignant neoplasms arising in polyposis syndromes such as Peutz-Jeghers, infectious processes, systemic sclerosis, and bowel obstruction.

Enteral Contrast Media

The main principle behind obtaining diagnostic small bowel images is good distension and opacification of the bowel lumen. There is still no consensus on the amount of oral contrast needed for an enterographic examination and timing of image acquisition. Kuehle et al. studied the effect of different types and volumes of oral contrast on bowel distension and timing of image acquisition and found that good distension of the bowel was achieved with 1,350 ml of contrast (1.2–2 % sorbitol solution and 0.2 % locust bean gum) and no additional diagnostic benefit was achieved by increasing the contrast volume to 1,800 ml [27]. Water was found to provide inadequate distension at all volumes. Ajaj reported no significant differences in bowel distension with either 1,000, 1,200, or 1,500 ml of mannitol solution [28]. The optimal time for imaging the entire small bowel has been reported to range between 50 and 60 min [1, 29].

Several enteral contrast agents have been described that include water, methylcellulose, or solutions containing locust bean gum, mannitol, polyethylene glycol, and superparamagnetic agents. Enteral contrast agents may be positive; that is, they produce increased signal intensity within the bowel lumen (e.g., gadolinium chelates), whereas negative agents cause a signal dropout (e.g., superparamagnetic particles). Biphasic agents (e.g., polyethylene glycol, mannitol solution) behave as positive or negative agents depending on the imaging sequence applied. Studies have reported different advantages and disadvantages for positive and negative contrast agents, although there does not seem to be any significant difference in terms of diagnostic accuracy [30].

At our institution, the oral contrast material is divided into two aliquots of 600–650 ml each, and the patient drinks one aliquot every 25–30 min. An oral suspension of 10 mg of metoclopramide is given with the first aliquot to promote gastric emptying. Continuous, steady ingestion of the oral contrast material over the allocated time promotes uniform and consistent filling of the proximal and distal small bowel [31]. Just before imaging, patients are asked to drink another 200 ml of contrast material to opacify the stomach and duodenum. The single most important factor for promoting enteral transit is a full stomach [28]. Therefore the addition of a second dose of oral contrast keeps the stomach full, promoting peristalsis and filling of the intestine. Once oral contrast reaches the ileocecal junction, it reduces peristalsis and bowel transit due to a neuronal and hormonal feedback mechanism. Therefore the administration of oral metoclopramide with the first aliquot (metoclopramide reaches its peak serum concentration at 20–30 min) acts in conjunction with the full stomach and further accentuates the gastric emptying during the latter half of contrast ingestion by overriding the neuronal feedback mechanism.

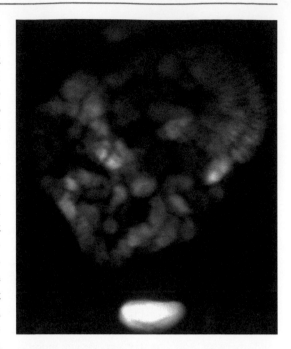

Fig. 5.1 Thick-slab HASTE image enteral contrast outlining the small bowel up to the ascending colon

MR Technique and Sequences

The author's specific protocol for MRE requires the patient to undertake a low-residue diet for the preceding 3 days and fast for 6 h before the procedure. The fasting decreases the possibility of food particles and debris being mistaken for mucosal abnormalities or polyps [25]. Patients who are acutely ill do not undergo the low-residue diet but are kept nil by mouth for 6 h prior to the MRE examination.

Firstly a thick-slab half-Fourier single-shot turbo spin-echo (HASTE) image is obtained to check progress of the contrast column at 50–55 min (Fig. 5.1). If on this sequence contrast is seen to have reached the ileocecal junction, an intravenous injection of antiperistaltic drugs (20 mg of hyoscine-N-butylbromide or 1 mg of glucagon) is administered and further imaging sequences are performed (Table 5.1). If contrast is not yet present at the ileocecal region, a further visit to the MR scanner is planned at subsequent 15–20 min until this region is filled with luminal contrast. Although the antiperistaltic effect of glucagon has been reported to be

significantly longer (18.3 ± 7 min) compared to hyoscine-N-butylbromide (6.8 ± 5.3 min), the author prefers the latter due to lower costs [25, 32]. Occasionally it may be necessary to administer a second dose of antiperistaltic drug prior to imaging the postcontrast sequences if the imaging has been delayed or prolonged (>15 min). Coronal and axial images are then obtained using true fast imaging with steady state with free precession (true-FISP) with and without fat suppression and HASTE sequences. These are contiguous images, 4 mm in thickness, and required breath holds of 18–22 s (Video 5.1). Three-dimension volumetric interpolated breath-hold examination (VIBE) sequences are then used to acquire postcontrast images.

If bowel obstruction is observed on the initial thick-slab HASTE images, MR fluoroscopy of the affected segment is performed to assess for inflammatory adhesions or strictures before injection of antiperistaltic drugs (Video 5.2).

Patients can be scanned in the supine or prone position. The author prefers to perform MR enterography in the supine position, as this is more comfortable for patients. Prone positioning is

Table 5.1 MRI sequences for enterography examination

	1	2	3	4	5
MR sequences	HASTE with fat saturation	True-FISP with and without fat saturation	HASTE with fat saturation	VIBE/FLASH 3D with fat saturation	High-resolution imaging True-FISP with fat saturation
Plane	Coronal	Coronal and axial	Coronal and axial	Coronal and axial	Coronal and axial
Breath hold	No	Yes	Yes	Yes (multi)	Yes
Timing				In last part of study (unenhanced and enhanced [60 s after contrast administration])	
No. of slices	1	19–25	19–25	60–80	12–15
Slice thickness (mm)	50	4	4	2.5	2
Slice distance		0	0	0	0
Field of view (mm^2)	512×512	Coronal: 512×400	Coronal: 512×512	Coronal: 280×320	160×160
		Axial: 350×240	Axial: 350×350	Axial: 350×262	160×160
TR (ms)	5,000	2.5–4.0	1,200	2.5–5.12	2.5–4.0
TE (ms)	1,000	1.6–1.8	80	1–2.5	1.6–1.8
Flip angle (°)	90–140	50–80	90–140	10–20	50–80

advocated by some studies as it provides compression of the bowel loops with better loop separation, although this has not been proven to provide any significant diagnostic advantages [29].

MRE Findings in Crohn's Disease

Ulcers and Intestinal Fold Abnormalities

Acute inflammation in CD is characterized by ulcers and mucosal fold abnormalities. Intestinal folds may also have a thickened or polypoid appearance and folds may be absent in the chronic phase of CD (Fig. 5.2). Edema within the mucosal folds is seen as hyperintense signal on HASTE and true-FISP sequences (Fig. 5.2). In patients with active CD, the bowel wall may have a higher signal intensity compared to non-affected bowel wall. Early ulcers (aphthous ulcers) may be seen as a ring of edema around a tiny ulcer crater (Fig. 5.3).

Fissuring ulcers initially manifest as areas of breakdown in the mucosal lining (Fig. 5.4). These ulcers may extend in the submucosal space and cause undermining of the mucosal lining. Larger transmural ulcers are outlined by luminal contrast and appear as linear, high signal intensity protrusions into the bowel wall (Fig. 5.5) [5, 6, 33]. Residual mucosal islands between ulcerated mucosa may have a polypoid appearance (pseudopolyps) (Fig. 5.3). Linear ulcers are pathognomonic for CD [26]. They typically run parallel to the mesenteric border and may cause fibrosis and rigidity of the bowel leading to obstructive symptoms (Fig. 5.6). Confluent, intersecting longitudinal and transverse ulceration with residual mucosal islands leads to the formation of a "cobblestone" appearance. The presence of aphthous ulceration in combination with thickened intestinal folds has high specificity for CD [1].

An ulceration pattern with edema within mucosal folds is more readily visible on MRE compared to CT, as generally MR imaging has higher tissue specificity than CT. T2-weighted

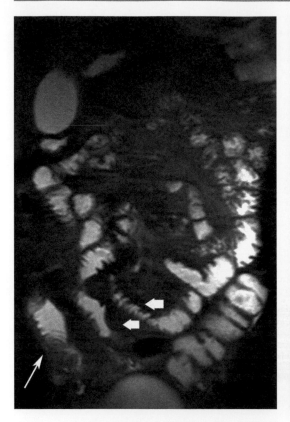 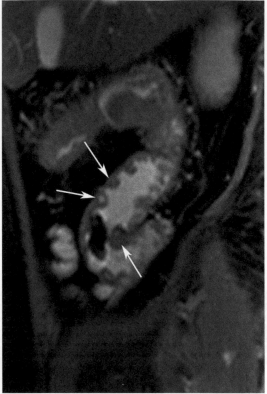

Fig. 5.2 Acute inflammatory CD. Thickened, distorted mucosal folds are readily visible against the bright signal from enteral contrast (*thick arrows*). Mural edema is seen as linear high signal (*thin arrow*)

Fig. 5.3 Ulcers. Sagittal true-FISP image shows multiple aphthous ulcers as high signal lesion surrounded by ring of edema (*arrows*). Note mural thickening and pseudopolypoid appearance of residual mucosa

sequences facilitate detection of ulcers due to high contrast obtained between luminal contrast and bowel wall. Abnormalities in the mucosal fold pattern can also be readily visualized on HASTE sequences against the background of the high signal from the luminal contrast.

Mural Thickening

Mural thickening is a significant feature of CD, although not entirely specific as several other disease entities can also cause bowel thickening. Mural thickness >3 mm should be considered to be abnormal and has been reported to have sensitivity and specificity ranges of 83–91 % and 86–100 %, respectively, in the detection of CD [1].

Good correlation between mural thickening and the CD activity index (CDAI) has been reported [34]. A recent comparative study of MRE and histopathology reported that using a mural thickness cutoff of >4.5 mm distinguished between severe and mild inflammation in CD [25].

Mural and Mesenteric Enhancement, Fibrofatty Proliferation

Engorged mesenteric vessels supplying inflamed bowel segments produce the "comb sign" on MRE examinations (Fig. 5.7) [35]. A secondary finding associated with bowel inflammation is "fat-wrapping" or "fat proliferation" around the inflamed bowel, which is a discriminating feature

Fig. 5.4 Ulcers. Coronal true-FISP image shows thickened terminal ileum with fissuring ulcers causing break in the mucosal outline (*arrow*). Note deeper ulcer (*thick arrow*) outlined by enteral contrast. Hypointense submucosa of the descending colon in quiescent phase of CD (*arrow*)

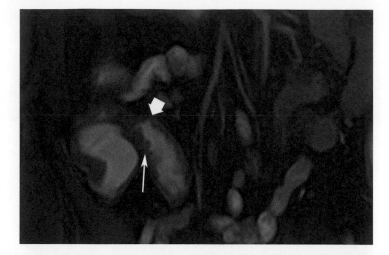

Fig. 5.5 Ulcers. Axial true-FISP image multiple transmural ulcers as linear high signal tracks traversing the inflamed bowel wall (*arrow*)

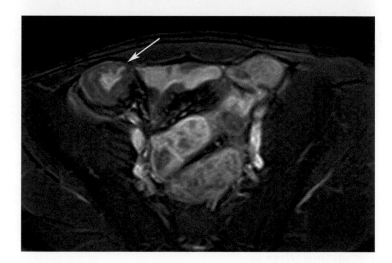

of CD [1, 36, 37]. Increased enhancement of the mesenteric fat around a bowel segment is a secondary sign of active bowel inflammation [38]. Active inflammation causes mucosal hyperemia that manifests as intense enhancement after intravenous contrast administration (Fig. 5.8). Increased mural enhancement has been reported to have good correlation with CDAI [25, 34, 39].

Enhancement can be homogeneous (all bowel wall enhancing equally), layered (both mucosal and serosal bowel wall layers enhancing with a central band of relatively reduced enhancement), or irregular. A layered pattern of bowel enhancement has good correlation with active inflammation, although an overlap exists, and this pattern may also be seen in chronic or inactive disease [25, 40].

A similar appearance may also be produced by a low signal intensity "halo" produced by fat hypertrophy and fibrosis of the submucosa in chronic inflammatory bowel disease (Fig. 5.9). In these cases the submucosa has a dark, hypointense signal, especially on fat-suppressed sequences.

Fibrotic strictures have been reported to demonstrate irregular or reduced mural enhancement [1]. This pattern of different enhancement has been attributed to differently expressed mediators in active and inactive CD [25]. MRE may be better suited to distinguish between a fibrotic stricture and one that is primarily due to acutely inflamed submucosa, as MR sequences can detect fibrotic change with greater facility than CT or ultrasound. Making the distinction between

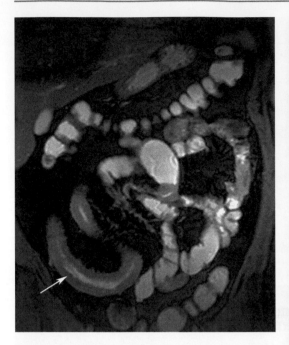

Fig. 5.6 Linear ulcer. Coronal true-FISP image shows inflamed ileum with a linear ulcer visible as high signal track along the bowel lumen (*arrow*)

inflammatory strictures with spasms and the fat-halo sign of fibrotic CD is important, as obstruction and spasm in active disease are best treated with medical therapy, whereas chronic strictures may require surgical intervention.

Fistulating Disease

In advanced inflammation, deep ulcers penetrate the intestinal wall and cause inflammation in the adjacent mesenteric tissue leading to formation of small peri-intestinal abscesses and blind-ending sinus tracts. Once these tracts perforate through the wall of an adjacent hollow organ a fistula is formed (Fig. 5.10). Sinus tracts manifest as nodular irregularities and spiculations adjacent to the serosal surface of the bowel and they are the precursors of fistulating disease [41]. Small sinus tracts may be better seen on high-resolution MR images and high-quality multiplanar reconstruction (MPR) images are useful in their assessment [25, 26]. Larger sinus tracts and fistulae may be outlined by enteral contrast and are seen as linear tracts of high signal intensity on MRE; however, the majority of fistulous tracts do not contain air or fluid within

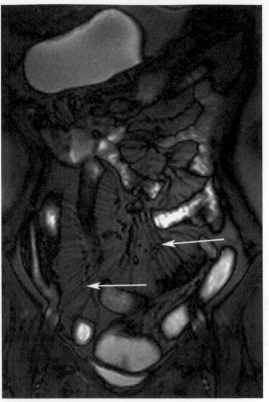

Fig. 5.7 Comb sign. Coronal true-FISP image shows engorged vessels as linear structures against background of mesenteric fat (*arrows*). Note extensive mesenteric fat proliferation surrounding inflamed bowel

their lumen [41]. Fistulas occur in up to one-third of patients with CD at some time during the course of their disease and the lifetime risk ranges from 20 to 40 % [41–43]. Internal fistulae are more common and enteroenteric fistulae are usually asymptomatic [44]. The most common location of fistulae is the perineal region (54 %). The reported sensitivity and specificity values of MRE for detection of internal fistulae range between 83.3–84.4 % and 100 %, respectively [30, 45, 46].

MR imaging has also been reported to be highly accurate for detection and depiction of perineal fistula. This is due to the inherent higher tissue contrast resolution of MR imaging. It is difficult to accurately assess perianal fistula on CT as the attenuation value and appearance of fistula tracts, fibrosis, and sphincter muscles are similar to each other. Furthermore, compared with endorectal ultrasound, MR imaging provides a wider field of view and is better suited for assessment of complex

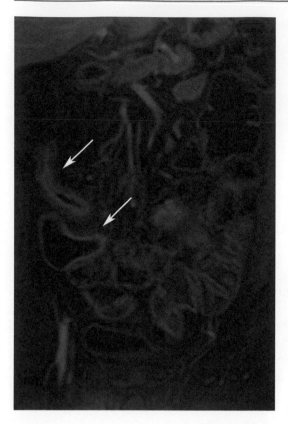

Fig. 5.8 Enhancement. Axial 3D VIBE image shows marked enhancement of inflamed ileum and cecum (*arrows*)

branching tracts, lateral extension, and extension above the levator muscles.

Surgical intervention may be required if fistulae cause recurrent infection or if they lead to significant malabsorption [47]. Fistulae may have a stellate ("star") appearance due to fibrotic and desmoplastic reaction in the mesentery around the inflamed fistulous tract (Fig. 5.11) [36]. Abdominal abscesses and inflammatory masses are less frequent than fistulae but are more likely to need intervention. Smaller abscesses may be treated with antibiotics or drained under imaging guidance, while larger ones may benefit from surgery.

Fibrostenotic Disease

Fibrostenotic disease typically presents with bowel obstruction. Fibrostenotic strictures are seen as a fixed narrowed segment of bowel with proximal bowel dilatation (Fig. 5.12). Chronic fibrotic strictures are typically hypointense on both T1- and T2-weighted sequences. Fibrotic strictures may show minor, inhomogeneous contrast enhancement without any evidence of edema or surrounding mesenteric inflammation or hyperemia. MR fluoroscopy can be used in conjunction with MRE to provide functional assessment of bowel obstruction and strictures similar to those obtained on enteroclysis with less patient discomfort [31].

Negaard et al. reported that the sensitivity for detecting stenosis of the terminal ileum on MRE was 86 % versus 100 % for MR enteroclysis, although the higher diagnostic accuracy was not statistically significant [3]. This higher accuracy is likely to be due to the better luminal distension in MR enteroclysis. However, in routine practice, symptomatic stenoses are easily detected on MRE as non-distending bowel segments with proximal dilatation.

Cancer in CD

There is an increased incidence of adenocarcinoma in intestinal segments affected with CD [48]. The risk for developing colorectal cancer in those with Crohn's colitis is between 4 and 20 times greater than in the general population [49, 50]. There is also an increased risk for developing cancer in excluded bowel segments [48]. Carcinoma in CD typically appears as a stricture, which may be difficult to differentiate from benign inflammatory strictures [50]. Some adverse features that may indicate underlying tumor are asymmetric mural thickening, shouldering, mesenteric infiltration, ascites, and lymphadenopathy (Fig. 5.13). Any bowel obstruction that does not resolve with conservative treatment and nasoenteric decompression should arouse the possibility of an underlying cancer. Imaging features that are out of keeping with clinical parameters should also raise concerns regarding an underlying tumor. Diffusion-weighted imaging may be a useful aide to differentiate between acute inflammatory strictures and underlying cancer [51].

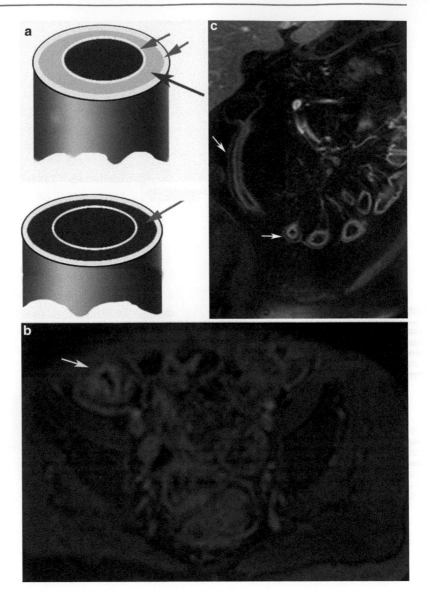

Fig. 5.9 Enhancement patterns. (**a**) Schematic diagram. (**b**) Layered enhancement shows enhancing serosa and mucosa and isointense submucosa (*arrow*). (**c**) Halo sign in chronic CD shows markedly hypointense submucosal layer between enhancing mucosa and serosa

MRE Findings in Other Small Intestinal Diseases and Disorders

Other clinical uses and roles for MRE are evolving and currently being investigated. There have been reports of the use of MRE in the evaluation of celiac disease, benign and malignant neoplasms arising in polyposis syndromes such as Peutz-Jeghers, and inflammatory conditions such as vasculitis, infectious processes, systemic sclerosis, and bowel obstruction [52, 53].

Tumors

High sensitivity and specificity have been reported in the detection of small-bowel neoplasms with MR enteroclysis on several studies [54, 55]. MRE has been reported to be a feasible alternative to capsule endoscopy for small-bowel surveillance in adults with Peutz-Jeghers and other familial polyposis syndromes [56, 57]. Benign tumors of the small intestine include leiomyomas, adenomas, lipomas, hemangiomas, inflammatory polyps, and hamartomas [58].

Fig. 5.10 Fistula. Axial
true-FISP image shows
multiple ileo-ileal fistulae
arising from inflamed ileal
segments (*arrow*)

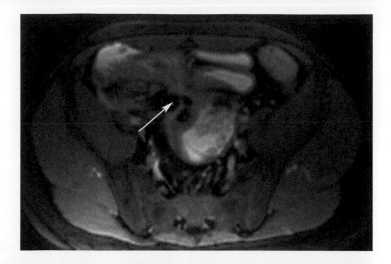

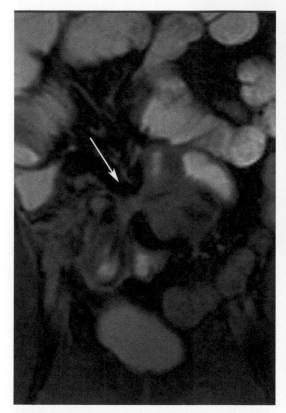

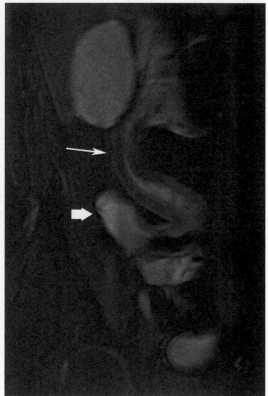

Fig. 5.11 Fistula. Coronal true-FISP image shows inter-
loop fistula forming the star sign (*arrow*)

Fig. 5.12 Stricture. Coronal true-FISP image shows
stricture in the distal ileum showing marked hypointensity
in the submucosal suggestive of fibrosis (*arrow*). *Thick
arrow* = distended proximal bowel segment

Benign tumors such as adenomas appear as
well-defined sessile or pedunculated lesions that
show homogeneous enhancement after intravenous contrast administration. Usually benign
tumors, such as adenomas, protrude into the

bowel lumen without causing obstruction and
have a smooth border with no mesenteric infiltration (Fig. 5.14) [59].

Fig. 5.13 Cancer in CD. Axial true-FISP image shows a thickened segment of distal ileum with fistulation into the sigmoid (*arrowhead*). The sigmoid thickening is eccentric with a shouldered appearance suggestive of a neoplastic growth (*arrow*). Adenocarcinoma was found at histology

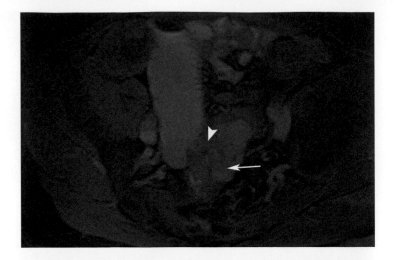

Fig. 5.14 Benign tumor. Coronal true-FISP image shows a small, well-defined polypoid lesion projecting into the bowel lumen of an ileo-anal pouch (*arrow*). This was a benign adenoma

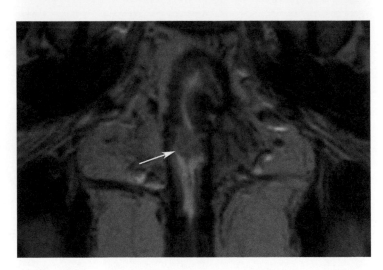

Malignant lesions include gastrointestinal stromal tumors (GISTs), adenocarcinomas, carcinoid tumors, lymphoma, sarcomas, and metastases. GISTs in the small bowel most often originate from the muscular layer and commonly demonstrate an exophytic growth. GISTs have a strong association with neurofibromatosis type 1 [60, 61]. Tumors usually show brisk enhancement. GISTs may be intraluminal, submucosal, or subserosal in location and appear as smooth, well-defined masses (Fig. 5.15). After intravenous contrast administration, GISTs are typically enhancing masses with areas of low attenuation from hemorrhage, necrosis, or cyst formation [61].

Adenocarcinomas are the most common primary malignancies of the small bowel. They most often arise in the duodenum (50 %), followed by the jejunum (30 %) and ileum (20 %) [59]. Adenocarcinomas typically show eccentric involvement of a short segment of bowel, and often lead to partial or complete bowel obstruction (Fig. 5.16). MRE findings of adenocarcinomas include annular or eccentric mural thickening with adjacent infiltration and lymphadenopathy. Adenocarcinomas typically demonstrate moderate enhancement [62]. Lymph node enlargement in metastatic adenocarcinoma is not as marked as in lymphomatous disease. Distant metastases from adenocarcinomas to the

Fig. 5.15 GIST. Axial true-FISP image shows a rounded, well-defined tumor with extra-serosal growth (*arrow*)

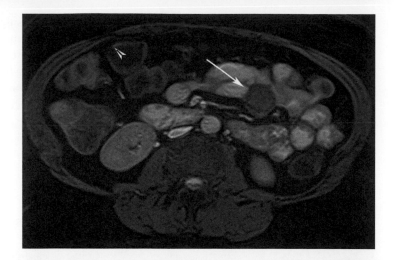

Fig. 5.16 Adenocarcinoma. Axial true-FISP image shows a concentric stricture in the jejunum (*arrow*) with lymphadenopathy and mesenteric invasion (*thick arrow*). Adenocarcinoma was found on histopathology

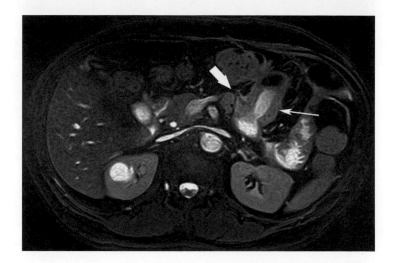

liver and peritoneum may also be depicted on MRE examinations [36, 51–53].

Most (50 %) carcinoid tumors occur in the appendix and about one-third (33 %) arise from the small bowel. One-tenth of patients develop carcinoid syndrome [54]. Carcinoids vary in appearance from small submucosal lesions to large ulcerating masses. These tumors often involve the adjacent mesentery, causing a desmoplastic reaction with in-drawing of adjacent bowel segments (Fig. 5.17). Carcinoid tumors are typically isointense to that in muscle on T1- and T2-weighted images, and sometimes exhibit radiating spicule-like strands of tissue.

On MRE, small intestinal lymphoma usually appears as circumferential bowel wall thickening involving a long segment. Extensive adjacent lymphadenopathy, aneurysmal dilatation, and lack of obstruction despite a large tumor mass are suggestive of lymphoma as the primary diagnostic consideration (Fig. 5.18).

Obstruction

MRE can be used in the diagnostic work-up of suspected small bowel obstruction. The diagnosis of a mechanical small bowel obstruction is based on the visualization of an abrupt change in bowel caliber without evidence of another cause of obstruction at the transition point from the dilated segment to the collapsed segment of bowel.

Adhesions and adhesive bands are not usually associated with thickening of the small-bowel wall [63] (Fig. 5.19). Occasionally adhesive bands, seen as hypointense linear structures, may be seen coursing through mesenteric fat on T2-weighted images. Clumping or kinking of bowel loops also may be seen [64].

MR imaging has been shown to have accuracy for the detection and characterization of malignant versus benign strictures in the small bowel [65]. Investigators have used MR imaging to map adhesions preoperatively using a visceral slide technique with a sensitivity of 87.5 % and a specificity of 92.5 % [66].

Celiac Disease

Celiac disease predominantly involves the duodenum and proximal jejunum [67, 68]. MRE findings in celiac disease include inflammatory thickening of the bowel wall, lymphadenopathy, and mesenteric vascular engorgement. Complications of the disease may include intussusception and extensive ulcerative jejunoileitis with marked, circumferential thickening of the small bowel (Fig. 5.20).

Infective Diseases and Disorders

MRE is not routinely indicated for the diagnosis of small intestinal infections. Usually, patients present with nausea, vomiting, and/or diarrhea and CT or ultrasonography is carried out in the acute phase [69, 70]. Infectious ileitis may manifest on MR images as nonspecific, segmental, or

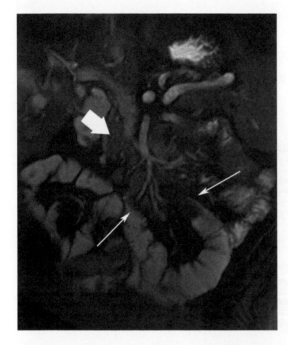

Fig. 5.17 Carcinoid tumor. Coronal true-FISP image shows an infiltrative mesenteric mass (*thick arrow*) causing in-drawing of surrounding bowel segments (*arrows*)

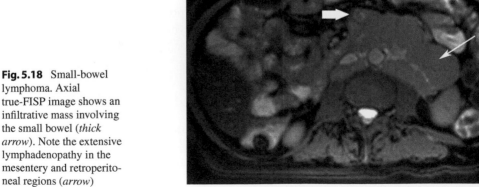

Fig. 5.18 Small-bowel lymphoma. Axial true-FISP image shows an infiltrative mass involving the small bowel (*thick arrow*). Note the extensive lymphadenopathy in the mesentery and retroperitoneal regions (*arrow*)

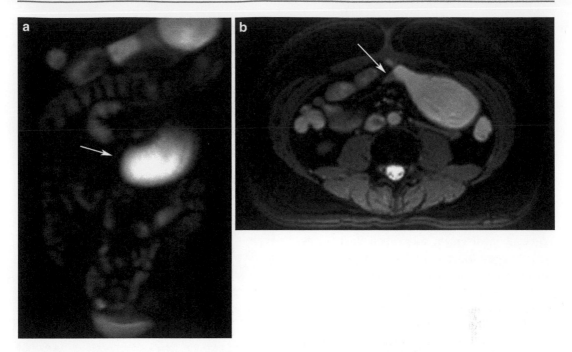

Fig. 5.19 Small-bowel obstruction. (**a**) HASTE image shows obstructed and dilated segment of proximal small intestine (*arrow*). (**b**) Axial true-FISP image shows the distended bowel loop and a kinked segment (*arrow*) caus-ing mechanical obstruction. Note lack of inflammation or any other finding at the site of obstruction. Adhesive band was found at surgery

Fig. 5.20 Celiac disease. Axial true-FISP image shows inflamed segment of jejunum with large ulcers (*arrow*) and lymphadenopathy (*thick arrow*). Ulcerative jejunitis was found at surgery

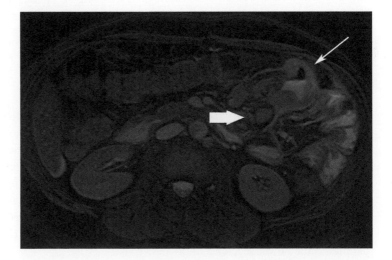

circumferential wall thickening of the terminal ileum and cecum with moderate or marked enlargement of the mesenteric lymph nodes [36].

GI tract tuberculosis typically involves the ileocecal region with the cecum and ascending colon usually involved to a greater degree than the terminal ileum [69]. Tuberculosis causes asymmetric thickening of the ileocecal valve and medial wall of the cecum with contraction of the cecum [69]. Enlarged lymph nodes with central areas of necrosis are often seen. Peritoneal disease and ascites are often associated with ileocecal tuberculosis [71]. The most common type of peritoneal disease called "wet-type" manifests as large amounts of viscous ascitic fluid that shows a high signal due to its high protein and cellular content.

It may be difficult to differentiate small-bowel tuberculosis from CD. Differentiating between these entities is important as corticosteroids are used for treating CD that can provoke fulminant, catastrophic infection in patients with tuberculosis. Ulcers in tuberculosis tend to be axial (girdle) or oval. Linear, longitudinal ulcers of CD are not seen. Contraction of the cecum and a prominence of cecal involvement more than ileal involvement suggest tuberculosis, whereas the ileum is predominantly involved in CD. Ascites and necrotic lymph nodes are commonly seen in tuberculous infections, but are uncommon in CD. Fat proliferation of the mesentery around the affected bowel is indicative of CD rather than tuberculosis.

Recent Advances

High-Resolution MR Enterography (HR-MRE)

High-resolution MR enterography (HR-MRE) has recently been reported as a refinement to the standard MRE technique [26]. High-resolution true-FISP images with fat suppression are acquired using contiguous thin slices (2–3 mm), using 160–250 mm field of view and matrix sizes of 128–256 × 128–256 providing in-plane resolution of 1–2 mm and small field of view [26]. HRE-MRE images are obtained after aligning the MR imaging plane either parallel or perpendicular to the affected bowel segment. Images aligned parallel to the bowel segments allow better visualization of mucosal irregularities and abnormalities. Images aligned perpendicular to the bowel provide accurate visualization of transmural ulcers, fistulae, sinus tracts, and para-intestinal abnormalities (Figs. 5.21 and 5.22) [38]. The higher in-plane resolution achieved on HR-MRE has been reported to be the main factor that increases the diagnostic accuracy. HR-MRE

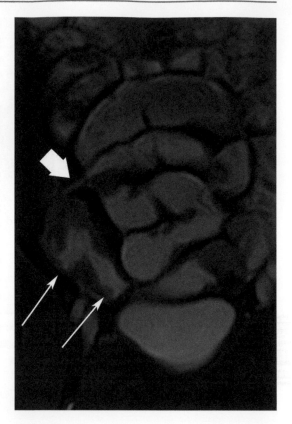

Fig. 5.21 High-resolution MRE. Coronal true-FISP image of the terminal ileum shows a marked mural thickening and transmural ulcers (*arrows*). Early ileo-ileal fistulation is also present (*thick arrow*). These changes were better visualized on HR-MRE compared to standard MRE imaging

images also allow high-quality MPR images that increase diagnostic confidence in the detection of smaller fistulae and ulceration. A comparative study has reported the sensitivities of MRE versus HR-MRE in the detection of superficial ulcers as (50 % versus 69 %) deep ulcers (69 % versus 94 %), fistulae (75 % versus 96 %), and abscesses (77 % versus 100 %), respectively [25].

Diffusion-Weighted MR Imaging (DW MR)

Diffusion-weighted MR (DW MR) imaging is emerging as an important tool in the diagnostic work-up of inflammatory bowel disease [51]. DW MR imaging can help in the assessment of

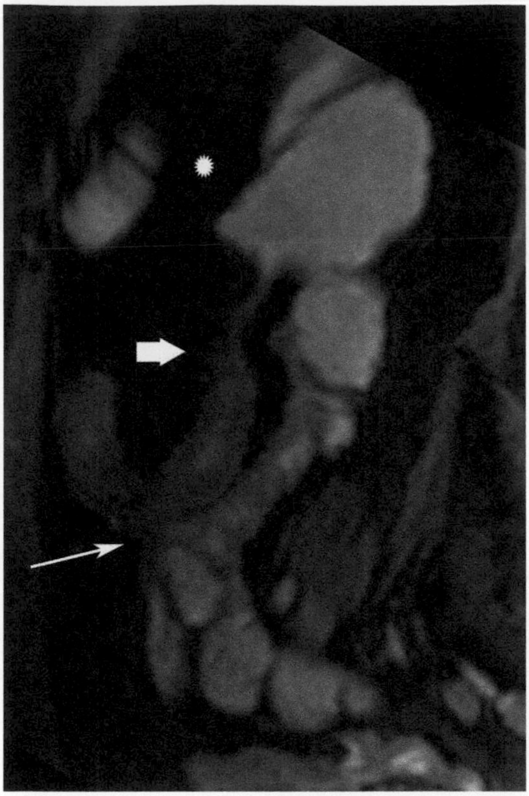

Fig. 5.22 High-resolution MRE. Sagittal true-FISP image shows a thickened segment of terminal ileum. Transmural disease with early sinus formation is present (*thick arrow*). There is also an ileo-ileal fistula (*arrow*). Note fat proliferation around the inflamed bowel (*asterisk*). HR-MRE provides excellent detail and allows far greater accuracy in assessment of the transmural changes in CD compared to standard imaging

inflammation, and complications such as abscesses and fistula formation, and also aid in monitoring of response to treatment. DW MR has also been reported to increase diagnostic confidence in the assessment of bowel abnormalities [72].

The advantages of DW MR imaging are its noninvasive nature and lack of exposure to ionizing radiation or contrast injection. As DW MR imaging can be integrated with standard MRE imaging, this does not require any additional equipment and can be easily added to a routine MR imaging protocol.

DW MR imaging uses the diffusion of water within biologic tissues to produce images. It therefore provides functional, quantitative information at the cellular level that can facilitate accurate assessment of inflammation and response to therapy.

As proposed by Albert Einstein in 1905, the random motion of molecules within a liquid depends on their inherent thermal energy [73]. Diffusion of water molecules within biological tissues is not completely free but restricted due to limitations of the cell membrane as compared to molecules in the extracellular or intravascular spaces [51]. Therefore an increase in total number of cells, such as inflammatory infiltrates, leads to an increase in overall restricted diffusion within a given volume of tissue [51, 74, 75].

Inflammatory CD leads to infiltration of the lamina propria and submucosa by inflammatory cells and lymphoid aggregates. This increased cellularity, viscosity, dilated lymphatic channels, and granulomas lead to increased restricted diffusion, which in turn leads to an increased signal on the DW images (Fig. 5.23) [74, 76]. Due to complete suppression of the signal from normal tissues, the abnormal tissues are easily visible as "hot spots" similar to nuclear imaging.

The level of diffusion weighting may be adjusted by changing a parameter called the b value with the following equation:

$$b = \gamma^2 G^2 \delta^2 \left(\Delta - \delta_{/3} \right),$$

where γ equals the gyromagnetic ratio of hydrogen; G equals the strength of the applied diffusion gradient; δ (*delta*) equals the duration of the gradient; and Δ (*Delta*) equals the time between the first and second gradients. By acquiring multiple DW images at different b values, an accurate diffusion coefficient may be calculated for each image voxel by plotting the signal intensity against the b value, which then yields an exponential value called the apparent diffusion coefficient (ADC). Apparent diffusion coefficient values can provide an objective measurement index that may be compared or followed over time.

ADC values measured from actively inflamed intestine have been reported to be significantly lower compared with normal bowel wall [74–76]. Overall, DW MR imaging has been reported to have high sensitivity and specificity in the

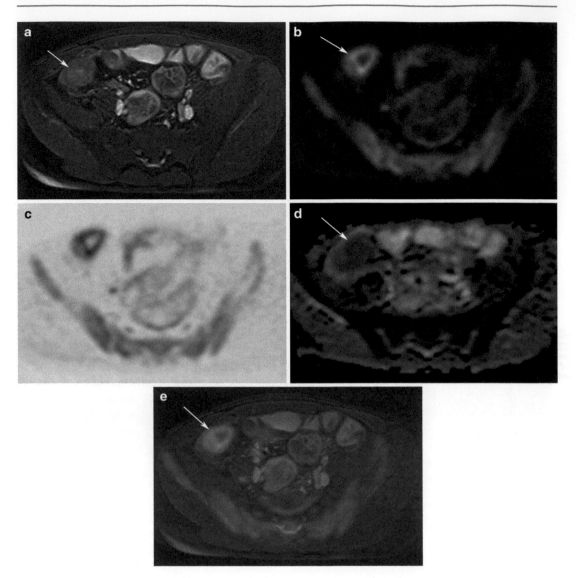

Fig. 5.23 Diffusion-weighted imaging. (**a**) Axial true-FISP image shows inflamed terminal ileum (*arrow*). (**b**) Diffusion-weighted MR image shows areas of high signal intensity in the inflamed segment (*arrow*). (**c**) Inverted grayscale diffusion-weighted MR image shows the abnormal bowel as a "hot spot" against suppressed signal from normal tissues. This presentation is similar to those seen at nuclear imaging. (**d**) ADC map shows an area of markedly low signal intensity (*arrow*) in the abnormal area confirming the restricted diffusion. (**e**) DW images can be color coded and fused with standard images (*arrow*) to match up the abnormal area with anatomy

detection of bowel inflammation (86–94 % and 81.4–84.8 %, respectively) [74, 77]. Using a threshold ADC value of 2.4×10^{-3} mm/s, Oto et al. reported differentiation between normal and inflamed colon with a sensitivity and specificity of 94 % and 88 %, respectively [75]. The hyperintense signal of the inflamed bowel segments against the suppressed signal of non-inflamed tissues on DW MR images makes their detection easier. Transmural inflammation is more typical of CD and manifests as high signal affecting the whole thickness of the bowel wall. There is good evidence that more advanced inflammation leads to lower ADC values [51, 74, 76, 78].

Transmural ulcers and sinuses may be seen as mural linear or nodular high signal changes traversing the bowel wall or the extramural tissues on DW imaging (Fig. 5.24).

DW MR imaging can also be particularly useful in patients in whom intravenous contrast cannot be administered due to allergy or renal

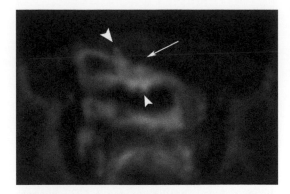

Fig. 5.24 Axial diffusion-weighted image shows abnormal signal involving the whole thickness of the bowel wall (*arrow*). Nodular and linear extensions of inflammation (*arrowheads*) suggest early sinus formation

impairment. In these particular cases DW MR imaging can quantify inflammation and complications despite lack of contrast enhancement findings (Fig. 5.25).

DW MR imaging has high accuracy for detection of fistulae and abdominal abscesses [37, 38]. Abscesses show restricted diffusion due to contained bacterial, inflammatory cells, and cellular debris [79, 80]. Finding of intra-abdominal abscesses is important, as they are a relative contraindication to the use of antitumor necrotic factor (anti-TNF) alpha agents (e.g., infliximab) [1, 36]. Intestinal fistulae complicating CD appear as hyperintense linear or serpiginous structures on the DW MR images connecting to separate bowel loops, communicating to the skin surface or other organs [81] (Fig. 5.26). The abnormal signal of fistulae on DW MR is due to the presence of pus, inflammatory cells, and debris within or around

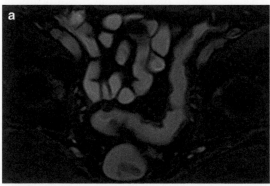
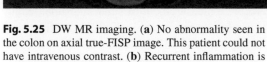
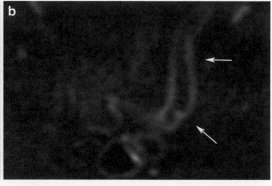

Fig. 5.25 DW MR imaging. (**a**) No abnormality seen in the colon on axial true-FISP image. This patient could not have intravenous contrast. (**b**) Recurrent inflammation is confirmed on DW MR image as hyperintense signal changes that form a double line or "tram-track" appearance (*arrows*)

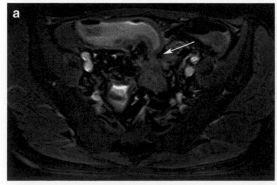
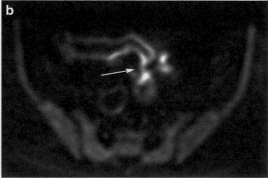

Fig. 5.26 DW MR imaging. (**a**) Axial true-FISP image shows inflamed ileum with an ileo-ileal fistula (*arrow*). (**b**) DW image confirms the fistula as a high signal track connecting the bowel lumen (*arrow*)

the fistula tract. The high viscosity of pus and inflammatory dense cellular composition lead to restricted diffusion and a resultant high signal on DW MR images [81]. Fibrotic strictures or adhesions do not show abnormal DW MR signal. Therefore lack of a high signal on DW MR imaging may help to distinguish between fibrotic and inflammatory strictures.

DW MR can be used in the detection of recurrent disease in patients with CD. In particular, early mucosal disease may not be clearly visualized on standard MR imaging as the high signal from the enteral contrast may mask mucosal changes. By nulling signal from all other tissues except for areas of inflammation, DW MR can help in diagnosing early mucosal recurrent disease. Early mucosal recurrent inflammation may be seen as high signal changes that form a double line or "tram-track" appearance (Fig. 5.25). Although the utility of DW MR imaging in the assessment of response to treatment has not been validated in large studies, the author's own experience suggests that DW MR provides useful information regarding treatment response in inflammatory bowel disease.

Currently DW MR imaging provides a useful adjunct to the standard MR imaging of the bowel. It is helpful in cases where intravenous contrast is a contraindication. Some studies have reported that the addition of DW MR imaging increased the radiologists' confidence in diagnosing abnormal bowel segments [78, 82]. In the author's experience, successful treatment is accompanied by a reduction in the DW MR signal and an increase in the ADC values of the affected segments.

Perfusion Imaging

There is scientific evidence that in active CD there is presence of microvascular ischemia in the affected bowel segment [83, 84]. The total volume of blood supplied to bowel segments with active CD is also reduced [85, 86]. However, the exact cause for this microvascular ischemia is yet to be determined. Potential factors include increased platelet aggregation and increased

platelet surface expression of P-selectin and GP53. These small studies with MRI have confirmed that mucosal perfusion is reduced in chronic CD, although larger studies are needed to validate these findings.

Bowel Peristalsis Assessment

Recently, work has been done on assessing small bowel motility and peristalsis in patients with active CD. During active CD there is inflammatory infiltration of the bowel wall, hypothesized to cause increased stiffness and therefore reduced peristalsis [87–89]. Some reported studies have shown reduced motility in active CD, whereas others have reported no differences between active and quiescent disease [87, 89]. Abnormal peristalsis or motility may help in detection of abnormal segments [90]. Assessment of motility changes appears promising but the difficulty in categorizing these changes due to subjective assessments makes this aspect of bowel imaging less useful. It is possible that in the future, peristaltic assessment may play a useful role in highlighting abnormal segments and distinguishing between fibrotic strictures and adhesions.

Bowel Length Measurement

Accurate measurement of small intestinal length is useful where multiple bowel resections are anticipated, such as in patients with CD. Therefore the functional outcome of extensive intestinal resection may depend on the length of remnant bowel. Patients with short intestinal length may develop "short-bowel syndrome" with significant nutritional deficiencies due to malabsorption of vitamins and minerals [91, 92]. Measurement of small intestinal length has been reported on barium follow-through examinations using an opisometer [93, 94]. However, this approach has inherent limitations as a two-dimensional image is used to measure an organ that typically has overlapping segments and loops.

There have been recent reports describing development of software for small-bowel length

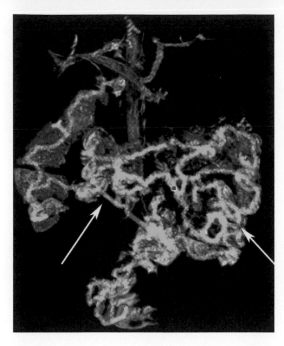

Fig. 5.27 Bowel length measurement. Coronal volume rendered image shows centerline plot for measuring bowel length

parameters such as mural edema and enhancement, which do not have any corresponding indices on histopathology or endoscopy.

Validated studies carried out by Rimola et al. concluded that for assessment of disease severity, the presence of edema and ulcerations must be evaluated in addition to mural thickness and contrast enhancement [102, 104]. The presence of ulcers was validated as direct evidence of active inflammation and the presence or absence of ulcers is of considerable clinical relevance in terms of disease course and surgical requirements [105].

Therefore, any grading system should include objective findings such as ulcers, mural thickening in combination with contrast enhancement, and bowel edema. Better resolution on MRE and objective measurements (e.g., T1 maps) may make future scoring systems even more accurate. It is quite likely that such comprehensive grading systems will be in use in the future and may provide an accurate noninvasive assessment of CD activity.

measurement [95]. These depend on employment of three-dimensional dynamic direction gradient vector flow snakes with centerline extraction [96–98]. A recent report has demonstrated the feasibility of mapping the small intestine on MR images with accurate assessment of bowel length to within 10 cm of in vivo measurement [99] (Fig. 5.27).

Grading of Crohn's Disease Activity

Several studies have been published on the value of MRI in detecting disease activity and assessing severity compared with colonoscopy or pathology data [100–103]. Grading systems have also been reported using MR parameters and good correlation has been shown between MR scoring and ileocolonoscopy. However, a significant drawback of most of these grading systems is that they do not evaluate complications such as fistulas or stenosis and many studies are not yet validated. Another major limitation of the current grading systems is that they rely on subjective

Disadvantages and Pitfalls of Enterography

Enterography is associated with less discomfort for patients, but it does not produce the same distension of the bowel as does the enteroclysis technique. The one area where enteroclysis technique is decidedly superior is in the diagnosis of strictures or obstruction secondary to CD. MRE may not provide adequate distension of the bowel to highlight partial or incipient strictures [106]. A "distension challenge" of the bowel as provided by an enteroclysis examination is better suited to highlight areas of partial narrowing or strictures [8, 25, 106]. Therefore, if obstruction or partial strictures are suspected then an enteroclysis examination should be the preferred diagnostic option. Compared to CT enterography, MRE is more costly, more time consuming, and less widely available. There is lower spatial resolution and there may be more variable image quality as compared to CT.

Enterography may not provide consistent distension of the proximal bowel loops, particularly the jejunum. However, isolated jejunal CD is very rare. In a large series and a meta-analysis, the incidence of isolated jejunal CD was estimated to be between 0.01 % and 0.03 % [107]. If there is strong clinical suspicion of CD despite a normal or suboptimal MRE examination, then MR enteroclysis or WCE should be considered for further evaluation.

Conclusion

An MRE examination can provide comprehensive diagnostic information regarding anatomic, pathophysiological, and cellular changes in the small bowel in a single, noninvasive procedure that is not possible with any other radiological modality. MRE examinations allow simultaneous diagnostic assessment of the luminal, mural, and extramural structures.

The advantages of MRE include its high sensitivity in the diagnosis of CD and its important role in the assessment of inflammatory activity. Recent advances in MRE technique have resulted in high diagnostic accuracy in detection of ulcers, mucosal fold abnormalities, and extraintestinal pathology. Its nonionizing nature is also a particular advantage in patients who undergo repeated imaging investigations. It is likely that MRE will play an important role in the diagnostic imaging of the small intestine in the future.

References

1. Sinha R, Murphy P, Hawker P, Sanders S, Rajesh A, et al. Role of MRI in Crohn's disease. Clin Radiol Clin Radiol. 2009;64(4):341–52.
2. Sinha R, Nwokolo C, Murphy PD. Magnetic resonance imaging in Crohn's disease. BMJ. 2008;336(7638):273–6.
3. Negaard A, Paulsen V, Sandvik L, Berstad AE, Borthne A, Try K, et al. A prospective randomized comparison between two MRI studies of the small bowel in Crohn's disease, the oral contrast method and MR enteroclysis. Eur Radiol. 2007;17:2294–301.
4. Negaard A, Sandvik L, Berstad AE, Paulsen V, Lygren I, Borthne A, et al. MRI of the small bowel with oral contrast or nasojejunal intubation in Crohn's disease: randomized comparison of patient acceptance. Scand J Gastroenterol. 2008;43(1):44–51.
5. Gourtsoyiannis N, Papanikolaou N, Grammatikakis J, Papamastorakis G, Prassopoulos P, Roussomoustakaki M. Assessment of Crohn's disease activity in the small bowel with MR and conventional enteroclysis: preliminary results. Eur Radiol. 2004;14(6):1017–24.
6. Masselli G, Casciani E, Polettini E, Lanciotti S, Bertini L, Gualdi G. Assessment of Crohn's disease in the small bowel: prospective comparison of magnetic resonance enteroclysis with conventional enteroclysis. Eur Radiol. 2006;16(12):2817–27.
7. Horsthuis K, Bipat S, Bennink RJ, Stoker J. Inflammatory bowel disease diagnosed with US, MR, scintigraphy, and CT: meta-analysis of prospective studies. Radiology. 2008;247(1):64–79.
8. Umschaden HW, Szolar D, Gasser J, Umschaden M, Haselbach H. Small-bowel disease: comparison of MR enteroclysis images with conventional enteroclysis and surgical findings. Radiology. 2000;215(3):717–25.
9. Frøkjaer JB, Larsen E, Steffensen E, Nielsen AH, Drewes AM. Magnetic resonance imaging of the small bowel in Crohn's disease. Scand J Gastroenterol. 2005;40(7):832–42.
10. Minordi LM, Vecchioli A, Guidi L, Mirk P, Fiorentini L, Bonomo L. Multidetector CT enteroclysis versus barium enteroclysis with methylcellulose in patients with suspected small bowel disease. Eur Radiol. 2006;16(7):1527–36.
11. Hassan C, Cerro P, Zullo A, Spina C, Morini S. Computed tomography enteroclysis in comparison with ileoscopy in patients with Crohn's disease. Int J Colorectal Dis. 2003;18(2):121–5.
12. Wold PB, Fletcher JG, Johnson CD, Sandborn WJ. Assessment of small bowel Crohn disease: noninvasive peroral CT enterography compared with other imaging methods and endoscopy–feasibility study. Radiology. 2003;229(1):275–81.
13. Maglinte D, Chernish S, Kelvin F, O'Connor K, Hage J. Crohn disease of the small intestine: accuracy and relevance of enteroclysis. Radiology. 1992;184(2):541–5.
14. Rajesh A, Sandrasegaran K, Jennings SG, Maglinte DDT, McHenry L, Lappas JC, et al. Comparison of capsule endoscopy with enteroclysis in the investigation of small bowel disease. Abdom Imaging. 2009;34(4):459–66.
15. Cirillo LC, Camera L, Della Noce M, Castiglione F, Mazzacca G, Salvatore M. Accuracy of enteroclysis in Crohn's disease of the small bowel: a retrospective study. Eur Radiol. 2000;10(12):1894–8.
16. Pera A, Bellando P, Caldera D, Ponti V, Astegiano M, Barletti C, et al. Colonoscopy in inflammatory bowel disease. Diagnostic accuracy and proposal of an endoscopic score. Gastroenterology. 1987;92(1):181–5.
17. Wilkins T, Jarvis K, Patel J. Diagnosis and management of Crohn's disease. Am Fam Physician. 2011;84(12):1365–75.
18. Desmond AN, O'Regan K, Curran C, McWilliams S, Fitzgerald T, Maher MM, et al. Crohn's disease:

factors associated with exposure to high levels of diagnostic radiation. Gut. 2008;57(11):1524–9.

19. Low RN, Francis IR. MR imaging of the gastrointestinal tract with i.v., gadolinium and diluted barium oral contrast media compared with unenhanced MR imaging and CT. AJR Am J Roentgenol. 1997; 169(4):1051–9.

20. Siddiki H, Fidler J, Fletcher J, Burton S, Huprich J, Hough D, et al. Prospective comparison of state-of-the-art MR enterography and CT enterography in small-bowel Crohn's disease. AJR Am J Roentgenol. 2009;193(1):113–21.

21. Fraquelli M, Colli A, Casazza G, Paggi S, Colucci A, Massironi S, et al. Role of US in detection of Crohn disease: meta-analysis. Radiology. 2005; 236(1):95–101.

22. Albert JG, Martiny F, Krummenerl A, Stock K, Lesske J, Göbel CM, et al. Diagnosis of small bowel Crohn's disease: a prospective comparison of capsule endoscopy with magnetic resonance imaging and fluoroscopic enteroclysis. Gut. 2005;54(12):1721–7.

23. Sandrasegaran K, Maglinte DDT, Jennings SG, Chiorean MV. Capsule endoscopy and imaging tests in the elective investigation of small bowel disease. Clin Radiol. 2008;63(6):712–23.

24. Maglinte D, Sandrasegaran K, Chiorean M, Dewitt J, McHenry L, Lappas J. Radiologic investigations complement and add diagnostic information to capsule endoscopy of small-bowel diseases. AJR Am J Roentgenol. 2007;189(2):306–12.

25. Sinha R, Murphy P, Sanders S, Ramachandran I, Hawker P, Rawat S, et al. Diagnostic accuracy of high-resolution MR enterography in Crohn's disease: comparison with surgical and pathological specimen. Clin Radiol. 2013;68(9):917–27.

26. Sinha R, Rajiah P, Murphy P, Hawker P, Sanders S. Utility of high-resolution MR imaging in demonstrating transmural pathologic changes in Crohn disease. RadioGraphics. 2009;29(6):1847–67.

27. Kuehle CA, Ajaj W, Ladd SC, Massing S, Barkhausen J, Lauenstein TC. Hydro-MRI of the small bowel: effect of contrast volume, timing of contrast administration, and data acquisition on bowel distention. AJR Am J Roentgenol. 2006; 187(4):375–85.

28. Ajaj W, Goehde SC, Schneemann H, Ruehm SG, Debatin JF, Lauenstein TC. Dose optimization of mannitol solution for small bowel distension in MRI. J Magn Reson Imaging. 2004;20(4):648–53.

29. Lohan D, Cronin C, Meehan C, Alhajeri AN, Roche C, Murphy J. MR small bowel enterography: optimization of imaging timing. Clin Radiol. 2007;62(8): 804–7.

30. Rieber A, Nüssle K, Reinshagen M, Brambs H-J, Gabelmann A. MRI of the abdomen with positive oral contrast agents for the diagnosis of inflammatory small bowel disease. Abdom Imaging. 2002; 27(4):394–9.

31. Sinha R, Rawat S. MRI enterography with divided dose oral preparation: effect on bowel distension and

diagnostic quality. Indian J Radiol Imaging. 2013; 23(1):86–91.

32. Froehlich JM, Daenzer M, von Weymarn C, Erturk SM, Zollikofer CL, Patak MA. Aperistaltic effect of hyoscine N-butylbromide versus glucagon on the small bowel assessed by magnetic resonance imaging. Eur Radiol. 2009;19(6):1387–93.

33. Negaard A, Sandvik L, Mulahasanovic A, Berstad AE, Klöw N-E. Magnetic resonance enteroclysis in the diagnosis of small-intestinal Crohn's disease: diagnostic accuracy and inter- and intra-observer agreement. Acta Radiol Stockh Swed 1987. 2006;47(10):1008–16.

34. Sempere G, Martinez Sanjuan V, Medina Chulia E, Benages A, Tome Toyosato A, Canelles P, et al. MRI evaluation of inflammatory activity in Crohn's disease. AJR Am J Roentgenol. 2005;184(6):1829–35.

35. Meyers MA, McGuire PV. Spiral CT demonstration of hypervascularity in Crohn disease: "vascular jejunization of the ileum" or the "comb sign.". Abdom Imaging. 1995;20(4):327–32.

36. Sinha R, Verma R, Verma S, Rajesh A. MR enterography of Crohn disease: part 2, imaging and pathologic findings. AJR Am J Roentgenol. 2011; 197(1):80–5.

37. Stange E, Travis S, Vermeire S, Beglinger C, Kupcinkas L, Geboes K, et al. European evidence based consensus on the diagnosis and management of Crohn's disease: definitions and diagnosis. Gut. 2006;55:1–15.

38. Peyrin-Biroulet L, Chamaillard M, Gonzalez F, Beclin E, Decourcelle C, Antunes L, et al. Mesenteric fat in Crohn's disease: a pathogenetic hallmark or an innocent bystander? Gut. 2007;56(4):577–83.

39. Florie J, Wasser M, Arts-Cieslik K, Akkerman E, Siersema P, Stoker J. Dynamic contrast-enhanced MRI of the bowel wall for assessment of disease activity in Crohn's disease. AJR Am J Roentgenol. 2006;186(5):1384–92.

40. Del Vescovo R, Sansoni I, Caviglia R, Ribolsi M, Perrone G, Leoncini E, et al. Dynamic contrast enhanced magnetic resonance imaging of the terminal ileum: differentiation of activity of Crohn's disease. Abdom Imaging. 2008;4:417–24.

41. Herrmann K, Michaely H, Zech C, Seiderer J, Reiser M, Schoenberg S. Internal fistulas in Crohn disease: magnetic resonance enteroclysis. Abdom Imaging. 2006;31(6):675–87.

42. Bell SJ, Williams AB, Wiesel P, Wilkinson K, Cohen RCG, Kamm MA. The clinical course of fistulating Crohn's disease. Aliment Pharmacol Ther. 2003; 17(9):1145–51.

43. Schwartz DA, Loftus EV, Tremaine WJ, Panaccione R, Harmsen WS, Zinsmeister AR, et al. The natural history of fistulizing Crohn's disease in Olmsted County, Minnesota. Gastroenterology. 2002;122(4):875–80.

44. Lichtenstein GR. Treatment of fistulizing Crohn's disease. Gastroenterology. 2000;119(4):1132–47.

45. Schreyer AG, Geissler A, Albrich H, Schölmerich J, Feuerbach S, Rogler G, et al. Abdominal MRI after

enteroclysis or with oral contrast in patients with suspected or proven Crohn's disease. Clin Gastroenterol Hepatol. 2004;2(6):491–7.

46. Fallis SA, Murphy P, Sinha R, Hawker P, Gladman L, Busby K, et al. Magnetic resonance enterography in Crohn's disease: a comparison with the findings at surgery. Colorectal Dis. 2013;15(10):1273–80.

47. Fichera A, Michelassi F. Surgical treatment of Crohn's disease. J Gastrointest Surg. 2007;11(6): 791–803.

48. Richards ME, Rickert RR, Nance FC. Crohn's disease-associated carcinoma. A poorly recognized complication of inflammatory bowel disease. Ann Surg. 1989;209(6):764–73.

49. Ribeiro MB, Greenstein AJ, Sachar DB, Barth J, Balasubramanian S, Harpaz N, et al. Colorectal adenocarcinoma in Crohn's disease. Ann Surg. 1996; 223(2):186–93.

50. Kerber GW, Frank PH. Carcinoma of the small intestine and colon as a complication of Crohn disease: radiologic manifestations. Radiology. 1984;150(3): 639–45.

51. Sinha R, Rajiah P, Ramachandran I, Sanders S, Murphy PD. Diffusion-weighted MR imaging of the gastrointestinal tract: technique, indications, and imaging findings. Radiographics. 2013;33(3):655–76.

52. Amzallag-Bellenger E, Oudjit A, Ruiz A, Cadiot G, Soyer PA, Hoeffel CC. Effectiveness of MR enterography for the assessment of small-bowel diseases beyond Crohn disease. Radiographics. 2012;32(5):1423–44.

53. Masselli G, Polettini E, Laghi F, Monti R, Gualdi G. Noninflammatory conditions of the small bowel. Magn Reson Imaging Clin N Am. 2014;22(1): 51–65.

54. Masselli G, Casciani E, Polettini E, Laghi F, Gualdi G. Magnetic resonance imaging of small bowel neoplasms. Cancer Imaging. 2013;13:92–9.

55. Van Weyenberg SJB, Bouman K, Jacobs MAJM, Halloran BP, Van der Peet DL, Mulder CJJ, et al. Comparison of MR enteroclysis with video capsule endoscopy in the investigation of small-intestinal disease. Abdom Imaging. 2013;38(1):42–51.

56. Maccioni F, Al Ansari N, Mazzamurro F, Barchetti F, Marini M. Surveillance of patients affected by Peutz-Jeghers syndrome: diagnostic value of MR enterography in prone and supine position. Abdom Imaging. 2012;37(2):279–87.

57. Caspari R, von Falkenhausen M, Krautmacher C, Schild H, Heller J, Sauerbruch T. Comparison of capsule endoscopy and magnetic resonance imaging for the detection of polyps of the small intestine in patients with familial adenomatous polyposis or with Peutz-Jeghers' syndrome. Endoscopy. 2004;36(12):1054–9.

58. Balthazar EJ, Herlinger H, Maglinte D, Birnbaum BA. Clinical imaging of the small intestine. 2nd ed. Berlin: Springer; 2001.

59. Ramachandran I, Sinha R, Rajesh A, Verma R, Maglinte D. Multidetector row CT of small bowel tumours. Clin Radiol. 2007;62(7):607–14.

60. Hartley N, Rajesh A, Verma R, Sinha R, Sandrasegaran K. Abdominal manifestations of neurofibromatosis. J Comput Assist Tomogr. 2008; 32(1):4–8.

61. Sinha R, Verma R, Kong A. Mesenteric gastrointestinal stromal tumor in a patient with neurofibromatosis. AJR Am J Roentgenol. 2004;183(6):1844–6.

62. Buckley J, Fishman E. CT evaluation of small bowel neoplasms: spectrum of disease. Radiographics. 1998;18(2):379–92.

63. Cronin CG, Lohan DG, Browne AM, Alhajeri AN, Roche C, Murphy JM. MR enterography in the evaluation of small bowel dilation. Clin Radiol. 2009;64(10):1026–34.

64. Fidler JL, Guimaraes L, Einstein DM. MR imaging of the small bowel. Radiographics. 2009;29(6): 1811–25.

65. Low RN, Chen SC, Barone R. Distinguishing benign from malignant bowel obstruction in patients with malignancy: findings at MR imaging. Radiology. 2003;228(1):157–65.

66. Lienemann A, Sprenger D, Steitz HO, Korell M, Reiser M. Detection and mapping of intraabdominal adhesions by using functional cine MR imaging: preliminary results. Radiology. 2000;217(2):421–5.

67. Masselli G, Picarelli A, Gualdi G. Celiac disease: MR enterography and contrast enhanced MRI. Abdom Imaging. 2010;35(4):399–406.

68. Paolantonio P, Tomei E, Rengo M, Ferrari R, Lucchesi P, Laghi A. Adult celiac disease: MRI findings. Abdom Imaging. 2007;32(4):433–40.

69. Sinha R, Rajesh A, Rawat S, Rajiah P, Ramachandran I. Infections and infestations of the gastrointestinal tract. Part 1: bacterial, viral and fungal infections. Clin Radiol. 2012;67(5):484–94.

70. Sinha R, Rajesh A, Rawat S, Rajiah P, Ramachandran I. Infections and infestations of the gastrointestinal tract. Part 2: parasitic and other infections. Clin Radiol. 2012;67(5):495–504.

71. Mitchell RS, Bristol LJ. Intestinal tuberculosis: an analysis of 346 cases diagnosed by routine intestinal radiography on 5,529 admissions for pulmonary tuberculosis, 1924–49. Am J Med Sci. 1954; 227(3):241–9.

72. Kinner S, Blex S, Maderwald S, Forsting M, Gerken G, Lauenstein TC. Addition of diffusion-weighted imaging can improve diagnostic confidence in bowel MRI. Clin Radiol. 2014;69(4):372–7.

73. Einstein A. Über die von der molekularkinetischen Theorie der Wärme geforderte Bewegung von in ruhenden Flüssigkeiten suspendierten Teilchen. Ann Phys. 1905;322(8):549–60.

74. Oto A, Zhu F, Kulkarni K, Karczmar GS, Turner JR, Rubin D. Evaluation of diffusion-weighted MR imaging for detection of bowel inflammation in patients with Crohn's disease. Acad Radiol. 2009;1 6(5):597–603.

75. Oto A, Kayhan A, Williams J, Fan X, Yun L, Arkani S, et al. Active Crohn's disease in the small bowel: evaluation by diffusion weighted imaging and

quantitative dynamic contrast enhanced MR imaging. J Magn Reson Imaging. 2011;33(3):615–24.

76. Oussalah A, Laurent V, Bruot O, Bressenot A, Bigard M, Régent D, et al. Diffusion-weighted magnetic resonance without bowel preparation for detecting colonic inflammation in inflammatory bowel disease. Gut. 2010;59(8):1056–65.

77. Kiryu S, Dodanuki K, Takao H, Watanabe M, Inoue Y, Takazoe M, et al. Free-breathing diffusion-weighted imaging for the assessment of inflammatory activity in Crohn's disease. J Magn Reson Imaging. 2009;29(4):880–6.

78. Tielbeek JAW, Ziech MLW, Li Z, Lavini C, Bipat S, Bemelman WA, et al. Evaluation of conventional, dynamic contrast enhanced and diffusion weighted MRI for quantitative Crohn's disease assessment with histopathology of surgical specimens. Eur Radiol. 2014;24(3):619–29.

79. Chan JH, Tsui EY, Luk SH, Fung AS, Yuen MK, Szeto ML, et al. Diffusion-weighted MR imaging of the liver: distinguishing hepatic abscess from cystic or necrotic tumor. Abdom Imaging. 2001;26(2):161–5.

80. Chan JH, Tsui EY, Luk SH, Fung SL, Cheung YK, Chan MS, et al. MR diffusion-weighted imaging of kidney: differentiation between hydronephrosis and pyonephrosis. Clin Imaging. 2001;25(2):110–3.

81. Schmid-Tannwald C, Agrawal G, Dahi F, Sethi I, Oto A. Diffusion-weighted MRI: role in detecting abdominopelvic internal fistulas and sinus tracts. J Magn Reson Imaging. 2012;35(1):125–31.

82. Hori M, Oto A, Orrin S, Suzuki K, Baron R. Diffusion-weighted MRI: a new tool for the diagnosis of fistula in ano. J Magn Reson Imaging. 2009;30(5):1021–6.

83. Danese S, Sans M, de la Motte C, Graziani C, West G, Phillips MH, et al. Angiogenesis as a novel component of inflammatory bowel disease pathogenesis. Gastroenterology. 2006;130(7):2060–73.

84. Thornton M, Solomon MJ. Crohn's disease: in defense of a microvascular aetiology. Int J Colorectal Dis. 2002;17(5):287–97.

85. Angerson WJ, Allison MC, Baxter JN, Russell RI. Neoterminal ileal blood flow after ileocolonic resection for Crohn's disease. Gut. 1993;34(11):1531–4.

86. Tateishi S, Arima S, Futami K. Assessment of blood flow in the small intestine by laser Doppler flowmetry: comparison of healthy small intestine and small intestine in Crohn's disease. J Gastroenterol. 1997;32(4):457–63.

87. Cullmann JL, Bickelhaupt S, Froehlich JM, Szucs-Farkas Z, Tutuian R, Patuto N, et al. MR imaging in Crohn's disease: correlation of MR motility measurement with histopathology in the terminal ileum. Neurogastroenterol Motil. 2013;25(9):749-e577.

88. Heye T, Stein D, Antolovic D, Dueck M, Kauczor H-U, Hosch W. Evaluation of bowel peristalsis by dynamic cine MRI: detection of relevant functional disturbances—initial experience. J Magn Reson Imaging. 2012;35(4):859–67.

89. Patak MA, Froehlich JM, von Weymarn C, Breitenstein S, Zollikofer CL, Wentz K-U. Non-invasive measurement of small-bowel motility by MRI after abdominal surgery. Gut. 2007;56(7):1023–5.

90. Froehlich JM, Waldherr C, Stoupis C, Erturk SM, Patak MA. MR motility imaging in Crohn's disease improves lesion detection compared with standard MR imaging. Eur Radiol. 2010;20(8):1945–51.

91. Lal S, Teubner A, Shaffer JL. Review article: intestinal failure. Aliment Pharmacol Ther. 2006;24(1):19–31.

92. O'Keefe SJD, Buchman AL, Fishbein TM, Jeejeebhoy KN, Jeppesen PB, Shaffer J. Short bowel syndrome and intestinal failure: consensus definitions and overview. Clin Gastroenterol Hepatol. 2006;4(1):6–10.

93. Nightingale JMD, Bartram CI, Lennard-Jones JE. Length of residual small bowel after partial resection: correlation between radiographic and surgical measurements. Gastrointest Radiol. 1991;16(1):305–6.

94. Shatari T, Clark MA, Lee JR, Keighley MRB. Reliability of radiographic measurement of small intestinal length. Colorectal Dis. 2004;6(5):327–9.

95. Fabbri R, Costa LDF, Torelli JC, Bruno OM. 2D Euclidean distance transform algorithms: a comparative survey. ACM Comput Surv. 2008;40(1):1–44.

96. Deschamps T, Cohen LD. Fast extraction of minimal paths in 3D images and applications to virtual endoscopy. Med Image Anal. 2001;5(4):281–99.

97. Wan M, Liang Z, Ke Q, Hong L, Bitter I, Kaufman A. Automatic centerline extraction for virtual colonoscopy. IEEE Trans Med Imaging. 2002;21:1450–60.

98. Harders M, Wildermuth S, Weishaupt D, Székely G. Improving virtual endoscopy for the intestinal tract. Lect Notes Comput Sci. 2002;2489:20–7.

99. Sinha R, Trivedi D, Murphy P, Fallis S. Small intestinal length measurement on MR enterography: comparison with in-vivo surgical measurement. AJR Am J Roentgenol. 2014;203(3):274–9.

100. Tielbeek JAW, Makanyanga JC, Bipat S, Pendsé DA, Nio CY, Vos FM, et al. Grading Crohn disease activity with MRI: interobserver variability of MRI features, MRI scoring of severity, and correlation with Crohn disease endoscopic index of severity. AJR Am J Roentgenol. 2013;201(6):1220–8.

101. Tielbeek JAW, Bipat S, Boellaard TN, Nio CY, Stoker J. Training readers to improve their accuracy in grading Crohn's disease activity on MRI. Eur Radiol. 2014;24(5):1059–67.

102. Rimola J, Ordás I, Rodriguez S, García-Bosch O, Aceituno M, Llach J, et al. Magnetic resonance imaging for evaluation of Crohn's disease: validation of parameters of severity and quantitative index of activity. Inflamm Bowel Dis. 2011;17(8):1759–68.

103. Girometti R, Zuiani C, Toso F, Brondani G, Sorrentino D, Avellini C, et al. MRI scoring system

including dynamic motility evaluation in assessing the activity of Crohn's disease of the terminal ileum. Acad Radiol. 2008;15(2):153–64.

104. Rimola J, Rodriguez S, García-Bosch O, Ordás I, Ayala E, Aceituno M, et al. Magnetic resonance for assessment of disease activity and severity in ileocolonic Crohn's disease. Gut. 2009;58(8):1113–20.

105. Allez M, Lemann M, Bonnet J, Cattan P, Jian R, Modigliani R. Long term outcome of patients with active Crohn's disease exhibiting extensive and deep ulcerations at colonoscopy. Am J Gastroenterol. 2002;97(4):947–53.

106. Kohli M, Maglinte D. CT enteroclysis in incomplete small bowel obstruction. Abdom Imaging. 2009; 34:321–7.

107. Farmer RG, Hawk WA, Turnbull Jr RB. Clinical patterns in Crohn's disease: a statistical study of 615 cases. Gastroenterology. 1975;68:627–35.

Video Legends

Video 5.1 - Coronal true-FISP images showing good distension and opacification of the small-bowel loops (MP4 1456 kb)

Video 5.2 - Coronal MR fluoroscopy performed to assess for obstruction (MP4 653 kb)

Part IV

Recent Endoscopic Advances: Technology and Techniques

Small Bowel Capsule Endoscopy

6

Otto S. Lin

Introduction

Since its introduction in 2001, capsule endoscopy has revolutionized the evaluation of the small bowel. In the past, options for visualization of the jejunum and ileum were limited. Push enteroscopy accessed only the duodenum and proximal edge of the jejunum; barium small bowel follow-through (SBFT) was labor intensive, uncomfortable, and inaccurate; computerized tomographic enterography (CTE) was limited by its inability to detect flat mucosal lesions; and intraoperative endoscopy—the ultimate technique for small bowel evaluation—was highly invasive and morbid. Fortunately, small bowel cancers are relatively uncommon. Nevertheless, there are situations in which accurate and complete evaluation of the small bowel is important, with obscure gastrointestinal bleeding (OGIB) being the most common such indication [1]. As a noninvasive, safe, and easily performed modality that visualizes the entire extent of the small intestines, capsule endoscopy has become increasingly popular in many countries.

Electronic supplementary material: The online version of this chapter (doi: 10.1007/978-3-319-14415-3_6) contains supplementary material, which is available to authorized users. Videos can also be accessed at http://link.springer.com/chapter/10.1007/978-3-319-14415-3_6.

O.S. Lin, M.D., M.Sc. (✉)
Digestive Diseases Institute, Virginia Mason Medical Center, Seattle, WA, USA
e-mail: Otto.Lin@vmmc.org

Technical Specifications

There are currently five small bowel video capsules available or in development (Fig. 6.1). Each system consists of a light-emitting diode light source, a lens, a camera based on complementary metal oxide semiconductor (CMOS) or charge-coupled device (CCS) technology, a battery, and (in most cases) a wireless transmitter [2, 3].

Table 6.1 lists some of the technical differences between the available capsules. The most commonly used capsule is the Pillcam SB series manufactured by Given Imaging (Yokneam, Israel) (Video 6.1). The most recent version, the SB3 (approved by the US Food and Drug Administration in 2013), weighs 3 g and measures 11 mm in diameter and 26 mm in length. It is equipped with a CMOS image sensor, a short focal length lens, four white light-emitting diodes for illumination, and an ultrahigh-frequency radio telemetry transmitter for communication of video data to a portable recorder worn by the patient. The angle of view is 156°, and the minimal detection size is estimated to be 0.07 mm. The capsule features "adaptive frame rate" technology, with video collection rates ranging from two to six frames per second depending on how fast the capsule is traveling. There are two versions of the battery, giving either 8 or 12 h of data collection time. The capsule is used with the RAPID Recorder DR3 and RAPID Sensor Belt SB3 accessories. There is an external real-time image viewer (RAPID Real Time Viewer), which

R. Kozarek and J.A. Leighton (eds.), *Endoscopy in Small Bowel Disorders*,
DOI 10.1007/978-3-319-14415-3_6, © Springer International Publishing Switzerland 2015

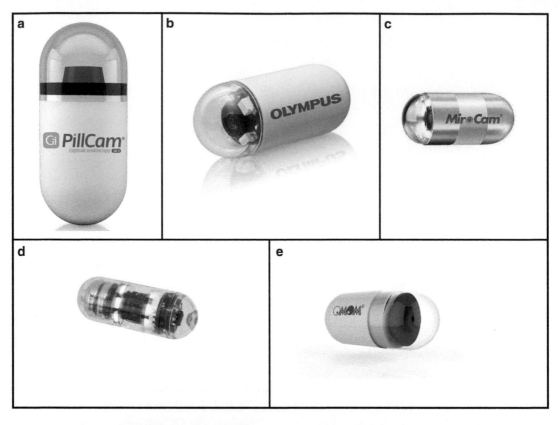

Fig. 6.1 (**a**) Pillcam SB3 (Given Imaging, Yokneam, Israel); (**b**) Endocapsule (Olympus Medical Systems Corporation, Tokyo, Japan); (**c**) Mirocam (IntroMedic Co., Ltd., Seoul, Korea); (**d**) Capsocam SV1 (Capsovision, Saratoga, USA); (**e**) OMOM capsule (Jinshan Science and Technology Co., Chongqing, China)

is helpful to determine if the capsule has reached the colon and whether the study can be terminated early. The software program has also undergone incremental improvements. The most recent version (RAPID Reader 8.0) includes an advanced A-mode feature for video compilation, as well as flexible spectral imaging color enhancement (FICE) contouring and a progress indicator, based on time elapsed, linear distance traveled, and capsule motion information, to assist in localizing lesions for therapeutic intervention. There is also a function to describe findings semiquantitatively using the Lewis Score [4]. Figures 6.2 and 6.3 show representative images of small bowel pathology by the Pillcam SB2 and SB3.

The Endocapsule EC-S10 (Olympus America, Allentown, Pennsylvania) is almost identical in size to the SB3, with a weight of 3.3 g. This

device captures two frames per second, using a supersensitive CCD image sensor with high resolution. In addition, the Endocapsule features automatic brightness adjustment capabilities similar to that used in Olympus endoscopes and has a battery life of 12 h. The accompanying software (Endocapsule Software 10) has red color detection and 3-dimensional tracking functions. A small study on patients with obscure small intestinal bleeding showed reasonably good agreement between slightly older versions of the Pillcam SB and Endocapsule, but did not demonstrate any definite superiority of one capsule over the other [5]. A previous European study also failed to show any significant difference in diagnostic yields between the two [6].

The Mirocam MC1000-W (Intromedic, Seoul, Korea) has recently been FDA approved but is not yet in widespread use in the USA. Small

Table 6.1 Current small bowel capsule endoscopes that are commercially available or in development

Capsule	Manufacturer	Dimensions (mm)	Angle of view (°)	Image capture rate (fps)	Battery life (h)	Data transmission technology
Pillcam SB3	Given Imaging	11×26	156	2–6	12	Radiofrequency
Endocapsule	Olympus	11×26	145	2	8	Radiofrequency
Mirocam	IntroMedic	10.8×24.5	170	3	12	Electrical field propagation
Capsocam SV1	Capsovision	11×31	360	12–20	15	Capsule retrieval/download
OMOM JS-ME-II	Jinshan	13×27.9	140	2	8	Radiofrequency

fps frames per second

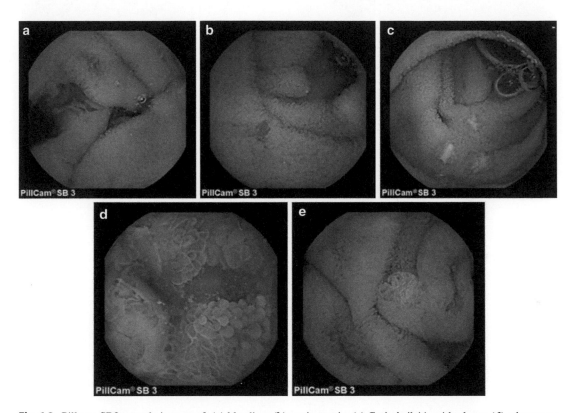

Fig. 6.2 Pillcam SB3 capsule images of: (**a**) bleeding; (**b**) angioectasia; (**c**) Crohn's ileitis with ulcers; (**d**) edematous villi; (**e**) normal papilla of Vater

comparative studies have reported equivalent outcomes between the Mirocam and Pillcam SB or Endocapsule in terms of yield and findings [7–10]. An associated model, the MC1000-WM, has limited ability to be steered in real time.

The Capsocam SV1 (Capsovision, Saratoga, California) features 360° panoramic viewing (via four cameras), capturing 20 frames per second (five for each camera) for the first 2 h followed by 12 frames per second for the remainder of the 15-h battery life. It is slightly larger than the other capsules, with dimensions of 11 mm by 31 mm. Its smart motion sense technology activates the cameras only when the capsule is in motion, limiting the number of redundant images and improving battery life. There are 16 white light-emitting diodes powered by an automatic light controller. However, unlike the other

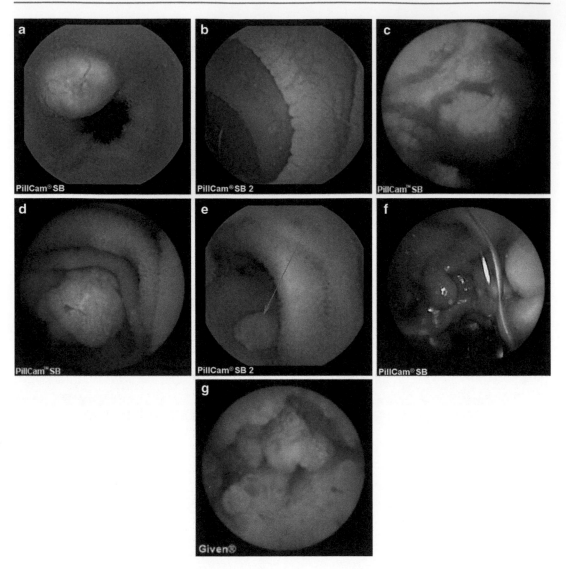

Fig. 6.3 Pillcam SB or SB2 capsule images of (**a**) carcinoid tumor; (**b**) celiac sprue; (**c**) cytomegalovirus enteritis; (**d**) small bowel polyp in the setting of familial adenomatous polyposis syndrome; (**e**) gastrointestinal stromal tumor with ulcer; (**f**) jejunal varices; (**g**) small bowel adenocarcinoma. Images courtesy of Dr. Michael Chiorean

capsules, the data are not wirelessly transmitted to a receiver; instead, the capsule must be retrieved after passage from the body and the data downloaded via a direct connection. This may potentially adversely affect patient acceptance. On the other hand, the presence of cardiac pacemakers or implanted defibrillators is not a listed contraindication, and there is no need for the patient to wear an external receiver. Small studies have shown comparable diagnostic yield and image quality between the Capsocam and Pillcam

SB, but reading time with the Capsocam was longer [11, 12]. Finally, the OMOM JS-ME-II capsule (Jinshan Science and Technology, Chongqing, China) is slightly larger than the Pillcam SB3, but other technical specifications are similar. An associated version, the OMOM JS-ME-III, is controllable in real time; this function is mainly intended to move the capsule around when examining the stomach. Uncontrolled studies have shown promising diagnostic yields and rates of complete small bowel examination [13, 14]. Currently, neither the Capsocam nor the OMOM capsule are approved by the FDA for use in the USA.

The following comments, unless otherwise specified, apply to the Pillcam SB series, the longest approved and most commonly used capsule endoscope in the USA.

Bowel Preparation and Procedure Protocol

The capsule is swallowed following an 8–12-h fast and, in many cases, some form of bowel preparation. Patients are typically allowed to drink clear liquids 2 h into the study, and to eat solid food 4 h after capsule ingestion. During the 8–12 h of battery life, the capsule passes through the gastrointestinal tract via peristalsis while images are recorded and transmitted wirelessly to an external recorder worn by the patient. The images are formatted into a video file that can be viewed on a computer using specialized software. For patients who are unable to swallow the capsule or suffer from delayed gastric emptying, the capsule can be deployed endoscopically in the duodenum or postoperative anatomy using a specially designed capsule holder fitted onto the tip of a conventional endoscope.

Currently, there is wide variation in the bowel preparation process used in different units. Various types of osmotic or stimulant laxatives, such as magnesium citrate or bisacodyl, and prokinetic agents, such as metoclopramide, may be used to prepare the small bowel for capsule endoscopy. Three meta-analyses have concluded that mucosal visualization was better when the bowel was prepared with sodium phosphate, polyethylene glycol, or erythromycin compared with clear liquid diet alone [15–17]. A 2 L polyethylene glycol preparation has been proven to be equally efficacious to a 4 L preparation in terms of mucosal visualization and capsule completion rate [18]. A score has been developed based upon the proportion of mucosa visualized and quantification of the degree of obscuration by bubbles, debris, or bile [19]. The interobserver agreement of this scale was shown to be good (k=0.8), although it has yet to be validated prospectively.

Diagnostic Yield for Obscure Bleeding and Anemia

The diagnostic yield (i.e., the percentage of capsule studies demonstrating clinically significant findings) varies considerably depending on indication and patient characteristics. Reported diagnostic yields are 36–92 % for obscure overt gastrointestinal bleeding, 41–63 % for occult bleeding, and 42–66 % for unexplained iron-deficiency anemia [20–33]. The most common finding explaining obscure bleeding is small bowel angioectasia. Serious findings in these studies were particularly common in young patients with unexplained anemia [34]. However, performing capsule endoscopy in patients who had only a positive fecal occult blood test (without anemia or visible bleeding) was not fruitful [35]. Most studies have not been able to report true accuracy data (such as sensitivity or specificity) due to the difficulty of establishing a reliable gold standard for obscure small bowel bleeding.

Several meta-analyses have summarized the data on comparative studies involving capsule endoscopy for small bowel evaluation [36–38]. For obscure bleeding, the diagnostic yield of capsule endoscopy proved superior to that of push enteroscopy (with a yield gain of 30 %), small bowel barium studies (gain of 36 %) [38], and magnetic resonance enteroclysis [39]. In fact, capsule endoscopy was almost as accurate as intraoperative endoscopy [38, 40]. Another meta-analysis concluded that capsule endoscopy had a higher yield than "unidirectional" double-balloon enteroscopy, but was inferior to "bidirectional" double-balloon enteroscopy; that is, when per-oral and per-rectal approaches were both used [41]. Since bleeding lesions (including tumors) can be missed by capsule endoscopy [42], repeat capsule endoscopy can be useful in a significant proportion of patients [43–45].

The clinical impact of capsule endoscopy on patient management is important, because nonspecific, clinically insignificant lesions are often found, even in asymptomatic individuals [46]. Studies have generally shown that capsule endoscopy often positively influences clinical management and outcomes, although some recent studies have raised doubts as to its clinical impact on long-term outcomes [47, 48]. For "positive" capsule studies for obscure bleeding, 44–82 % lead to specific therapeutic interventions or changes in management, and 63–83 % are associated with cessation of bleeding [21, 24–26, 49, 50]. Some studies have reported that negative capsule studies can predict a lower risk of rebleeding [51–54], although data have been discordant in other studies [55–57]. For iron-deficiency anemia, the medium-term impact has proven modest despite relatively high diagnostic yields [28, 58, 59]. In the acute setting, immediate capsule endoscopy has been shown to be more useful than angiography [60].

Diagnostic Yield for Crohn's Disease and Other Non-bleeding Indications

In up to one-third of patients with Crohn's disease, inflammation is confined to the small intestine, and beyond the reach of the push enteroscope or colonoscope [61, 62]. Barium small bowel follow-through examinations have limited ability to detect mild mucosal inflammation in early Crohn's disease [37, 63], and have been supplanted by computerized tomographic enterography (CTE) and magnetic resonance enterography (MRE), which can also demonstrate extraluminal disease such as abscesses or fistulae. However, capsule endoscopy is probably superior to CTE or MRE for detecting superficial mucosal ulcerations. The diagnostic yield of capsule endoscopy, CTE, and MRE were compared in a meta-analysis of 12 trials [64]. Capsule endoscopy enjoyed significant incremental yield over that of ileocolonoscopy (22 % gain) and CTE (47 %). A subsequent study on suspected or newly diagnosed Crohn's disease compared capsule endoscopy against CTE and MRE [65]. Patients underwent ileocolonoscopy, CTE, or MRE, followed by capsule endoscopy. The sensitivity and specificity for the diagnosis of terminal ileitis were 100 % and 91 % for capsule endoscopy, compared with 81 % and 86 % for MRE, and 76 % and 85 % for CTE.

In patients with symptoms suspicious for Crohn's disease, the combination of capsule endoscopy and ileocolonoscopy identified 97 % of all small bowel inflammatory lesions, while small bowel follow-through and ileocolonoscopy detected only 57 %. Of the patients ultimately found to have small bowel Crohn's disease, 55 % were diagnosed by capsule endoscopy alone [61]. It should, however, be noted that small bowel erosions seen on capsule endoscopy may be non-specific or due to the use of nonsteroidal anti-inflammatory drugs (NSAIDs); furthermore, there have been well-documented cases of small bowel ulcers being identified even in "normal" individuals [46, 66].

Capsule endoscopy can also be helpful in monitoring the extent and severity of inflammation in patients with established Crohn's disease [67]. In persistently symptomatic patients, capsule endoscopy identified active inflammation in 82 % of patients, compared with only 49 % detected by ileocolonoscopy [68]. In another study, 56 % of subjects were noted on capsule endoscopy to have jejunal ulcerations not seen on CTE [69, 70]. Capsule endoscopy is also useful for documenting mucosal healing after treatment [1–3, 67, 71]. In a prospective study, capsule endoscopy performed before and after treatment demonstrated a significant reduction in the number of small bowel ulcers, and mucosal healing correlated with other measures such as the Crohn's Disease Activity Index, Inflammatory Bowel Disease Questionnaire, and C reactive protein values [72]. Lastly, capsule endoscopy can be used to screen for anastomotic recurrence of Crohn's disease after surgical therapy [73, 74].

In 4–10 % of patients with inflammatory bowel disease involving the colon, distinguishing ulcerative colitis from Crohn's disease is not possible with just ileocolonoscopy and imaging [2, 75]. In some situations, establishing this distinction has important implications for medical and particularly surgical treatment. By providing direct visualization of the entire small bowel, capsule endoscopy can often clarify the diagnosis in patients initially presenting with indeterminate colitis. Studies have shown that capsule endoscopy altered the diagnosis in 29–40 % of such patients [62, 76–78].

Capsule endoscopy has also been useful for the assessment of other non-bleeding indications such as celiac sprue [79–81], small bowel tumors [82–84], and lymphomas [85]. A tentative scoring system has been proposed to help diagnose small bowel tumors on capsule endoscopy [86].

Capsule Endoscopy Scoring Systems for Crohn's Findings

Currently, there are two validated scoring systems available to describe the extent and severity of Crohn's disease seen on capsule endoscopy. The Capsule Endoscopy Crohn's Disease Activity Index (CECDAI) is based on the severity of inflammation, extent of disease, and the presence or absence of strictures. The score ranges between 0 and 36, with higher numbers representing more severe disease [87, 88]. The Lewis Index is based on villous edema, mucosal ulceration, and luminal stenosis [4]. A score of <135 is normal, while a score of ≥790 denotes moderate to severe inflammation [89]. However, studies have suggested that correlation is poor between the CECDAI and fecal calprotectin, while the Lewis score only correlates with low calprotectin levels [90, 91]. Correlation is mediocre between the CECDAI and C-reactive protein levels [92].

Comparison of Capsule Endoscopy and Deep Enteroscopy

Double- or single-balloon-assisted enteroscopy, also termed deep enteroscopy, is an alternative means for evaluating the entire small bowel that has become available in the last decade. This method is somewhat limited by the special training required and the frequent need for extended procedure times and anesthesia support, but sometimes can detect lesions missed by capsule endoscopy [93]. A meta-analysis reported diagnostic yields of 57 % with capsule endoscopy and 60 % with deep enteroscopy. Stratified analysis looking at vascular lesions, inflammatory changes, and small bowel polyps/tumors all showed comparable yields between capsule endoscopy and deep enteroscopy [94]. More recent meta-analyses also concluded that the two

modalities were comparable and complementary [95, 96], although deep enteroscopy had an increased yield when performed after a positive capsule endoscopy. Similarly, intraoperative enteroscopy also had an increased yield if performed after a positive capsule endoscopy [97]. In general, capsule endoscopy would be recommended as the initial test of choice in the evaluation of small bowel disease, and can be followed up by deep enteroscopy if indicated. Intraoperative enteroscopy is the test of last resort in extremely recalcitrant obscure bleeding patients.

Contraindications and Complications

Contraindications to capsule endoscopy are few and the complication rate is low [98, 99]. The most important potential complication is capsule impaction in the small bowel. According to guidelines, capsule impaction is defined as retention of the capsule in the small bowel for longer than 2 weeks [100]. Capsule impaction should be distinguished from type 1 regional transit abnormality, in which the capsule stays at the same point for more than 60 min (but less than 2 weeks) with no abnormality visible on the capsule video image [101, 102], or type 2 regional transit abnormality (previously termed transient capsule retention), in which the capsule stays at the same point for >60 min (but less than 2 weeks) with a visible abnormality such as a stricture [103]. Regional transit abnormalities are fairly common, with reported incidence rates of 5.7–13.3 % [104]. Capsule impaction is much less common, with occurrence rates influenced by the indication and patient characteristics. A systematic review reported capsule retention rates of 1.2 % for obscure bleeding, 2.6 % for Crohn's disease, and 2.1 % for small bowel tumors [105]. There have been no reported cases of capsule impaction occurring in a normal small intestine [46]. Capsule impaction usually occurs at sites of structural abnormality in the small bowel, such as ulcers, masses, strictures, or surgical anastomoses [106].

Most cases of capsule impaction are asymptomatic, even when the capsule remains impacted for very long periods (as long as 2.5 years) [104, 107]. There have been only a few reported cases of symptomatic capsule retention, including capsule entrapment in a Meckel's diverticulum [108], acute obstruction in a Crohn's disease patient [109], capsule impaction in the appendix leading to appendicitis [110], and intestinal perforation [111, 112]. Once diagnosed, options to treat capsule retention include endoscopic retrieval or, in the majority of cases, surgery. Capsule retention helps to localize the site of the pathology, allowing the surgeon to target his or her intervention and potentially remove the offending lesion at the same time as the impacted capsule [100].

Radiographic studies can identify possible obstructive intestinal lesions, but cannot reliably predict capsule impaction [98, 107]. The capsule has been known to pass normally even in patients with radiographically evident strictures [113]. Nevertheless, in some situations, small bowel follow-through, and more recently CTE or MRE, may be helpful if performed before capsule endoscopy in patients at increased risk for obstruction.

Another predictive tool is the Pillcam Patency Capsule (Given Imaging, Yokneam, Israel), which is a radio-opaque, self-dissolving capsule made of lactose and barium with two side timer plugs with exposed windows. It is the same size and shape as the Pillcam SB3 and contains a radiofrequency identification tag that allows it to be detected by an external scanning device before it disintegrates 30 h after ingestion [106, 113–115]. In patients with known or suspected small bowel strictures, the patency capsule had a 91 % negative predictive value for capsule retention [116]. In one study, in which only those patients successfully passing the patency capsule were selected for capsule endoscopy, the capsule retention rate was zero [114]. Overall, the patency capsule seems to be a useful tool for assessing certain high-risk patients prior to capsule endoscopy [117]. Rare complications from the patency capsule, such as transient intestinal occlusion and abdominal discomfort, have been reported [114, 118].

The radiofrequency waves used by the capsule endoscope to transmit data to the recorder can pose a theoretical risk of interference with implanted electronic devices. Based on this concern, the FDA and the manufacturer, Given Imaging, list the presence of cardiac pacemakers or defibrillators as a contraindication to capsule endoscopy. However, data from a number of studies have demonstrated that capsule endoscopy does not result in any cardiac arrhythmias or alteration of implanted electronic device function [119–123]. A brief lapse in capsule image acquisition (less than 2 min) was noted in only two patients, who remained asymptomatic and had no adverse events. Such data suggest that capsule endoscopy is probably safe to perform in patients with implanted electronic devices.

Current Limitations

Capsule endoscopy, in its present form, still suffers from several limitations. Some problems are logistical, such as difficulties with insurance coverage, reimbursement for capsule study interpretation, and training and quality control. However, capsule endoscopy has inherent technical limitations as well. One of the most important drawbacks is its inability to precisely localize detected lesions in order to target further therapy. The temporal relationship of visualized lesions with the pyloric channel and ileocecal valve gives the examiner an approximate idea of where the lesion is, but this can be misleading because the speed of capsule movement along the small bowel is not constant. The capsule also lacks the ability to mark the location of detected lesions (such as with a tattoo), a function that would be helpful for subsequent endoscopic or surgical therapy. Furthermore, delayed gastric emptying and slow small bowel transit can lead to exhaustion of the battery before the cecum is reached. In some older studies, this occurred in up to 20 % of capsules deployed, although longer battery life and adaptive frame collection technology in the Pillcam SB3 may alleviate this problem in the future [124]. Reducing the frame rate in OMOM capsules has been shown to improve complete small bowel examination rate without adversely affecting diagnostic yield [125, 126].

Capsule endoscopy visualization can be impaired by the presence of bubbles, food materials, suboptimal lighting, or resolution problems. The capsule examiner can repeatedly scrutinize video frames of interest, but cannot retroactively obtain better images; in contrast, during standard endoscopy the examiner can scrutinize the area of interest repeatedly in real time, maneuver the endoscope to adjust perspective, angle or distance, and perform flushing, suctioning, or air insufflation as needed. Because the movement of the capsule through the intestines is entirely passive, there is no way to control capsule movement in real time to improve the image quality in areas of interest. The random motion of the capsule means that in some frames only part of the 360° circumference of the small bowel is visible. Capsules with an extremely wide angle of view using multiple cameras, such as the Capsocam, may address this issue in the future. Finally, current capsules are purely diagnostic and have no capability to obtain biopsies or intervene therapeutically.

Conclusion

Future Directions

Since its advent, most of the advances in capsule technology have been evolutionary in nature. Further improvements in resolution, brightness control, and angle and depth of view will undoubtedly occur, but their impact will be limited. On the other hand, breakthroughs in lesion localization and therapeutic intervention, when they occur, will be revolutionary [124]. Some of the possible future roles for capsule endoscopy include the performance of biopsies, medication injection, tattooing, capsule ultrasonography, and argon plasma coagulation. Most of these capabilities require real-time imaging and the ability to control the capsule. Already there are capsules in development with limited steering capabilities, such as some versions of the Capsocam and OMOM capsule. The most recent versions of the Pillcam SB and Endocapsule both feature a limited real-time imaging function. In the emergency room, capsule endoscopy can be used to rule out upper gastrointestinal bleeding in real time in order to assist triage. Preliminary studies have

shown that capsule endoscopy in the acute setting is feasible and useful [127–130].

In the future, true real-time control capabilities may become technically feasible, but there are still some logistical challenges. Since the small intestinal transit time can range from 30 min to 12 h, it would not be practical to perform real-time imaging for all capsule studies. A more realistic approach would be for all patients to first undergo diagnostic capsule endoscopy with retroactive examination of the video recording, similar to what is currently done. If a lesion is potentially amenable to capsule treatment, then the patient can be referred for a more involved therapeutic capsule procedure performed with real-time control. Continuous advances in capsule technology are taking place, with capsule endoscopes for evaluation of the esophagus and colon making their appearance in the commercial market in the last few years. Small bowel capsule endoscopy has already been shown to be safe and cost effective [131], and the learning curve for reading capsule endoscopy is relatively modest [132]. It is likely that the scope of capsule endoscopy will continue to expand. We look forward to a day when we can finally examine the darkest recesses of the small bowel with the same accuracy and ease that we currently enjoy for the stomach and colon.

References

1. Swain P, Adler D, Enns R. Capsule endoscopy in obscure intestinal bleeding. Endoscopy. 2005;37(7):655–9.
2. Bourreille A, Ignjatovic A, Aabakken L, Loftus Jr EV, Eliakim R, Pennazio M, et al. Role of small-bowel endoscopy in the management of patients with inflammatory bowel disease: an international OMED-ECCO consensus. Endoscopy. 2009;41(7): 618–37.
3. Eliakim R. Video capsule endoscopy of the small bowel. Curr Opin Gastroenterol. 2013;29(2):133–9.
4. Gralnek IM, Defranchis R, Seidman E, Leighton JA, Legnani P, Lewis BS. Development of a capsule endoscopy scoring index for small bowel mucosal inflammatory change. Aliment Pharmacol Ther. 2008;27(2):146–54.
5. Cave DR, Fleischer DE, Leighton JA, Faigel DO, Heigh RI, Sharma VK, et al. A multicenter random-

ized comparison of the endocapsule and the pillcam sb. Gastrointest Endosc. 2008;68(3):487–94.

6. Hartmann D, Eickhoff A, Damian U, Riemann JF. Diagnosis of small-bowel pathology using paired capsule endoscopy with two different devices: a randomized study. Endoscopy. 2007;39(12):1041–5.

7. Pioche M, Gaudin JL, Filoche B, Jacob P, Lamouliatte H, Lapalus MG, et al. Prospective, randomized comparison of two small-bowel capsule endoscopy systems in patients with obscure GI bleeding. Gastrointest Endosc. 2011;73(6):1181–8.

8. Choi EH, Mergener K, Semrad C, Fisher L, Cave DR, Dodig M, et al. A multicenter, prospective, randomized comparison of a novel signal transmission capsule endoscope to an existing capsule endoscope. Gastrointest Endosc. 2013;78(2):325–32.

9. Kim HM, Kim YJ, Kim HJ, Park S, Park JY, Shin SK, et al. A pilot study of sequential capsule endoscopy using MiroCam and PillCam SB devices with different transmission technologies. Gut Liver. 2010;4(2):192–200.

10. Dolak W, Kulnigg-Dabsch S, Evstatiev R, Gasche C, Trauner M, Puspok A. A randomized head-to-head study of small-bowel imaging comparing mirocam and endocapsule. Endoscopy. 2012;44(11):1012–20.

11. Pioche M, Vanbervliet G, Jacob P, de Duburque C, Gincul R, Filoche B, et al. Prospective randomized comparison between axial- and lateral-viewing capsule endoscopy systems in patients with obscure digestive bleeding. Endoscopy. 2014;46(6):479–84.

12. Friedrich K, Gehrke S, Stremmel W, Sieg A. First clinical trial of a newly developed capsule endoscope with panoramic side view for small bowel: a pilot study. J Gastroenterol Hepatol. 2013;28(9):1496–501.

13. Liao Z, Gao R, Li F, Xu C, Zhou Y, Wang JS, et al. Fields of applications, diagnostic yields and findings of OMOM capsule endoscopy in 2400 Chinese patients. World J Gastroenterol. 2010;16(21):2669–76.

14. Li CY, Zhang BL, Chen CX, Li YM. OMOM capsule endoscopy in diagnosis of small bowel disease. J Zhejiang Univ Sci B. 2008;9(11):857–62.

15. Niv Y. Efficiency of bowel preparation for capsule endoscopy examination: a meta-analysis. World J Gastroenterol. 2008;14(9):1313–7.

16. Rokkas T, Papaxoinis K, Triantafyllou K, Pistiolas D, Ladas SD. Does purgative preparation influence the diagnostic yield of small bowel video capsule endoscopy? A meta-analysis. Am J Gastroenterol. 2009;104(1):219–27.

17. Belsey J, Crosta C, Epstein O, Fischbach W, Layer P, Parente F, et al. Meta-analysis: efficacy of small bowel preparation for small bowel video capsule endoscopy. Curr Med Res Opin. 2012;28(12):1883–90.

18. Kantianis A, Karagiannis S, Liatsos C, Galanis P, Psilopoulos D, Tenta R, et al. Comparison of two schemes of small bowel preparation for capsule endoscopy with polyethylene glycol: a prospective, randomized single-blind study. Eur J Gastroenterol Hepatol. 2009;21(10):1140–4.

19. Park SC, Keum B, Hyun JJ, Seo YS, Kim YS, Jeen YT, et al. A novel cleansing score system for capsule endoscopy. World J Gastroenterol. 2010;16(7):875–80.

20. Rastogi A, Schoen RE, Slivka A. Diagnostic yield and clinical outcomes of capsule endoscopy. Gastrointest Endosc. 2004;60(6):959–64.

21. Pennazio M, Santucci R, Rondonotti E, Abbiati C, Beccari G, Rossini FP, et al. Outcome of patients with obscure gastrointestinal bleeding after capsule endoscopy: report of 100 consecutive cases. Gastroenterology. 2004;126(3):643–53.

22. Apostolopoulos P, Liatsos C, Gralnek IM, Giannakoulopoulou E, Alexandrakis G, Kalantzis C, et al. The role of wireless capsule endoscopy in investigating unexplained iron deficiency anemia after negative endoscopic evaluation of the upper and lower gastrointestinal tract. Endoscopy. 2006;38(11):1127–32.

23. Estevez E, Gonzalez-Conde B, Vazquez-Iglesias JL, de Los Angeles Vazquez-Millan M, Pertega S, Alonso PA, et al. Diagnostic yield and clinical outcomes after capsule endoscopy in 100 consecutive patients with obscure gastrointestinal bleeding. Eur J Gastroenterol Hepatol. 2006;18(8):881–8.

24. Delvaux M, Fassler I, Gay G. Clinical usefulness of the endoscopic video capsule as the initial intestinal investigation in patients with obscure digestive bleeding: validation of a diagnostic strategy based on the patient outcome after 12 months. Endoscopy. 2004;36(12):1067–73.

25. Viazis N, Papaxoinis K, Theodoropoulos I, Sgouros S, Vlachogiannakos J, Pipis P, et al. Impact of capsule endoscopy in obscure small-bowel bleeding: defining strict diagnostic criteria for a favorable outcome. Gastrointest Endosc. 2005;62(5):717–22.

26. Neu B, Ell C, May A, Schmid E, Riemann JF, Hagenmuller F, et al. Capsule endoscopy versus standard tests in influencing management of obscure digestive bleeding: results from a German multicenter trial. Am J Gastroenterol. 2005;100(8): 1736–42.

27. Carey EJ, Leighton JA, Heigh RI, Shiff AD, Sharma VK, Post JK, et al. A single-center experience of 260 consecutive patients undergoing capsule endoscopy for obscure gastrointestinal bleeding. Am J Gastroenterol. 2007;102(1):89–95.

28. Tong J, Svarta S, Ou G, Kwok R, Law J, Enns R. Diagnostic yield of capsule endoscopy in the setting of iron deficiency anemia without evidence of gastrointestinal bleeding. Can J Gastroenterol. 2012;26(10):687–90.

29. Calabrese C, Liguori G, Gionchetti P, Rizzello F, Laureti S, Di Simone MP, et al. Obscure gastrointestinal bleeding: single centre experience of capsule endoscopy. Intern Emerg Med. 2013;8(8):681–7.

30. Goenka MK, Majumder S, Kumar S, Sethy PK, Goenka U. Single center experience of capsule endoscopy in patients with obscure gastrointestinal bleeding. World J Gastroenterol. 2011;17(6): 774–8.

31. van Turenhout ST, Jacobs MA, van Weyenberg SJ, Herdes E, Stam F, Mulder CJ, et al. Diagnostic yield of capsule endoscopy in a tertiary hospital in patients with obscure gastrointestinal bleeding. J Gastrointestin Liver Dis. 2010;19(2):141–5.

32. Riccioni ME, Urgesi R, Spada C, Cianci R, Pelecca G, Bizzotto A, et al. Unexplained iron deficiency anaemia: is it worthwhile to perform capsule endoscopy? Dig Liver Dis. 2010;42(8):560–6.

33. Muhammad A, Pitchumoni CS. Evaluation of iron deficiency anemia in older adults: the role of wireless capsule endoscopy. J Clin Gastroenterol. 2009;43(7):627–31.

34. Koulaouzidis A, Yung DE, Lam JH, Smirnidis A, Douglas S, Plevris JN. The use of small-bowel capsule endoscopy in iron-deficiency anaemia alone; be aware of the young anemic patient. Scand J Gastroenterol. 2012;47(8–9):1094–100.

35. Chiba H, Sekiguchi M, Ito T, Tsuji Y, Ohata K, Ohno A, et al. Is it worthwhile to perform capsule endoscopy for asymptomatic patients with positive immunochemical faecal occult blood test? Dig Dis Sci. 2011;56(12):3459–62.

36. Triester SL, Leighton JA, Leontiadis GI, Fleischer DE, Hara AK, Heigh RI, et al. A meta-analysis of the yield of capsule endoscopy compared to other diagnostic modalities in patients with obscure gastrointestinal bleeding. Am J Gastroenterol. 2005;100(11):2407–18.

37. Marmo R, Rotondano G, Piscopo R, Bianco MA, Cipolletta L. Meta-analysis: capsule enteroscopy vs. conventional modalities in diagnosis of small bowel diseases. Aliment Pharmacol Ther. 2005;22(7):595–604.

38. Leighton JA, Triester SL, Sharma VK. Capsule endoscopy: a meta-analysis for use with obscure gastrointestinal bleeding and Crohn's disease. Gastrointest Endosc Clin N Am. 2006;16(2):229–50.

39. Wiarda BM, Heine DG, Mensink P, Stolk M, Dees J, Hazenberg HJ, et al. Comparison of magnetic resonance enteroclysis and capsule endoscopy with balloon-assisted enteroscopy in patients with obscure gastrointestinal bleeding. Endoscopy. 2012;44(7):668–73.

40. Hartmann D, Schmidt H, Bolz G, Schilling D, Kinzel F, Eickhoff A, et al. A prospective two-center study comparing wireless capsule endoscopy with intraoperative enteroscopy in patients with obscure GI bleeding. Gastrointest Endosc. 2005;61(7):826–32.

41. Chen X, Ran ZH, Tong JL. A meta-analysis of the yield of capsule endoscopy compared to double-balloon enteroscopy in patients with small bowel diseases. World J Gastroenterol. 2007;13(32):4372–8.

42. Zagorowicz ES, Pietrzak AM, Wronska E, Pachlewski J, Rutkowski P, Kraszewska E, et al. Small bowel tumors detected and missed during capsule endoscopy: single center experience. World J Gastroenterol. 2013;19(47):9043–8.

43. Jones BH, Fleischer DE, Sharma VK, Heigh RI, Shiff AD, Hernandez JL, et al. Yield of repeat wireless video capsule endoscopy in patients with obscure gastrointestinal bleeding. Am J Gastroenterol. 2005;100(5):1058–64.

44. Svarta S, Segal B, Law J, Sandhar A, Kwok R, Jacques A, et al. Diagnostic yield of repeat capsule endoscopy and the effect on subsequent patient management. Can J Gastroenterol. 2010;24(7):441–4.

45. Min BH, Chang DK, Kim BJ, Lee IS, Choi MG. Does back-to-back capsule endoscopy increase the diagnostic yield over a single examination in patients with obscure gastrointestinal bleeding? Gut Liver. 2010;4(1):54–9.

46. Goldstein JL, Eisen GM, Lewis B, Gralnek IM, Zlotnick S, Fort JG. Video capsule endoscopy to prospectively assess small bowel injury with celecoxib, naproxen plus omeprazole, and placebo. Clin Gastroenterol Hepatol. 2005;3(2):133–41.

47. Min YW, Kim JS, Jeon SW, Jeen YT, Im JP, Cheung DY, et al. Long-term outcome of capsule endoscopy in obscure gastrointestinal bleeding: a nationwide analysis. Endoscopy. 2014;46(1):59–65.

48. Laine L, Sahota A, Shah A. Does capsule endoscopy improve outcomes in obscure gastrointestinal bleeding? Randomized trial versus dedicated small bowel radiography. Gastroenterology. 2010;138(5):1673–80. e1671; quiz e1611–72.

49. Saurin JC, Delvaux M, Vahedi K, Gaudin JL, Villarejo J, Florent C, et al. Clinical impact of capsule endoscopy compared to push enteroscopy: 1-year follow-up study. Endoscopy. 2005;37(4):318–23.

50. Leighton JA, Sharma VK, Hentz JG, Musil D, Malikowski MJ, McWane TL, et al. Capsule endoscopy versus push enteroscopy for evaluation of obscure gastrointestinal bleeding with 1-year outcomes. Dig Dis Sci. 2006;51(5):891–9.

51. Riccioni ME, Urgesi R, Cianci R, Rizzo G, D'Angelo L, Marmo R, et al. Negative capsule endoscopy in patients with obscure gastrointestinal bleeding reliable: recurrence of bleeding on long-term follow-up. World J Gastroenterol. 2013;19(28):4520–5.

52. Iwamoto J, Mizokami Y, Shimokobe K, Yara S, Murakami M, Kido K, et al. The clinical outcome of capsule endoscopy in patients with obscure gastrointestinal bleeding. Hepato-Gastroenterology. 2011;58(106):301–5.

53. Lorenceau-Savale C, Ben-Soussan E, Ramirez S, Antonietti M, Lerebours E, Ducrotte P. Outcome of patients with obscure gastrointestinal bleeding after negative capsule endoscopy: results of a one-year follow-up study. Gastroenterol Clin Biol. 2010;34(11):606–11.

54. Macdonald J, Porter V, McNamara D. Negative capsule endoscopy in patients with obscure GI bleeding predicts low rebleeding rates. Gastrointest Endosc. 2008;68(6):1122–7.

55. Koh SJ, Im JP, Kim JW, Kim BG, Lee KL, Kim SG, et al. Long-term outcome in patients with obscure gastrointestinal bleeding after negative capsule endoscopy. World J Gastroenterol. 2013;19(10):1632–8.

56. Kim JB, Ye BD, Song Y, Yang DH, Jung KW, Kim KJ, et al. Frequency of rebleeding events in obscure gastrointestinal bleeding with negative capsule endoscopy. J Gastroenterol Hepatol. 2013;28(5):834–40.

57. Park JJ, Cheon JH, Kim HM, Park HS, Moon CM, Lee JH, et al. Negative capsule endoscopy without subsequent enteroscopy does not predict lower long-term rebleeding rates in patients with obscure GI bleeding. Gastrointest Endosc. 2010;71(6):990–7.

58. Holleran GE, Barry SA, Thornton OJ, Dobson MJ, McNamara DA. The use of small bowel capsule endoscopy in iron deficiency anaemia: Low impact on outcome in the medium term despite high diagnostic yield. Eur J Gastroenterol Hepatol. 2013;25(3):327–32.

59. Sheibani S, Levesque BG, Friedland S, Roost J, Gerson LB. Long-term impact of capsule endoscopy in patients referred for iron-deficiency anemia. Dig Dis Sci. 2010;55(3):703–8.

60. Leung WK, Ho SS, Suen BY, Lai LH, Yu S, Ng EK, et al. Capsule endoscopy or angiography in patients with acute overt obscure gastrointestinal bleeding: a prospective randomized study with long-term follow-up. Am J Gastroenterol. 2012;107(9):1370–6.

61. Leighton JA, Gralnek IM, Cohen SA, Toth E, Cave DR, Wolf DC, et al. Capsule endoscopy is superior to small-bowel follow-through and equivalent to ileocolonoscopy in suspected Crohn's disease. Clin Gastroenterol Hepatol. 2014;12(4):609–15.

62. Doherty GA, Moss AC, Cheifetz AS. Capsule endoscopy for small-bowel evaluation in Crohn's disease. Gastrointest Endosc. 2011;74(1):167–75.

63. Lewis BS, Eisen GM, Friedman S. A pooled analysis to evaluate results of capsule endoscopy trials. Endoscopy. 2005;37(10):960–5.

64. Dionisio PM, Gurudu SR, Leighton JA, Leontiadis GI, Fleischer DE, Hara AK, et al. Capsule endoscopy has a significantly higher diagnostic yield in patients with suspected and established small-bowel Crohn's disease: a meta-analysis. Am J Gastroenterol. 2010;105(6):1240–8. quiz 1249.

65. Jensen MD, Nathan T, Rafaelsen SR, Kjeldsen J. Diagnostic accuracy of capsule endoscopy for small bowel Crohn's disease is superior to that of MR enterography or ct enterography. Clin Gastroenterol Hepatol. 2011;9(2):124–9.

66. Maiden L, Thjodleifsson B, Seigal A, Bjarnason II, Scott D, Birgisson S, et al. Long-term effects of nonsteroidal anti-inflammatory drugs and cyclooxygenase-2 selective agents on the small bowel: a cross-sectional capsule enteroscopy study. Clin Gastroenterol Hepatol. 2007;5(9):1040–5.

67. Legnani P, Abreu MT. Use of capsule endoscopy for established Crohn's disease. Gastrointest Endosc Clin N Am. 2006;16(2):299–306.

68. Dubcenco E, Jeejeebhoy KN, Petroniene R, Tang SJ, Zalev AH, Gardiner GW, et al. Capsule endoscopy findings in patients with established and suspected small-bowel Crohn's disease: correlation with radiologic, endoscopic, and histologic findings. Gastrointest Endosc. 2005;62(4):538–44.

69. Flamant M, Trang C, Maillard O, Sacher-Huvelin S, Le Rhun M, Galmiche JP, et al. The prevalence and outcome of jejunal lesions visualized by small bowel capsule endoscopy in Crohn's disease. Inflamm Bowel Dis. 2013;19(7):1390–6.

70. Dussault C, Gower-Rousseau C, Salleron J, Vernier-Massouille G, Branche J, Colombel JF, et al. Small bowel capsule endoscopy for management of Crohn's disease: a retrospective tertiary care centre experience. Dig Liver Dis. 2013;45(7):558–61.

71. Calabrese C, Gionchetti P, Rizzello F, Liguori G, Gabusi V, Tambasco R, et al. Short-term treatment with infliximab in chronic refractory pouchitis and ileitis. Aliment Pharmacol Ther. 2008;27(9):759–64.

72. Efthymiou A, Viazis N, Mantzaris G, Papadimitriou N, Tzourmakliotis D, Raptis S, et al. Does clinical response correlate with mucosal healing in patients with Crohn's disease of the small bowel? A prospective, case-series study using wireless capsule endoscopy. Inflamm Bowel Dis. 2008;14(11):1542–7.

73. Pons Beltran V, Nos P, Bastida G, Beltran B, Arguello L, Aguas M, et al. Evaluation of postsurgical recurrence in Crohn's disease: a new indication for capsule endoscopy? Gastrointest Endosc. 2007;66(3):533–40.

74. Bourreille A, Jarry M, D'Halluin PN, Ben-Soussan E, Maunoury V, Bulois P, et al. Wireless capsule endoscopy versus ileocolonoscopy for the diagnosis of postoperative recurrence of Crohn's disease: a prospective study. Gut. 2006;55(7):978–83.

75. de Melo Jr SW, Di Palma JA. The role of capsule endoscopy in evaluating inflammatory bowel disease. Gastroenterol Clin N Am. 2012;41(2):315–23.

76. Mehdizadeh S, Chen GC, Barkodar L, Enayati PJ, Pirouz S, Yadegari M, et al. Capsule endoscopy in patients with Crohn's disease: diagnostic yield and safety. Gastrointest Endosc. 2010;71(1):121–7.

77. Maunoury V, Savoye G, Bourreille A, Bouhnik Y, Jarry M, Sacher-Huvelin S, et al. Value of wireless capsule endoscopy in patients with indeterminate colitis (inflammatory bowel disease type unclassified). Inflamm Bowel Dis. 2007;13(2):152–5.

78. Lopes S, Figueiredo P, Portela F, Freire P, Almeida N, Lerias C, et al. Capsule endoscopy in inflammatory bowel disease type unclassified and indeterminate colitis serologically negative. Inflamm Bowel Dis. 2010;16(10):1663–8.

79. Katsinelos P, Tziomalos K, Fasoulas K, Paroutoglou G, Koufokotsios A, Mimidis K, et al. Can capsule endoscopy be used as a diagnostic tool in the evaluation of nonbleeding indications in daily clinical practice? A prospective study. Med Princ Pract. 2011;20(4):362–7.

80. Kurien M, Evans KE, Aziz I, Sidhu R, Drew K, Rogers TL, et al. Capsule endoscopy in adult celiac disease: a potential role in equivocal cases of celiac disease? Gastrointest Endosc. 2013;77(2):227–32.

81. Rokkas T, Niv Y. The role of video capsule endoscopy in the diagnosis of celiac disease: a meta-analysis. Eur J Gastroenterol Hepatol. 2012;24(3):303–8.

82. Urgesi R, Riccioni ME, Bizzotto A, Cianci R, Spada C, Pelecca G, et al. Increased diagnostic yield of small bowel tumors with pillcam: the role of capsule endoscopy in the diagnosis and treatment of gastrointestinal stromal tumors (gists). Italian single-center experience. Tumori. 2012;98(3):357–63.

83. Cheung DY, Lee IS, Chang DK, Kim JO, Cheon JH, Jang BI, et al. Capsule endoscopy in small bowel tumors: a multicenter Korean study. J Gastroenterol Hepatol. 2010;25(6):1079–86.

84. Trifan A, Singeap AM, Cojocariu C, Sfarti C, Stanciu C. Small bowel tumors in patients undergoing capsule endoscopy: a single center experience. J Gastrointestin Liver Dis. 2010;19(1):21–5.

85. Akamatsu T, Kaneko Y, Ota H, Miyabayashi H, Arakura N, Tanaka E. Usefulness of double balloon enteroscopy and video capsule endoscopy for the diagnosis and management of primary follicular lymphoma of the gastrointestinal tract in its early stages. Dig Endosc. 2010;22(1):33–8.

86. Shyung LR, Lin SC, Shih SC, Chang WH, Chu CH, Wang TE. Proposed scoring system to determine small bowel mass lesions using capsule endoscopy. J Formos Med Assoc. 2009;108(7):533–8.

87. Gal E, Geller A, Fraser G, Levi Z, Niv Y. Assessment and validation of the new capsule endoscopy Crohn's disease activity index (CECDAI). Dig Dis Sci. 2008;53(7):1933–7.

88. Niv Y, Ilani S, Levi Z, Hershkowitz M, Niv E, Fireman Z, et al. Validation of the capsule endoscopy Crohn's disease activity index (CECDAI or Niv score): a multicenter prospective study. Endoscopy. 2012;44(1):21–6.

89. Rosa B, Moreira MJ, Rebelo A, Cotter J. Lewis score: a useful clinical tool for patients with suspected Crohn's disease submitted to capsule endoscopy. J Crohns Colitis. 2012;6(6):692–7.

90. Langhorst J, Elsenbruch S, Koelzer J, Rueffer A, Michalsen A, Dobos GJ. Noninvasive markers in the assessment of intestinal inflammation in inflammatory bowel diseases: performance of fecal lactoferrin, calprotectin, and pmn-elastase, crp, and clinical indices. Am J Gastroenterol. 2008;103(1):162–9.

91. Koulaouzidis A, Douglas S, Plevris JN. Lewis score correlates more closely with fecal calprotectin than capsule endoscopy Crohn's disease activity index. Dig Dis Sci. 2012;57(4):987–93.

92. Yang L, Ge ZZ, Gao YJ, Li XB, Dai J, Zhang Y, et al. Assessment of capsule endoscopy scoring index, clinical disease activity, and c-reactive protein in small bowel Crohn's disease. J Gastroenterol Hepatol. 2013;28(5):829–33.

93. Ross A, Mehdizadeh S, Tokar J, Leighton JA, Kamal A, Chen A, et al. Double balloon enteroscopy detects small bowel mass lesions missed by capsule endoscopy. Dig Dis Sci. 2008;53(8):2140–3.

94. Pasha SF, Leighton JA, Das A, Harrison ME, Decker GA, Fleischer DE, et al. Double-balloon enteroscopy and capsule endoscopy have comparable diagnostic yield in small-bowel disease: a meta-analysis. Clin Gastroenterol Hepatol. 2008;6(6):671–6.

95. Zhang Q, He Q, Liu J, Ma F, Zhi F, Bai Y. Combined use of capsule endoscopy and double-balloon enteroscopy in the diagnosis of obscure gastrointestinal bleeding: meta-analysis and pooled analysis. Hepato-Gastroenterology. 2013;60(128):1885–91.

96. Teshima CW, Kuipers EJ, van Zanten SV, Mensink PB. Double balloon enteroscopy and capsule endoscopy for obscure gastrointestinal bleeding: an updated meta-analysis. J Gastroenterol Hepatol. 2011;26(5):796–801.

97. Douard R, Wind P, Berger A, Maniere T, Landi B, Cellier C, et al. Role of intraoperative enteroscopy in the management of obscure gastrointestinal bleeding at the time of video-capsule endoscopy. Am J Surg. 2009;198(1):6–11.

98. Rondonotti E, Herrerias JM, Pennazio M, Caunedo A, Mascarenhas-Saraiva M, de Franchis R. Complications, limitations, and failures of capsule endoscopy: a review of 733 cases. Gastrointest Endosc. 2005;62(5):712–6. quiz 752, 754.

99. Li F, Gurudu SR, De Petris G, Sharma VK, Shiff AD, Heigh RI, et al. Retention of the capsule endoscope: a single-center experience of 1000 capsule endoscopy procedures. Gastrointest Endosc. 2008;68(1):174–80.

100. Sidhu R, Sanders DS, Morris AJ, McAlindon ME. Guidelines on small bowel enteroscopy and capsule endoscopy in adults. Gut. 2008;57(1):125–36.

101. Tang SJ, Zanati S, Dubcenco E, Christodoulou D, Cirocco M, Kandel G, et al. Capsule endoscopy regional transit abnormality: a sign of underlying small bowel pathology. Gastrointest Endosc. 2003;58(4):598–602.

102. Tang SJ, Zanati S, Dubcenco E, Monkewich G, Arya N, Cirocco M, et al. Capsule endoscopy regional transit abnormality revisited. Gastrointest Endosc. 2004;60(6):1029–32.

103. Sears DM, Avots-Avotins A, Culp K, Gavin MW. Frequency and clinical outcome of capsule retention during capsule endoscopy for GI bleeding of obscure origin. Gastrointest Endosc. 2004;60(5):822–7.

104. Cave D, Legnani P, de Franchis R, Lewis BS. ICCE consensus for capsule retention. Endoscopy. 2005;37(10):1065–7.

105. Liao Z, Gao R, Xu C, Li ZS. Indications and detection, completion, and retention rates of small-bowel capsule endoscopy: a systematic review. Gastrointest Endosc. 2010;71(2):280–6.

106. Delvaux M, Ben Soussan E, Laurent V, Lerebours E, Gay G. Clinical evaluation of the use of the m2a patency capsule system before a capsule endoscopy procedure, in patients with known or suspected intestinal stenosis. Endoscopy. 2005;37(9):801–7.

107. Buchman AL, Miller FH, Wallin A, Chowdhry AA, Ahn C. Videocapsule endoscopy versus barium con-

trast studies for the diagnosis of Crohn's disease recurrence involving the small intestine. Am J Gastroenterol. 2004;99(11):2171–7.

108. Yu WK, Yang RD. M2A video capsule lodged in the Meckel's diverticulum. Gastrointest Endosc. 2006;63(7):1071–2. discussion 1072.

109. Baichi MM, Arifuddin RM, Mantry PS. What we have learned from 5 cases of permanent capsule retention. Gastrointest Endosc. 2006;64(2):283–7.

110. Matta A, Koppala J, Reddymasu SC, Lanspa S. Acute appendicitis: a potential complication of video capsule endoscopy. BMJ Case Rep. 2014. doi:10.1136/bcr-2014-204240.

111. Lin OS, Brandabur JJ, Schembre DB, Soon MS, Kozarek RA. Acute symptomatic small bowel obstruction due to capsule impaction. Gastrointest Endosc. 2007;65(4):725–8.

112. Um S, Poblete H, Zavotsky J. Small bowel perforation caused by an impacted endocapsule. Endoscopy. 2008;40 Suppl 2:E122–3.

113. Spada C, Spera G, Riccioni M, Biancone L, Petruzziello L, Tringali A, et al. A novel diagnostic tool for detecting functional patency of the small bowel: the given patency capsule. Endoscopy. 2005;37(9):793–800.

114. Herrerias JM, Leighton JA, Costamagna G, Infantolino A, Eliakim R, Fischer D, et al. Agile patency system eliminates risk of capsule retention in patients with known intestinal strictures who undergo capsule endoscopy. Gastrointest Endosc. 2008;67(6):902–9.

115. Boivin ML, Lochs H, Voderholzer WA. Does passage of a patency capsule indicate small-bowel patency? A prospective clinical trial? Endoscopy. 2005;37(9):808–15.

116. Yadav A, Heigh RI, Hara AK, Decker GA, Crowell MD, Gurudu SR, et al. Performance of the patency capsule compared with nonenteroclysis radiologic examinations in patients with known or suspected intestinal strictures. Gastrointest Endosc. 2011;74(4):834–9.

117. Zhang W, Han Z, Cheng Y, Xu Y, Xiao K, Li A, et al. The value of the patency capsule in pre-evaluation for capsule endoscopy in cases of intestinal obstruction: a meta-analysis. J Dig Dis. 2014;15(7):345–51.

118. Gay G, Delvaux M, Laurent V, Reibel N, Regent D, Grosdidier G, et al. Temporary intestinal occlusion induced by a "patency capsule" in a patient with Crohn's disease. Endoscopy. 2005;37(2):174–7.

119. Payeras G, Piqueras J, Moreno VJ, Cabrera A, Menendez D, Jimenez R. Effects of capsule endoscopy on cardiac pacemakers. Endoscopy. 2005;37(12):1181–5.

120. Harris LA, Hansel SL, Rajan E, Srivathsan K, Rea R, Crowell MD, et al. Capsule endoscopy in patients with implantable electromedical devices is safe. Gastroenterol Res Pract. 2013;2013:959234.

121. Leighton JA, Srivathsan K, Carey EJ, Sharma VK, Heigh RI, Post JK, et al. Safety of wireless capsule endoscopy in patients with implantable cardiac defibrillators. Am J Gastroenterol. 2005;100(8):1728–31.

122. Leighton JA, Sharma VK, Srivathsan K, Heigh RI, McWane TL, Post JK, et al. Safety of capsule endoscopy in patients with pacemakers. Gastrointest Endosc. 2004;59(4):567–9.

123. Bandorski D, Lotterer E, Hartmann D, Jakobs R, Bruck M, Hoeltgen R, et al. Capsule endoscopy in patients with cardiac pacemakers and implantable cardioverter-defibrillators—a retrospective multicenter investigation. J Gastrointestin Liver Dis. 2011;20(1):33–7.

124. Lin OS. Breaching the final frontier: the future of small-intestinal capsule endoscopy. Gastrointest Endosc. 2008;68(3):495–8.

125. Liao Z, Xu C, Li ZS. Completion rate and diagnostic yield of small-bowel capsule endoscopy: 1 vs. 2 frames per second. Endoscopy. 2010;42(5):360–4.

126. Liao Z, Li ZS, Xu C. Reduction of capture rate in the stomach increases the complete examination rate of capsule endoscopy: a prospective randomized controlled trial. Gastrointest Endosc. 2009;69(3 Pt 1):418–25.

127. Gralnek IM, Ching JY, Maza I, Wu JC, Rainer TH, Israelit S, et al. Capsule endoscopy in acute upper gastrointestinal hemorrhage: a prospective cohort study. Endoscopy. 2013;45(1):12–9.

128. Meltzer AC, Pinchbeck C, Burnett S, Buhumaid R, Shah P, Ding R, et al. Emergency physicians accurately interpret video capsule endoscopy findings in suspected upper gastrointestinal hemorrhage: a video survey. Acad Emerg Med. 2013;20(7):711–5.

129. Meltzer AC, Ali MA, Kresiberg RB, Patel G, Smith JP, Pines JM, et al. Video capsule endoscopy in the emergency department: a prospective study of acute upper gastrointestinal hemorrhage. Ann Emerg Med. 2013;61(4):438–43. e431.

130. Rubin M, Hussain SA, Shalomov A, Cortes RA, Smith MS, Kim SH. Live view video capsule endoscopy enables risk stratification of patients with acute upper GI bleeding in the emergency room: a pilot study. Dig Dis Sci. 2011;56(3):786–91.

131. Leighton JA, Gralnek IM, Richner RE, Lacey MJ, Papatheofanis FJ. Capsule endoscopy in suspected small bowel Crohn's disease: economic impact of disease diagnosis and treatment. World J Gastroenterol. 2009;15(45):5685–92.

132. Korean Gut Image Study Group, Lim YJ, Joo YS, Jung DY, Ye BD, Kim JH, et al. Learning curve of capsule endoscopy. Clin Endosc. 2013;46(6):633–6.

Video Legends

Video 6.1 - Brief video comparing resolution differences between Pillcam SB1, SB2 and SB3 capsules visualizing normal small intestinal mucosa.

Balloon Enteroscopy

7

Klaus Mönkemüller, John Ospina Nieto,
Shabnam Sarker, and Lucia Fry

Introduction

The advent of double-balloon enteroscopy (DBE) a decade ago was a major breakthrough for the diagnosis and treatment of small bowel disorders [1–4]. Soon thereafter single-balloon enteroscopy (SBE) was introduced [5–8]. Both DBE and SBE have replaced push enteroscopy as the methods of

Electronic supplementary material: The online version of this chapter (doi: 10.1007/978-3-319-14415-3_7) contains supplementary material, which is available to authorized users. Videos can also be accessed at http://link.springer.com/chapter/10.1007/978-3-319-14415-3_7.

K. Mönkemüller, M.D., Ph.D., F.A.S.G.E (✉)
Division of Gastroenterology, University of Alabama at Birmingham, 1808 7th Avenue South, 380 BDB, Birmingham, AL 35249, USA
e-mail: klaus1@uab.edu

J. Ospina Nieto, M.D., M.S.C.C., M.S.C.H., M.A.S.G.E
Unidad de Estudios Digestivos, UNESDI,
Carrera 2E#19-50, Chía, Bogotá, Colombia
e-mail: endoscopiaterapeutica@yahoo.com

S. Sarker, M.D.
Department of Internal Medicine, University of Alabama at Birmingham, 1808 7th Avenue South, 380 BDB, Birmingham, AL 35249, USA
e-mail: ssarker@uabmc.edu

L. Fry, M.D., Ph.D, F.A.S.G.E
Division of Gastroenterology, Hepatology and Infectious Diseases, Otto-von-Guericke University, Leipzigerstr 44, Magdeburg 39120, Germany
e-mail: luciafry@yahoo.com

choice to perform deep enteroscopy. Both techniques of SBE and DBE, similar to push enteroscopy, use the principle of the push-and-pull technique: The endoscope is first advanced (pushed) into the small bowel and this is followed by advancement of the overtube toward the tip of the endoscope. Then both the endoscope and overtube are pulled back together, pleating the small bowel over the scope. Hence the concept of "push and pull" [9]. However, when performing SBE and DBE, the major factor governing the maneuverability and depth of insertion of the enteroscope is the presence of a balloon on the distal end of the flexible overtube. Therefore, we proposed to call this technique "balloon-assisted" enteroscopy (BAE) [10]. This terminology also allows one to include the through-the-scope balloon into the spectrum of BAE [11].

In the meantime another overtube-based spiral enteroscopy device was developed [12]. The principle of spiral enteroscopy is based on the use of an overtube, which has a screwlike tubing covering it. This configuration allows for "screwing" the overtube and the endoscope into the jejunum [12, 13]. Because all modern deep enteroscopy methods rely on some sort of device, the term "device-assisted enteroscopy" was coined [14]. However, spiral enteroscopy did not gain the expected popularity and utility and is currently unavailable in most parts of the world. In addition, a new disposable device, the NaviAid™ AB (AB = advancing balloon), also called BGE device (balloon-guided endoscopy), has been developed [15]. The NaviAid™ system can be used with standard endoscopes, consisting of a catheter with an inflatable balloon attached at the distal end. Once advanced through the working channel, the balloon can be inflated and used for anchoring, allowing the advancement of the endoscope. In this chapter we present the technical aspects of performing BAE, focusing on advances of the technique, equipment, and indications.

Definition of Balloon-Assisted Enteroscopy

BAE is the performance of either diagnostic or therapeutic interventions of the small bowel using a balloon-catheter or balloon-overtube. Currently there are three types of BAE: DBE, SBE, and balloon-catheter-guided enteroscopy (BGE). Both DBE and SBE use an overtube with a balloon attached at the distal part of the overtube. The main difference between SBE and DBE

is the presence of a second balloon attached to the scope (Figs. 7.1 and 7.2). Deep enteroscopy performed with a through-the-scope balloon catheter is known as balloon-guiding endoscopy (BGE, NaviAid®) [15] (Fig. 7.2). For easiness and clear understanding of the methods used, we prefer to specifically state whether the BAE was performed using an overtube with a single balloon (SBE) or double balloon (DBE), or if an on-the-scope balloon technique (BGE) was employed.

Indications

The indications for BAE have increased significantly since its introduction in 2004. Currently, BAE techniques are not only used to perform deep enteroscopy, but the equipment can also be used for endoscopic retrograde cholangiopancreatography (ERCP), incomplete colonoscopies, or exploring the gastrointestinal tract of patients with surgically deranged anatomy [16–28]

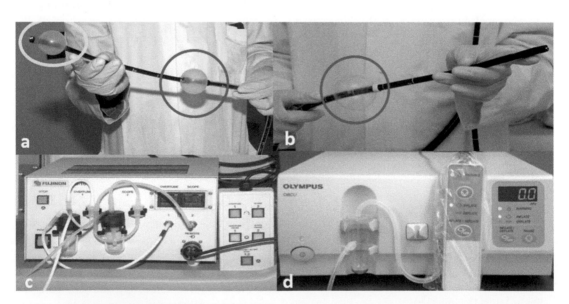

Fig. 7.1 Balloon-assisted enteroscopy. (**a**) Double-balloon enteroscope. (**b**) Single-balloon enteroscope. The major similitude is the overtube with the balloon (*red circle*). In double-balloon enteroscopy there is an additional balloon on top of the scope (*yellow oval*). Note balloon insufflators for Fujinon (**c**) and Olympus systems (**d**), respectively

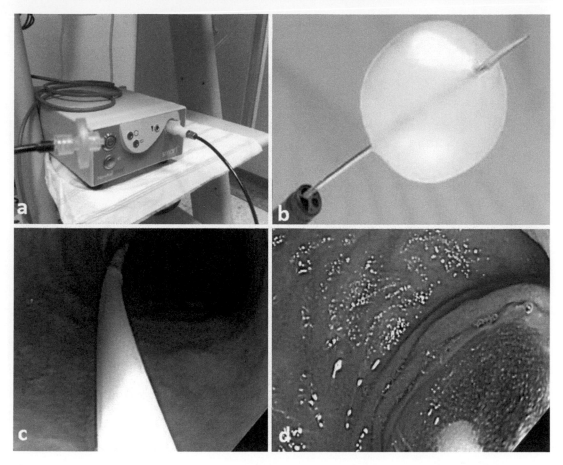

Fig. 7.2 Balloon-guided enteroscopy (BGE). The BGE device is attached to the scope. (**a**) Inflation device. (**b**) Advancing balloon. (**c**) Endoscopic view of advancing catheter. (**d**) Endoscopic view of advancing balloon

(Fig. 7.3). Table 7.1 lists indications for BAE. Furthermore, BAE has become an important tool to deliver various types of endoscopic therapies during deep enteroscopy, but also for many other gastrointestinal problems, such as insertion of self-expanding metal stents into the small bowel or into the stomach in patients with deranged anatomy [22–26] (Table 7.1, Figs. 7.4 and 7.5).

Equipment

We will separately describe the equipment and technique used for overtube-based BAE and through-the-scope balloon-guided enteroscopy.

Overtube-Assisted BAE

Currently there are two types of balloon enteroscopes: DBE (Fujifilm, Japan) and SBE (Olympus Optical Co, Ltd, Tokyo, Japan) [1–8, 13, 29, 30] (Fig. 7.1). The enteroscopes used to perform DBE come in various lengths and diameters (Table 7.2). This variety allows one to choose the scope for different conditions. The diagnostic or small-diameter enteroscope is potentially useful for narrowed luminal diameter, significant adhesions, and/or performing incomplete colonoscopy [13, 30]. However, the small working channel of this enteroscope limits the therapeutic capabilities, as there are few accessories that can be easily

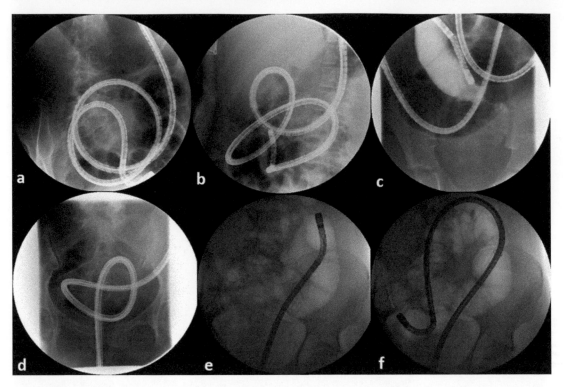

Fig. 7.3 Fluoroscopy during balloon-assisted enteroscopy (BAE). The images show (**a**) antegrade (oral) BAE, (**b**) looping of bowel due to adhesions during an oral BAE, (**c**) use of contrast to delineate a stricture in a patient with Crohn's disease, (**d**) "pretzel" configuration of the scope in a patient with previously failed colonoscopy, (**e**) retrograde (anal) BAE, and (**f**) passing of a long and floppy splenic flexure during anal BAE

Table 7.1 Indications and potential therapeutic interventions using the balloon-assisted enteroscopy

Small bowel bleeding
Hemostasis
- Argon plasma coagulation
- Injection of diluted epinephrine (1:100,000)
- Sclerotherapy (cyanoacrylate injection, Dermabond®, Histoacryl®)
- Placement of clips (standard hemoclips or over-the-scope clips)

Crohn's disease
Balloon dilation of strictures
Retrieval of retained small bowel capsule

NSAID enteropathy
Balloon dilation of strictures

Malabsorption syndromes

Celiac disease (surveillance)

Polyposis syndromes (surveillance)

Polypectomy

Endoscopic mucosal resection

Tumors (adenocarcinoma, gastrointestinal stromal tumors, search for primary neuroendocrine tumors)

Submucosal injection with India ink

Removal of foreign bodies (e.g., capsule endoscope, pins, dentures, needles, coins)

Colonoscopy
Complete a previously failed colonoscopy
Stent placement

Percutaneous endoscopic jejunostomy in normal and altered bowel anatomy (gastric bypass, Roux-en-Y)

Biliary interventions
ERCP
- Cholangiogram
- Pancreatogram
- Sphincterotomy
- Precut sphincterotomy
- Papillectomy
- Balloon dilation
- Stone removal
- Stent placement/removal (plastic and metal stents)
- Removal of dislocated metal stent

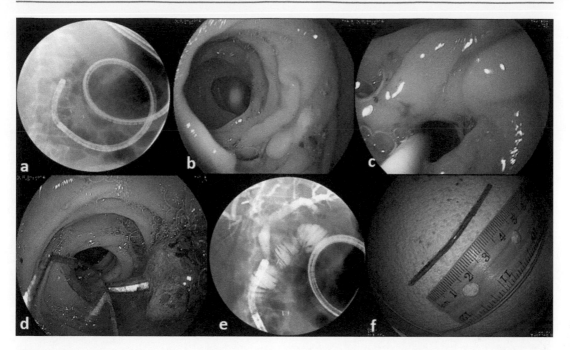

Fig. 7.4 BAE-ERCP in a patient with Whipple operation and hepaticojejunostomy with Roux-en-Y anastomosis. (**a**) Scope in biliodigestive limb. (**b**) The hepaticojejunostomy is often difficult to find. Here it is located at the 6 o'clock position. (**c**) Cannulation of the hepaticojejunostomy. (**d**) Removal of sludge and an inwardly migrated plastic stent with a basket. (**e**) Cholangiography. (**f**) Removed stent

advanced through this 2.2 mm channel. For this reason, most experts prefer the "therapeutic" enteroscope, which has a larger diameter and wider working channel (2.8 mm) [29, 30] (Table 7.2, Video 7.1). The single-balloon enteroscope (SIF Q260) has a 200 cm working length, a 9.2 mm outer diameter, and a 2.8 mm working channel [5–8]. This enteroscope from Olympus and the "diagnostic" and "therapeutic" enteroscopes from Fujifilm have the same length, in contrast to the short enteroscopes from Fujifilm (Table 7.2) [1–8, 13, 24]. The advantage of the shorter enteroscope is its utility for ERCP [27, 28, 30]. To simplify the definitions, we call the long enteroscopes "standard" length scopes and the shorter scopes "short enteroscopes." In addition, the reader should know that the DBE scopes could also be used to perform SBE [29]. In this instance, no balloon is attached to the endoscope itself.

Both standard DBE enteroscopes and their respective overtubes have the same length (enteroscope 200 cm, overtube 1,450 mm), but the external diameters of both the endoscope and the overtube are different. The diagnostic DBE (EN-450P5, Fujinon, Saitama, Japan) has an external diameter of 8.5 mm and the overtube has a diameter of 12.2 mm, whereas the therapeutic DBE (EN-450T5) has an external diameter of 9.4 mm and the overtube has a diameter of 13.2 mm [13, 24, 30]. The diameter of the working channel of the therapeutic DBE is 2.8 mm whereas the diagnostic one is 2.2 mm wide [13, 24, 29, 30]. Thus, careful attention should be paid when choosing accessories, as these must be long enough to exit the scope and also have an external diameter that permits their insertion and pushing through the respective working channels. In our endoscopy unit we keep a list of the

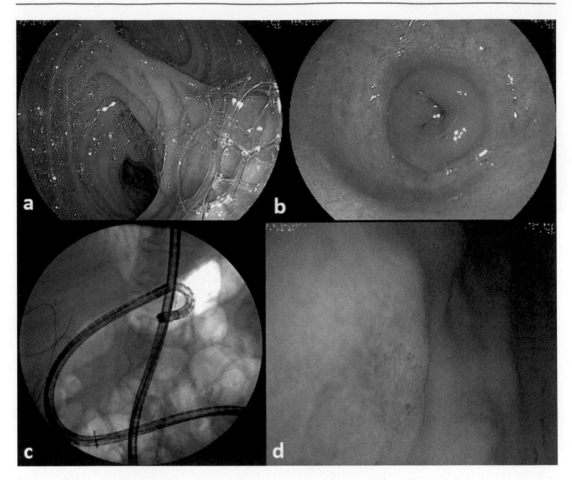

Fig. 7.5 BAE in a patient with Roux-en-Y gastric bypass. (**a**) Recognition of the afferent loop is facilitated by the presence of many small and large yellowish air bubbles, which result from the presence of bile. (**b**) Pylorus viewed from the "back." (**c**) Retroflexion of the enteroscope inside of the excluded stomach. The retroflexion was performed to visualize the antrum. (**d**) Multiple ulcers and erosions were seen

sizes, diameters, lengths, and working channel capabilities of all the endoscopes we use. These tables are posted on the wall of each room and serve as a quick reference. The lengths and sizes of the overtubes are also specified in Table 7.2.

Technique of Balloon-Assisted Enteroscopy

We prefer to use general anesthesia when performing oral (antegrade) BAE. When using general anesthesia we prefer to place the patient on their back (i.e., supine). This position will also allow for easy external manual compression when this is needed to improve advancement of the scope. When conscious sedation is utilized, left-lateral decubitus positions are mandatory, so that the patient's secretions can be managed properly and thus aspiration avoided [13]. We use moderate sedation for the majority of our patients undergoing anal (retrograde) BAE.

Both techniques of SBE and DBE, similar to overtube-assisted push enteroscopy, use the principle of the push-and-pull technique using the overtube: The endoscope is first inserted (pushed) into the small bowel, then the overtube is advanced toward the tip of the endoscope, and then both endoscope and overtube are pulled back; hence the name "push and pull" (Fig. 7.6) [13].

Table 7.2 Enteroscopy device specifications

Scopes	Scope working length (cm)	Scope diameter (mm)	Specifications Channel diameter (mm)	Overtube length (cm)	Overtube outer diameter (mm)
SBE (Olympus, SIF-Q180)	200	9.2	2.8	140	13.2
DBE (Fujinon, EN-450PS/20)	200	8.5	2.2	145	12.2
DBE (Fujinon, EN-450T5)	200	9.4	2.8	145	13.2
DBE (Fujinon, EC-450BI5)	152	9.4	2.8	105	13.2
Pentax VSB-3,430 K	220	11.6	3.8		
SE Spirus medical, discovery SB	a	a	a	118	16

DBE double-balloon enteroscopy, *SB* small bowel, *SE* spiral enteroscopy, *SBE* single-balloon enteroscopy
[a]Either the Fujinon DBE enteroscope or the Olympus SBE enteroscope can be used to perform SE with a spiral enteroscopy overtube

Fig. 7.6 Key elements of double-balloon enteroscopy. (**a**) Both the overtube and scope are pulled back (*red arrow*) to straighten the bowel and retract the proximal bowel on top of the overtube. (**b**) The balloon of the overtube is kept inflated (keeping the retracted bowel in place) and the balloon of the scope is deflated. The inflated balloon prevents the intestine to slide forward, keeping it "shortened" while the scope is being pushed or advanced forward (*green arrow* shows direction of scope)

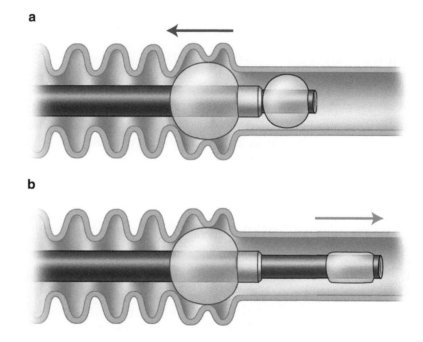

This standard approach to BAE requires two people, the operator and an assistant. The assistant holding the overtube plays a crucial role, as a stable overtube will positively influence the depth of insertion and the maneuverability of the scope [13]. When using SBE and DBE, the major factor governing the depth of insertion of the enteroscope is the presence of the balloon on the distal end of the flexible overtube. The overtube stabilizes the intestine, preventing it from bending or looping [13, 30]. Although, the overtube stabilizes the intestine, preventing it from bending or looping, the key action of the inflated overtube balloon is to shorten the small bowel proximally (Fig. 7.6a). The inflated balloon prevents the intestine from sliding forward while the scope is being pushed or advanced forward (Fig. 7.6b) [13, 30]. This allows the endoscopist to firmly push on the enteroscope, effectively transmitting forces to the distal end of the endoscope and hence permitting the advancement of the enteroscope deeper into the small bowel without looping or stretching of the proximal intestine [1–8, 10, 13, 30]. The key steps and aspects of BAE are listed in Table 7.3 and shown in Fig. 7.6 and Video 7.2.

Table 7.3 Key technical steps used to perform double-balloon enteroscopy

Step 1	The scope and overtube are advanced into the intestine (large bowel or small bowel).
Step 2	The balloon of the overtube is inflated.
Step 3	The scope is advanced (pushed) forward into the small bowel.
Step 4	The balloon of the scope is inflated, anchoring the bowel.
Step 5	The balloon of the overtube is deflated.
Step 6	The overtube is advanced (slid) toward the tip of the scope.
Step 7	The balloon of the overtube is inflated. Now both the scope and overtube balloons are inflated.
Step 8	Both the overtube and scope are pulled back to straighten the bowel and retract and pleat the proximal bowel onto the overtube.
Step 9	The balloon of the overtube is kept inflated (keeping the retracted bowel in place) and the balloon of the scope is deflated.

At this level the procedure continues with step 3 (see above).

Single-balloon enteroscopy follows exactly the same principles, with the exception of not inflating any balloon on the scope. In SBE, the scope tip needs to bend to anchor the intestine. Therefore step 4 is bending of the tip of the scope instead of inflating a balloon

The insertion method for both SBE and DBE is similar (Table 7.3, Fig. 7.6, Video 7.2). The main difference between the SBE and DBE technique is the approach of holding the small intestine in place while the overtube is advanced [13, 30]. When using the SBE technique, after the endoscope is inserted maximally, the tip of the endoscope is bent to form a hook shape, holding the small intestine in a stable position (Video 7.2), instead of the inflated balloon on the tip in DBE technique. When the sliding overtube is advanced to the tip of the scope, the overtube balloon is then inflated to hold and stabilize the intestine [13, 30]. After returning the tip of the endoscope to the neutral position to avoid mucosal injury, both the scope and the sliding tube are simultaneously withdrawn, thus pleating and shortening the intestine over the scope. By repeating these maneuvers, the endoscope can be inserted into the deep small bowel.

For performing ERCP in patients with a Roux-en-Y anastomosis or surgically altered upper gastrointestinal tract anatomy we recommend the use of the therapeutic DBE with a working channel of 2.8 mm or the short enteroscopes (Fig. 7.4) [30]. These therapeutic scopes have better maneuverability than the smaller diameter enteroscopes. In addition, the working channel is larger, allowing for an easier introduction of the diagnostic and therapeutic accessories. Although we have performed several cases of DB-ERCP utilizing only the balloon of the overtube ("single-balloon ERCP"), we still recommend attaching the balloons to both the scope and the overtube and we use the double-balloon push-and-pull technique to advance through the small bowel [30].

Balloon-Guided Enteroscopy

The BGE is made of disposable device consisting of a two-balloon element and an air supply unit to control the operation of the balloons (Fig. 7.2) [14]. The catheter length is 190 cm and the balloon diameter is 40 mm. The BGE device is compatible with scopes ranging from 10 to 13 mm in diameter. The BGE device is mounted on the scope, with a stabilizing balloon at the distal end of the scope and an advancing balloon, sheltered within the stabilizing balloon [14]. The advancing balloon is advanced or retracted manually ahead of the scope by a flexible advancing tube, which passes through a dedicated external channel, leaving the working channel of the scope free for accessory usage. BGE is performed in a similar fashion to DBE [14]. Once the scope has been positioned in the intestine (step 1), the stabilizing balloon is inflated and the anchoring balloon is advanced into the intestine (step 2), ahead of the scope. Once it has been advanced, it is inflated to anchor the intestine (step 3). Then the stabilizing balloon at the scope tip is deflated and the scope is again inserted toward the inflated anchoring balloon (step 4). Then the stabilizing balloon is inflated as well (step 5) and with both balloons inflated, the scope is pulled back and the intestine is straightened (step 6). Then the advancing balloon is deflated and advanced, beginning with step 2.

Use of Fluoroscopy

We recommend the availability and/or use of fluoroscopy when performing the BAE (Figs. 7.3, 7.4, and 7.5, Video 7.3). Fluoroscopy may help estimate the depth of insertion, and scope positioning, and minimize the formation of figure-eight loops [13]. Whereas fluoroscopy is not always needed during a standard oral or retrograde BAE, it is mandatory to use it for planned therapeutic procedures, in patients with surgically altered anatomy and those with abdominal scarring and bowel adhesions (Figs. 7.4 and 7.5). Previous abdominal surgery may make BAE more difficult. Adhesions may limit the mobility of the intestine and make insertion of the BAE more cumbersome. The most important aspect to remember is to be patient and not to advance the scope and or overtube forcefully. In addition, careful attention should be paid to avoiding excessive air insufflation while advancing the endoscope as the bowel gets distended and further advancement is thus hampered. The use of carbon dioxide (CO_2) instead of air allows for deeper intubation and bowel visualization [31, 32]. In addition, patients experience less pain due to abdominal distention when using CO_2 [31]. Changing the patient's position or applying external abdominal pressure may help. Thus, it is evident that fluoroscopy can be very helpful in situations when advancement is limited, as it permits one to estimate the degree of looping present as well as to visualize the direction that the scope is taking.

Sedation and Anesthesia

BAE has been traditionally performed using conscious sedation [1–8]. However, these procedures are lengthy and physically demanding on both the patient and endoscopy team. The risk of aspiration and desaturation is high [32, 33]. Therefore, currently we perform the majority of BAE with the patient under general anesthesia [34]. Despite the procedures under general anesthesia needing additional time for preparation, we prefer this option to perform anterograde enteroscopies as well as therapeutic BAE and BAE-ERCP in patients with surgically altered upper GI tract anatomy [30, 32–34]. Conscious sedation may be used when retrograde BAE is performed.

Determination of the Primary Route of Insertion of BAE (Oral or Antegrade Versus Anal or Retrograde)

Oral or antegrade BAE allows for a median investigation of 250–300 cm of small bowel, whereas retrograde or anal enteroscopy permits depths of investigation of about 100–200 cm [1–8, 13]. When both routes are used successively a "total" small bowel enteroscopy can be achieved in 10–70 % of patients [1–8, 13]. In the ideal world, a total enteroscopy should be achieved using either route. But this is still not possible in the majority of cases. Thus, whenever a patient with a suspected small bowel disorder presents to us for small bowel investigation, the choice for either the oral ("antegrade") or the anal ("retrograde") route will depend on the suspected location of the lesion within the small bowel based on the clinical manifestations, as well as the results of laboratory, radiological, and capsule endoscopic examinations [1–10, 13]. When achieving total enteroscopy is desired, a second procedure in the opposite direction is scheduled.

Imaging and Advanced Imaging

Small bowel endoscopic imaging comprises techniques such as high-definition white light, standard white light with chromoendoscopy, virtual chromoendoscopy, magnification, as well as endomicroscopy for the evaluation of the gastrointestinal mucosa [29] (Table 7.4, Fig. 7.7). The concept of using more than one imaging method when performing endoscopy is currently called multimodal endoscopy [29]. For example, using a combination of standard white light and chromoendoscopy is an example of bimodal endoscopy.

Table 7.4 Standard and advanced endoscopic imaging during balloon-assisted enteroscopy

Standard white light endoscopy
High-definition white light endoscopy
Water immersion technique
Dye-based chromoendoscopy • Methylene blue • Indigo carmine
Dye-less chromoendoscopy ("virtual" chromoendoscopy) • Fujinon intelligent chromoendoscopy (FICE) • i-Scan • Narrow-band imaging (NBI)
Zoom and magnification endoscopy
Endocytoscopy
Confocal laser endomicroscopy

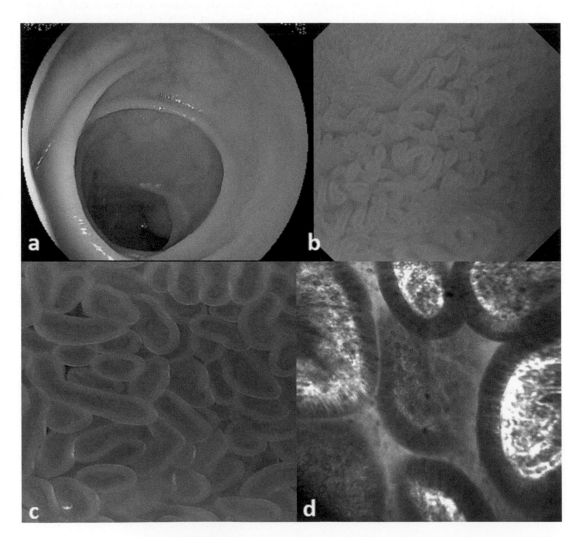

Fig. 7.7 Advanced imaging during BAE. Normal small bowel mucosa. (**a**) High-definition white light. (**b**) Magnification endoscopy. (**c**) FICE and magnification endoscopy. (**d**) Confocal endomicroscopy

When using three methods the terminology changes to advanced trimodal imaging and so forth [29, 35, 36]. The most common methods used are high-definition white light, water immersion technique, and "dye-less" virtual chromoendoscopy [29, 35, 36]. The water immersion technique is very useful when mucosal atrophy is suspected. We utilize immersion technique every time when investigating patients for celiac disease and malabsorption syndromes [29]. Virtual chromoendoscopy is technically very simple, without the burden of the standard chromoendoscopy, and is also beneficial to demarcate lesions as well as identify disease activity and mucosal healing in inflammatory bowel disease [29, 35]. However, we prefer to use standard dye-based methods using indigo carmine or methylene blue when evaluating polyposis syndromes and during endoscopic resection [36].

Conclusion

This chapter reviews and demonstrates the indications, principles, and techniques of device-assisted enteroscopy. It is clear that device-assisted enteroscopy has become the primary method to perform deep enteroscopy and to perform diagnostic and therapeutic pancreatobiliary interventions in patients with surgically distorted small bowel anatomy such as Roux-en-Y anastomosis with hepaticojejunostomy. We expect further refinements of the endoscope such as increase in the working channel and innovations of the interventional accessories that will result in more possibilities to better treat patients who have small bowel disorders and those with complex postsurgical anatomy.

References

1. Yamamoto H, Kita H, Sunada K, Hayashi Y, Sato H, Yano T, Iwamoto M, Sekine Y, Miyata T, Kuno A, Ajibe H, Ido K, Sugano K. Clinical outcomes of double-balloon endoscopy for the diagnosis and treatment of small-intestinal diseases. Clin Gastroenterol Hepatol. 2004;2:1010–6.
2. Mönkemüller K, Weigt J, Treiber G, Kolfenbach S, Kahl S, Röcken C, Ebert M, Fry LC, Malfertheiner P. Diagnostic and therapeutic impact of double-balloon enteroscopy. Endoscopy. 2006;38:67–72.
3. Bellutti M, Fry LC, Schmitt J, Seemann M, Klose S, Malfertheiner P, Mönkemüller K. Detection of neuroendocrine tumors of the small bowel by double balloon enteroscopy. Dig Dis Sci. 2009;54:1050–8.
4. Fry LC, Neumann H, Kuester D, Kuhn R, Bellutti M, Malfertheiner P, Monkemuller K. Small bowel polyps and tumours: endoscopic detection and treatment by double-balloon enteroscopy. Aliment Pharmacol Ther. 2009;29:135–42.
5. Upchurch BR, Sanaka MR, Lopez AR, et al. The clinical utility of single-balloon enteroscopy: a single-center experience of 172 procedures. Gastrointest Endosc. 2010;71:1218–23.
6. Tsujikawa T, Saitoh Y, Andoh A, Imaeda H, Hata K, Minematsu H, Senoh K, Hayafuji K, Ogawa A, Nakahara T, Sasaki M, Fujiyama Y. Novel single-balloon enteroscopy for diagnosis and treatment of the small intestine: preliminary experiences. Endoscopy. 2008;40:11–5.
7. Kawamura T, Yasuda K, Tanaka K, Uno K, Ueda M, Sanada K, Nakajima M. Clinical evaluation of a newly developed single-balloon enteroscope. Gastrointest Endosc. 2008;68:1112–6.
8. Katsinelos P, Chatzimavroudis G, Zavos C, Fasoulas K, Kountouras J. Single-balloon enteroscopy in life-threatening small-intestine hemorrhage. Endoscopy. 2010;42:88.
9. Mönkemüller K, Fry LC, Malfertheiner P. Double-balloon enteroscopy: beyond feasibility, what do we do now? Endoscopy. 2007;39:229–31.
10. Mönkemüller K, Fry LC, Bellutti M, Malfertheiner P. Balloon-assisted enteroscopy: unifying double-balloon and single-balloon enteroscopy. Endoscopy. 2008;40:537.
11. Adler SN, Bjarnason I, Metzger YC. New balloon-guided technique for deep small-intestine endoscopy using standard endoscopes. Endoscopy. 2008;40:502–5.
12. Akerman PA, Agrawal D, Chen W, Cantero D, Avila J, Pangtay J. Spiral enteroscopy: a novel method of enteroscopy by using the Endo-Ease Discovery SB overtube and a pediatric colonoscope. Gastrointest Endosc. 2009;69:327–32.
13. Mönkemüller K, Bellutti M, Fry LC, Malfertheiner P. Enteroscopy. Best Pract Res Clin Gastroenterol. 2008;22:789–811.
14. Elena RM, Riccardo U, Rossella C, Bizzotto A, Domenico G, Guido C. Current status of device-assisted enteroscopy: technical matters, indication, limits and complications. World J Gastrointest Endosc. 2012;4:453–61.
15. Tontini GE, Grauer M, Akin H, Vieth M, Tasdelen H, Vecchi M, Neurath MF, Neumann H. Extensive small-bowel diverticulosis identified with the newly introduced On Demand Enteroscopy system. Endoscopy. 2013;45 Suppl 2 UCTN:E350-1.
16. Mönkemüller K, Knippig C, Rickes S, Fry LC, Schulze A, Malfertheiner P. Use of the double-balloon intestinoscope to perform complete colonoscopy in

patients with previously failed colonoscopy. Scand J Gastroenterol. 2007;42:277–8.

17. Sakai P, Kuga R, Saftle-Ribeiro AV, Faintuch J, Gama-Rodrigues JJ, Ishida RK, Furuya CK, Yamamoto H, Ishioka S. Is it feasible to reach the bypassed stomach after roux-en-Y gastric bypass for morbid obesity? the use of the double balloon enteroscope. Endoscopy. 2005;37:566–9.

18. Pasha SF, Harrison ME, Das A, Corrado CM, Arnell KN, Leighton JA. Utility of double-balloon colonoscopy for completion of colon examination after incomplete colonoscopy with conventional colonoscope. Gastrointest Endosc. 2007;65:848–53.

19. Mönkemüller K, Fry LC, Bellutti M, Neumann H, Malfertheiner P. ERCP with the double balloon enteroscope in patients with Roux-en-Y anastomosis. Surg Endosc. 2009;2:1961–7.

20. Neumann H, Fry LC, Meyer F, Malfertheiner P, Monkemuller K. Endoscopic retrograde cholangiopancreatography using the single balloon enteroscope technique in patients with Roux-en-Y anastomosis. Digestion. 2009;80:52–7.

21. Skinner M, Peter S, Wilcox CM, Mönkemüller K. Diagnostic and therapeutic utility of double-balloon enteroscopy for obscure GI bleeding in patients with surgically altered upper GI anatomy. Gastrointest Endosc. 2014;80:181–6.

22. Jovanovic I, Vormbrock K, Zimmermann L, Djuranovic S, Ugljesic M, Malfertheiner P, Fry LC, Mönkemüller K. Therapeutic double-balloon enteroscopy: a binational, three-center experience. Dig Dis. 2011;29 Suppl 1:27–31.

23. Ross AS, Semrad C, Alverdy J, Waxman I, Dye C. Use of double-balloon enteroscopy to perform PEG in the excluded stomach after Roux-en-Y gastric bypass. Gastrointest Endosc. 2006;64:797–800.

24. Skinner M, Popa D, Neumann H, Wilcox CM, Mönkemüller K. ERCP with the overtube-assisted enteroscopy technique: a systematic review. Endoscopy. 2014;46:560–72.

25. Neumann H, Wilcox CM, Mönkemüller K. Balloon overtube-assisted placement of self-expanding metal stents. Endoscopy. 2013;45 Suppl 2 UCTN:E369-70.

26. Popa D, Ramesh J, Peter S, Wilcox CM, Mönkemüller K. Small bowel stent-in-stent placement for malignant small bowel obstruction using a balloon-assisted overtube technique. Clin Endosc. 2014;47:108–11.

27. Shimatani M, Takaoka M, Ikeura T, Mitsuyama T, Okazaki K. Evaluation of endoscopic retrograde cholangiopancreatography using a newly developed short-type single-balloon endoscope in patients with altered gastrointestinal anatomy. Dig Endosc. 2014;26 Suppl 2:147–55.

28. Kawamura T, Uno K, Suzuki A, Mandai K, Nakase K, Tanaka K, Yasuda K. Clinical usefulness of a short-type, prototype single-balloon enteroscope for endoscopic retrograde cholangiopancreatography in patients with altered gastrointestinal anatomy: preliminary experiences. Dig Endosc. 2014;4.

29. Mönkemüller K, Neumann H, Fry LC. Enteroscopy: advances in diagnostic imaging. Best Pract Res Clin Gastroenterol. 2012;26:221–33.

30. Skinner M, Velázquez-Aviña J, Mönkemüller K. Using balloon-overtube-assisted enteroscopy for postoperative endoscopic retrograde cholangiopancreatography. Therap Adv Gastroenterol. 2014;7:269–79.

31. Domagk D, Bretthauer M, Lenz P, Aabakken L, Ullerich H, Maaser C, Domschke W, Kucharzik T. Carbon dioxide insufflation improves intubation depth in double-balloon enteroscopy: a randomized, controlled, double-blind trial. Endoscopy. 2007;39:1064–7.

32. Zubek L, Szabo L, Lakatos PL, Papp J, Gal J, Elo G. Double balloon enteroscopy examinations in general anesthesia. World J Gastroenterol. 2010;16:3418–22.

33. Lara LF, Ukleja A, Pimentel R, Charles RJ. Effect of a quality program with adverse events identification on airway management during overtube-assisted enteroscopy. Endoscopy. 2014;46:927–32.

34. Phillips MC, Mönkemüller K. Anesthesia for complex endoscopy: a new paradigm. Endoscopy. 2014;46:919–21.

35. Neumann H, Fry LC, Bellutti M, Malfertheiner P, Mönkemüller K. Double-balloon enteroscopy-assisted virtual chromoendoscopy for small-bowel disorders: a case series. Endoscopy. 2009;41:468–71.

36. Mönkemüller K, Fry LC, Ebert M, Bellutti M, Venerito M, Knippig C, Rickes S, Muschke P, Röcken C, Malfertheiner P. Feasibility of double-balloon enteroscopy-assisted chromoendoscopy of the small bowel in patients with familial adenomatous polyposis. Endoscopy. 2007;39:52–7.

Video Legends

Video 7.1 - Therapeutic DBE.

Video 7.2 - DBE technique step by step.

Video 7.3 - SBE with fluoroscopy.

Spiral Enteroscopy and "On Demand" Enteroscopy

Michael V. Chiorean

Background, Instruments, Technique, and Indications

Spiral or rotational enteroscopy is a device-assisted technique for the endoscopic evaluation of the small bowel. It applies the same principle of pleating the small bowel as the double- and single-balloon enteroscopy. However, instead of sequential push–pull maneuvers it uses a rotational spiral overtube similar to a corkscrew in order to convert rotational motion into linear force that will fold the small bowel, thus "advancing" an endoscope that is threaded through the overtube [1]. The procedure can be performed either anterograde or retrograde using two different overtubes. The anterograde overtube has an overall length of 118 cm, outer diameter of 14.5 mm, internal diameter of 9.8 mm, spiral height 5.5 mm, and spiral length 22 cm (Fig. 8.1). The retrograde overtube is shorter at 100 cm and has a larger

Electronic supplementary material: The online version of this chapter (doi: 10.1007/978-3-319-14415-3_8) contains supplementary material, which is available to authorized users. Videos can also be accessed at http://link.springer.com/chapter/10.1007/978-3-319-14415-3_8.

M.V. Chiorean, M.D. (✉)
Inflammatory Bowel Disease Center of Excellence, Department of Gastroenterology, Digestive Disease Institute, Virginia Mason Medical Center, 1100 Ninth Ave, C3-GAS, Seattle, WA 98101, USA
e-mail: michael.chiorean@vmmc.org; Michael.Chiorean@virginiamason.org

external and internal diameter (18 mm and 13 mm respectively) and a shorter spiral length (20 cm) (Fig. 8.2) (Spirus Medical LLC, West Bridgewater, MA). Both devices are single use, latex free, and can accommodate a variety of small bowel enteroscopes and some pediatric colonoscopes.

Two operators are usually required to perform the spiral enteroscopy technique given the fact that both the overtube and the instrument have to be manipulated during the procedure. The overtube is installed on the enteroscope using an interlocking device, which can switch between a longitudinal (advance-withdrawal) and rotational axis of freedom for the scope within the overtube. The procedure can be performed with moderate sedation, monitored anesthesia care (deep sedation), or with general anesthesia depending on patient, indication, and operator variables. If general anesthesia is used for anterograde procedures, it is advisable to deflate the endotracheal balloon while the spiral is advanced through the upper esophagus to avoid trauma. Infrequently, in patients with significant cervical spine disease or cervical osteophytes, the overtube cannot be advanced past the upper esophagus and an alternative enteroscopy method has to be employed [2]. Once past the upper esophageal sphincter, the fixed overtube–enteroscope unit is carefully advanced through steady rotation through the stomach into the duodenum, keeping in mind the possibility of occult strictures. Nonobstructive esophageal Schatzki's rings are usually inconsequential, but strictures less than 15 mm in diameter should be traversed with caution. Once the overtube engages the pylorus and duodenum, the scope–overtube unit usually advances fairly

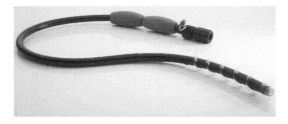

Fig. 8.1 The anterograde Spirus EndoEase Discovery SB overtube utilized primarily for anterograde deep enteroscopy. The same overtube can be used for retrograde procedures but only with a small bowel enteroscope. Reprinted with permission of Spirus Medical LLC

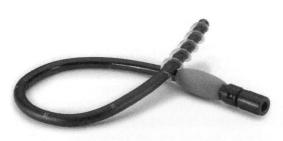

Fig. 8.2 The retrograde Spirus EndoEase Vista overtube is shorter and wider than its anterograde counterpart. It can be used with all small bowel enteroscopes as well as some pediatric colonoscopes with diameter <11 mm. Reprinted with permission of Spirus Medical LLC

easily with steady clockwise rotation into the small bowel. When the entire effective part of the overtube has been inserted and rotational advancement stops or when the operator encounters unusual rotational resistance, the unit can be unlocked again and the scope advanced independently in the small bowel to the maximal point of insertion or until pathology is found.

For the retrograde approach, the overtube serves primarily to "splint" the endoscope (usually an enteroscope) during insertion into the colon and avoid looping (Fig. 8.3). The retrograde spiral overtube can rarely be engaged through the ileocecal valve. Instead, in a relatively straight configuration and under favorable valve orientation, the enteroscope itself can be advanced relatively easily in the ileum (Video 8.1). In a small study, the terminal ileum was intubated in 100 % of patients and the depth of insertion past the ileocecal valve was estimated at 100 cm (range 50–150 cm) [3]. Controlled visualization and endoscopic therapy take place during withdrawal, which is essentially the reverse of the process described previously (i.e., counter-clockwise rotation of the overtube with the scope either in "locked" or "free" position). In order to increase the traction of the overtube on the small bowel, only the minimum amount of gas (air or CO_2) is insufflated during advancement.

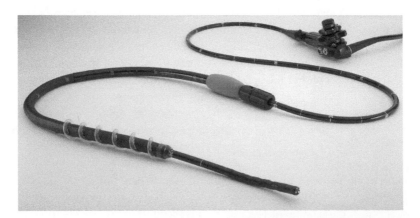

Fig. 8.3 The retrograde Spirus Vista overtube assembled on a 250 cm enteroscope. Note that the distal 20 cm of the scope are extending outside of the overtube during insertion to allow mobility of the scope and avoid excessive tension on the bowel wall. Some endoscopists prefer to have the overtube withdrawn all the way to the scope hub when they introduce the instrument through the rectum. After the scope is introduced for at least 60–70 cm, the colon loops are straightened and the overtube is advanced through the anus by gentle rotation while the colon lumen is kept in the field of view of the scope. Reprinted with permission of Spirus Medical LLC

A more detailed description of the procedure is available [1].

Spiral enteroscopy has the same indications as other device-assisted enteroscopies. In addition, it has the advantage of being a latex-free device and thus it can be utilized safely in patients with known latex allergy. Although no definite contraindications have been formulated, patients with severe luminal strictures (including surgical anastomoses, Crohn's disease, radiation enteropathy) esophageal varices, pregnancy, or severe coagulopathy have been excluded from most studies [2, 4].

Technical Success

The technical success rate, defined as the ability of the instrument to advance past the proximal jejunum in patients with normal anatomy, is approximately 95 % [2]. The most common reasons for failure are luminal strictures, abnormal or unusual anatomy (J-shaped stomach or narrow duodenal sweep) and anesthesia instability [2]. The maximal depth of insertion using spiral enteroscopy is on average 200–250 cm post-pyloric (range 10–600) and roughly corresponds to an area between the distal jejunum and proximal ileum, although these measurements have not been adequately validated [2, 5–7]. No clear predictors of the depth of insertion have been identified, although this is an important aspect of these procedures [8]. The average time to reach the maximum depth of insertion is variable, but in general it is shorter than either single- or double-balloon enteroscopy [4, 9, 10]. Akerman et al. reported an average insertion time of 18.7 min and total procedure time of 29 min [5]. In a US multicenter trial, the maximal extent was reached in an average of 22.1 ± 11.5 min and the mean total procedure time was 34.4 ± 10.1 min for diagnostic enteroscopies and 11.4 min longer (range 0–73 min) for those involving therapeutic interventions [2]. However, the depth of insertion and the rate of complete or panenteroscopy achieved with spiral enteroscopy appears to be inferior to that of double-balloon enteroscopy. In a small study using a combined anterograde and retrograde approach, panenteroscopy was accomplished in only 8 % of patients using spiral enteroscopy versus 92 % with DBE [4]. Spiral enteroscopy can be used successfully to access bypassed areas of the intestine in patients with altered anatomy such as Roux-en-Y anastomoses. In a small retrospective study, there was no difference in the diagnostic and therapeutic yield of spiral enteroscopy and SBE when both were used as platforms to perform endoscopic retrograde cholangiopancreatography (ERCP) in patients with altered anatomy including gastric bypass [11].

The learning curve with spiral enteroscopy seems to be relatively short. A selected group of experienced gastroenterologists was able to acquire the skills for spiral enteroscopy with fewer than ten procedures in a dedicated training environment [12].

Diagnostic and Therapeutic Yield

The diagnostic and therapeutic yield of spiral enteroscopy in patients with suspected small bowel disorders is similar to other device-assisted deep enteroscopy techniques. Significant small bowel abnormalities are found in 33–75 % of symptomatic patients [2, 9, 10, 13]. Selecting patients via preliminary noninvasive studies such as capsule endoscopy increases the yield [2, 7, 9]. Diagnostic and therapeutic interventions can be performed in over 70 % of patients with positive findings [2, 9]. One potential advantage of spiral enteroscopy over other methods is that the endoscope can be withdrawn completely from the patient while maintaining the overtube in a stable position, thus allowing repetitive maneuvers such as piecemeal polypectomy or foreign body retrieval.

Comparison with Other Deep Enteroscopy Techniques

Several small studies compared the technical performance and diagnostic yield of spiral enteroscopy with double-balloon (DBE) or single-balloon enteroscopy (SBE) [4, 9, 14, 15]. The only randomized trial including 26 patients found that the depth of insertion and the ability to perform

Table 8.1 Performance comparison of the three most popular deep enteroscopy techniques

	Spiral enteroscopy[a]	Single balloon	Double balloon
Depth of insertion	Medium	Shorter	Best
Procedure duration	Shortest	Medium	Longest
Bidirectional approach	Fair	Fair	Best
Ease of use	Fair	Easiest	Easy
Platform used	Any	Olympus	Fuji
Diagnostic yield	Good	Good	Good
Therapeutic yield	Good	Good	Good
Ability to remove the scope	Good	Good	Poor
Complication rate	Lower	Average	Average
Investment cost	Lowest	Medium	High

[a]Includes the need for two trained operators

Table 8.2 The rate of mucosal trauma with spiral enteroscopy

n=141 procedures	Minimal or no trauma (%)	Moderate erythema (%)	Mucosal disruption
Proximal esophagus	85	15	1.4 %
Distal esophagus	66	34	0
Lesser curve, stomach	93	6.7	0.7 %
Pylorus	75	25	2.1 %
Duodenum	80	20	0
Angle of Treitz	84	16	1.4 %
Small bowel	79	21	0

Adapted from ref. [2]

bidirectional panenteroscopy (combining oral and anal approaches) was significantly higher with DBE compared to spiral enteroscopy (92 % versus 8 %, $p=0.002$) but at the expense of a longer procedure time. However, the diagnostic and therapeutic yields were similar [4]. In contrast, a multicenter larger prospective cohort study found no difference in insertion depth, procedure duration, diagnostic and therapeutic yield between the two techniques. Panenteroscopy was not attempted in this study [9]. In a retrospective single-center study, the average depth of maximal insertion was found to be higher with spiral enteroscopy than SBE (301 cm versus 222 cm, $p<0.001$) but procedure duration and diagnostic yield were not significantly different, although there was a trend for longer procedure time with SBE [10]. A comparison of the three most popular deep enteroscopy modalities is provided in Table 8.1. Overall it appears that spiral enteroscopy is faster than either balloon-assisted procedure, but the depth of insertion is less than that of DBE and may be superior to that of SBE.

Complications of Spiral Enteroscopy

Despite its unique characteristics, spiral enteroscopy appears to be very safe with a complication rate similar to other deep enteroscopy techniques [2, 3, 16]. Although mucosal trauma or disruption

is not uncommon (see Table 8.2), perforations are infrequent. In the largest, single endoscopist experience with the anterograde procedure encompassing 1,750 patients, the rate of severe complications was 0.4 %. Of the seven patients with complications, 6 were perforations of which, interestingly, half involved the duodenum [16]. All perforations in this series occurred during scope advancement and not overtube torsion. Intestinal perforations have also been reported in patients with preexistent bowel pathology such as radiation injury or altered anatomy [4, 17]. No cases of pancreatitis have been described in multiple series but hyperamylasemia is common [18]. Very limited data exists regarding the safety of retrograde enteroscopy [3, 4].

On-Demand or Through the Scope Enteroscopy

A new on-demand enteroscopy device (ODE, NaviAid AB, Smart Medical Systems Ltd., Ra'anana, Israel) is the most recent addition to the armamentarium of the small bowel endoscopist. As opposed to the more established DBE, SBE, and spiral enteroscopy, ODE is a simpler technique, which requires a relatively modest investment in infrastructure. It is performed by using a balloon catheter that is advanced through the operative channel of an adult colonoscope (Fig. 8.4). The balloon is inflated using a barostat pump, several centimeters in front of the instru-

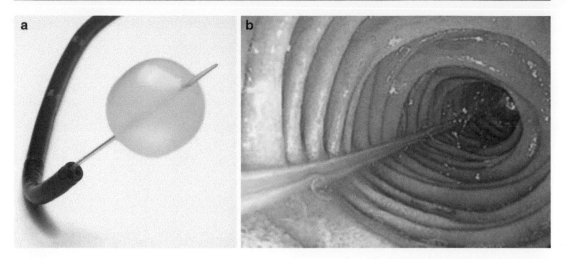

Fig. 8.4 (a) The NaviAid AB device with the balloon seen protruding through the tip of a scope. (b) The NaviAid AB balloon is advanced in the small bowel in front of the endoscope and inflated in position to "grasp" the bowel wall. Figures reprinted with permission from Smart Medical Systems Ltd., Ra'anana, Israel

ment, and it is used to "grasp" the small bowel wall in advance of the scope. Once the balloon is inflated in position, the scope and balloon are brought together through a push–pull technique, thus pleating the small bowel on the scope shaft. These steps can be repeated sequentially until the maximal extent of insertion is reached. Frequently the balloon catheter is advanced blindly in front of the scope as it bends around the curves in the small bowel outside of the depth of view. To prevent trauma or perforations, the catheter is fitted with a soft silicone tip, which bends easily under pressure. Given that the advancing platform utilizes the operative channel, the balloon has to be removed each time a therapeutic intervention is performed, which can be an inconvenience. The procedure can be performed both anterograde and retrograde, but it requires an endoscope with a 3.7 mm channel (usually only available in adult colonoscopes). Only limited data regarding the performance of ODE are available. In a small retrospective single-center series, the depth of maximal insertion was 120 cm for the anterograde and 110 cm for the retrograde approach with a mean procedure time of 15–20 min [19]. It is unclear if the insertion depth assessed with this method correlates with that of other techniques. No complications were reported using this approach in a two small series [19, 20].

Conclusion

In conclusion, spiral enteroscopy is an effective and safe method of small bowel endoscopy with a technical performance comparable to that of DBE and SBE but with significantly shorter procedure times. The major drawback of spiral enteroscopy in comparison to balloon-assisted enteroscopy is the requirement for two skilled operators.

Through-the-scope balloon enteroscopy is a relatively simple technique with limited depth of insertion in the small bowel, but is more suitable for on-demand enteroscopy.

References

1. Akerman PA, Cantero D. Spiral enteroscopy and push enteroscopy. Gastrointest Endosc Clin N Am. 2009; 19(3):357–69.
2. Morgan D, Upchurch B, Draganov P, Binmoeller KF, Haluszka O, Jonnalagadda S, et al. Spiral enteroscopy: prospective U.S. Multicenter study in patients with small-bowel disorders. Gastrointest Endosc. 2010;72(5):992–8.
3. Nagula S, Gaidos J, Draganov PV, Bucobo JC, Cho B, Hernandez Y, et al. Retrograde spiral enteroscopy: feasibility, success, and safety in a series of 22 patients. Gastrointest Endosc. 2011;74(3):699–702.

4. Messer I, May A, Manner H, Ell C. Prospective, randomized, single-center trial comparing double-balloon enteroscopy and spiral enteroscopy in patients with suspected small-bowel disorders. Gastrointest Endosc. 2013;77(2):241–9.

5. Akerman PA, Agrawal D, Cantero D, Pangtay J. Spiral enteroscopy with the new DSB overtube: a novel technique for deep peroral small-bowel intubation. Endoscopy. 2008;40(12):974–8.

6. May A, Nachbar L, Schneider M, Neumann M, Ell C. Push-and-pull enteroscopy using the double-balloon technique: method of assessing depth of insertion and training of the enteroscopy technique using the erlangen endo-trainer. Endoscopy. 2005; 37(1):66–70.

7. Buscaglia JM, Richards R, Wilkinson MN, Judah JR, Lam Y, Nagula S, et al. Diagnostic yield of spiral enteroscopy when performed for the evaluation of abnormal capsule endoscopy findings. J Clin Gastroenterol. 2011;45(4):342–6.

8. Chiorean M, Upchurch B, Draganov P, Morgan D, Binmoeller KF, Haluszka O, et al. Spiral enteroscopy: Predictors of depth of insertion from the prospective multicenter U.S. study. Gastroenterology. 2009; 136(S1):S1514.

9. Rahmi G, Samaha E, Vahedi K, Ponchon T, Fumex F, Filoche B, et al. Multicenter comparison of double-balloon enteroscopy and spiral enteroscopy. J Gastroenterol Hepatol. 2013;28(6):992–8.

10. Khashab MA, Lennon AM, Dunbar KB, Singh VK, Chandrasekhara V, Giday S, et al. A comparative evaluation of single-balloon enteroscopy and spiral enteroscopy for patients with mid-gut disorders. Gastrointest Endosc. 2010;72(4):766–72.

11. Lennon AM, Kapoor S, Khashab M, Corless E, Amateau S, Dunbar K, et al. Spiral assisted ERCP is equivalent to single balloon assisted ERCP in patients with Roux-en-Y anatomy. Dig Dis Sci. 2012;57(5):1391–8.

12. Buscaglia JM, Dunbar KB, Okolo III PI, Judah J, Akerman PA, Cantero D, et al. The spiral enteroscopy training initiative: results of a prospective study evaluating the discovery sb overtube device during small bowel enteroscopy (with video). Endoscopy. 2009; 41(3):194–9.

13. Akerman PA, Agrawal D, Chen W, Cantero D, Avila J, Pangtay J. Spiral enteroscopy: a novel method of enteroscopy by using the endo-ease discovery sb overtube and a pediatric colonoscope. Gastrointest Endosc. 2009;69(2):327–32.

14. May A, Manner H, Aschmoneit I, Ell C. Prospective, cross-over, single-center trial comparing oral double-balloon enteroscopy and oral spiral enteroscopy in patients with suspected small-bowel vascular malformations. Endoscopy. 2011;43(6):477–83.

15. Frieling T, Heise J, Sassenrath W, Hulsdonk A, Kreysel C. Prospective comparison between double-balloon enteroscopy and spiral enteroscopy. Endoscopy. 2010;42(11):885–8.

16. Akerman PA, Cantero D. Severe complications of spiral enteroscopy in the first 1750 patients. Gastrointest Endosc. 2009;69:127. (DDW09):Abstract.

17. Welch AR, Moyer MT, Dye CE, Skonier-Baer H, Mathew A. A single-center experience with spiral enteroscopy: a note of caution. Gastrointest Endosc. 2012;75(5):1125–6.

18. Teshima CW, Aktas H, Kuipers EJ, Mensink PB. Hyperamylasemia and pancreatitis following spiral enteroscopy. Can J Gastroenterol. 2012;26(9): 603–6.

19. Kumbhari V, Storm AC, Khashab MA, Canto MI, Saxena P, Akshintala VS, et al. Deep enteroscopy with standard endoscopes using a novel through-the-scope balloon. Endoscopy. 2014;46(8):685–9.

20. Rubin DT, Goeppinger SR. Initial experience of a through-the-scope balloon device for ileal intubation in crohn's disease. Gastrointest Endosc. 2013;78(4): 669–70.

Video Legends

Video 8.1 - Endoscopic view of the small bowel during antegrade spiral enteroscopy. Note the steady progression of the scope with minimal gas distention to allow a good grasp of the spiral on the bowel wall to facilitate advancement. Water can also be injected through the channel when more luminal distention is desired. Video used with permission of Spirus Medical LLC.

Part V

Small Bowel Imaging: Outcomes, Results, and Therapy

Obscure Gastrointestinal Bleeding

Christopher Teshima

Introduction

Obscure gastrointestinal bleeding (OGIB) is by far the most common indication for small bowel endoscopy, since a presumed bleeding source is usually attributed to the small intestine after negative esophagogastroduodenoscopy (EGD) and colonoscopy. In the first decade after the advent of video capsule endoscopy (VCE) and balloon-assisted enteroscopy (BAE), most research studies focused on "diagnostic yield" as the outcome of interest, which essentially translates into the proportion of cases in which a probable bleeding source was visualized during the procedure as determined by the endoscopist performing that procedure. The inherent limitation with using "diagnostic yield" is the lack of any gold standard to validate whether in fact the presumed source of bleeding is in fact the true source of bleeding, and whether treatment of that lesion actually results in an improvement in the patient's condition.

Electronic supplementary material: The online version of this chapter (doi: 10.1007/978-3-319-14415-3_9) contains supplementary material, which is available to authorized users. Videos can also be accessed at http://link.springer.com/chapter/10.1007/978-3-319-14415-3_9.

C. Teshima, M.D., M.Sc., Ph.D., F.R.C.P.C. (✉)
Division of Gastroenterology, St. Michael's Hospital, University of Toronto, 30 Bond Street, Toronto, ON, Canada M5B 1W8
e-mail: teshimac@smh.ca

Unfortunately, the majority of the small bowel endoscopy research literature is hamstrung by this limitation. Some investigators have attempted to circumvent this challenge by instead reporting whether a particular small bowel investigation led to a specific change in a patient's management, but it is likely dubious at best to consider "change in management" a clinically meaningful outcome. Recently, increasing attention has focused on the study of actual clinical outcomes determined by long-term follow-up after VCE, BAE and other small bowel imaging modalities, which provide a much more relevant picture of the impact of these investigations on patient care. It is these results from clinical outcomes studies in OGIB that are the focus of this chapter.

Immediate Endoscopic Results

Despite the limitations of much of the existing literature described previously, it is nonetheless informative to briefly consider the extensive research that has examined the immediate endoscopic results in the diagnosis and treatment of OGIB with VCE and with BAE, of which the latter relates primarily to double balloon endoscopy (DBE). Most of these findings are neatly summarized by recent systematic reviews of VCE [1] and DBE [2] that include nearly 300 studies and more than 30,000 procedures. Two-thirds of VCE procedures have been performed to investigate

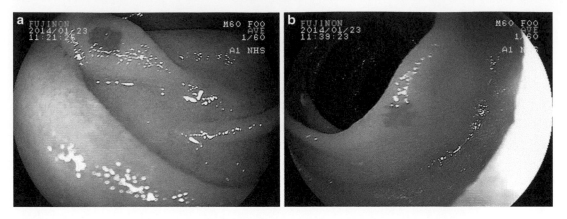

Fig. 9.1 (**a** and **b**) Angiodysplasia in jejunum

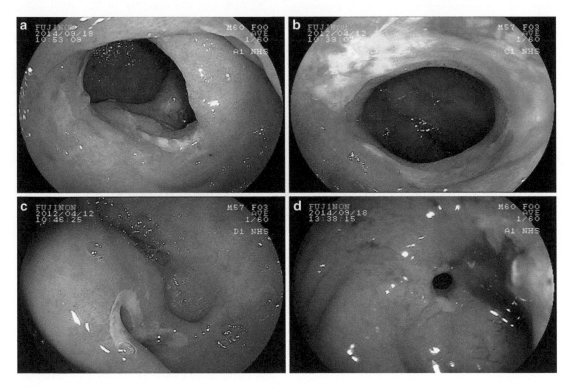

Fig. 9.2 (**a**) Ulcer due to ileal Crohn's disease (CD). (**b**) Ulceration due to recurrent CD in neo-terminal ileum. (**c**) Ulcer at ileal–ileal anastomosis post-ileal resection. (**d**) Ileal stricture due to CD

OGIB, resulting in a pooled diagnostic yield of 61 % [1]. The most common findings are angiodysplasias (50 %) (see Fig. 9.1), ulcers or other inflammatory lesions (27 %) (Fig. 9.2), and small bowel tumors (9 %) (Fig. 9.3). The rate of small bowel retention of the capsule endoscope is 1.2 % among OGIB patients. Similarly, 63 % of patients who have undergone DBE have done so because

of OGIB, achieving a pooled diagnostic yield of 68 % [2]. Angiodysplasias (40 %), inflammatory lesions (30 %), neoplasms (22 %), and diverticula (5 %) (Fig. 9.4) remain the most common abnormalities found on DBE, yet with striking differences between different regions of the world. In Europe, North America, and Australia, vascular lesions represent a clear majority of bleeding

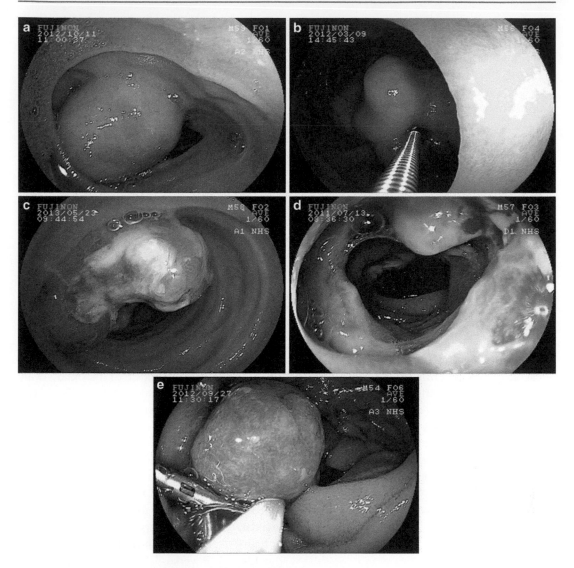

Fig. 9.3 (**a**) Ileal gastrointestinal stromal tumor (GIST). (**b**) GIST in jejunum. (**c**) Metastatic melanoma. (**d**) Enteropathy-associated T-cell lymphoma. (**e**) Juvenile polyp

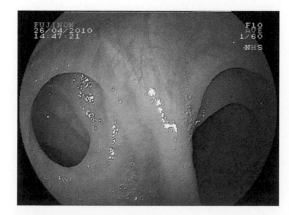

Fig. 9.4 Meckel's diverticulum

sources, usually in the proximal small bowel, whereas in Asia it is more evenly divided among vascular, neoplastic, and inflammatory causes. However, these conclusions are limited by heterogeneity of the data, which include both prospective and retrospective studies, utilize inconsistent outcome definitions, and that for the most part make no distinction between patients with overt and with occult manifestations of OGIB, which are likely dramatically different patient populations. In terms of head-to-head comparisons, unfortunately there are no randomized controlled trials comparing VCE to BAE for the evaluation of OGIB. However, there are three meta-analyses that have analyzed prospective, comparative studies looking at VCE and DBE; the first two [3, 4] included all indications for small bowel endoscopy and the most recent and largest focused specifically on OGIB [5]. In this latest meta-analysis that included 650 patients, a similar diagnostic yield was obtained for both VCE (62 %) and for DBE (56 %) ($p=0.16$). However, VCE was performed prior to DBE in most of the included studies, resulting in DBE having the benefit of being guided by the VCE results, likely creating a detection bias in favor of DBE and against VCE. An important result from this meta-analysis was the observation that the diagnostic yield from DBE was significantly higher when performed after a previously positive VCE (75 %) than for all DBE cases (56 %) ($p=0.02$) [5]. Therefore, while the consensus is that VCE and DBE are complementary tests, there is a general tendency to first perform VCE to optimize the selection of patients most likely to benefit from the more invasive DBE procedure, and to guide the direction of DBE insertion (oral versus rectal) [6, 7]. Furthermore, negative VCE identifies a group of patients who can likely undergo conservative management, since the rate of rebleeding at 1 year after negative VCE has usually been low [8–10].

Factors Predictive of a Positive Study

Given the time, cost, and potential adverse events related to VCE and DBE, it is important to understand the variables that are associated with an increased likelihood of a positive small bowel study in order to optimize the performance of these tests (see Table 9.1). Patients presenting with overt rather than with occult bleeding [11, 12], as well as those with ongoing overt bleeding rather than overt bleeding that has stopped [13, 14], are more likely to have a positive VCE. Similar superiority has been observed when DBE is performed for patients with overt bleeding who continue to bleed compared to those with inactive overt bleeding or occult bleeding [15]. Furthermore, there is a

Table 9.1 Factors predictive of a positive small bowel study

Initial small bowel study for OGIB	Repeat study performed for recurrent bleeding
• Active overt > inactive overt bleeding	• Previously positive BAE
• Overt > occult presentation	• Decline in hemoglobin >4 g/dL
• Short interval from bleeding episode to investigation	• Change in presentation from occult to overt bleeding
• Severe anemia/increased blood transfusion requirements • Multiple bleeding episodes • Anterograde > retrograde BAE insertion	• Iron deficiency anemia with hemoglobin decrease to <10 g/dL

BAE balloon-assisted enteroscopy

consistent pattern demonstrating increased diagnostic yield with earlier administration of VCE, speaking to the importance of the timely evaluation of patients with suspected small intestinal bleeding. The source of bleeding is more likely to be identified if VCE is performed within 2 weeks [14], within 1 week [16] and even more so within 48 h of the bleeding presentation, with the latter group having a particularly high diagnostic yield of 75 % [17]. In a study that examined patients admitted to hospital with an overt OGIB, those who underwent VCE within 3 days of admission had significantly higher diagnostic yields (44 % versus 28 %), increased rates of subsequent therapeutic intervention (19 % versus 7 %) and shorter lengths of hospital stay (6 versus 10 days) than those who had VCE beyond day 3 of hospitalization [18]. Furthermore, the patients who underwent delayed VCE in hospital had no better diagnostic or therapeutic rates compared to patients evaluated in an outpatient setting, suggesting that the benefit of inpatient workup for OGIB is lost if the necessary small bowel tests are not performed as soon as possible. All of this speaks to the importance of having OGIB protocols in place that enable referring physicians to have patients access tertiary centers performing small bowel endoscopy in a rapid fashion.

In addition to the timing of the investigations, there are a number of clinical factors that predict the likelihood of a positive result on VCE or DBE, including more severe anemia [19–21], increased transfusion requirements [19, 22, 23], multiple bleeding episodes [24], and increased number of previous endoscopies [23], as well as some conflicting data regarding associated medical conditions such as chronic kidney disease [25]. From a purely technical perspective, the diagnostic and therapeutic yield of BAE is superior when performed via the anterograde rather than the retrograde approach, especially when done without the benefit of a previously abnormal VCE or computed tomography (CT) scan [26]. However, this study was performed in the USA, and its finding of a preponderance of proximal bleeding sources may not necessarily hold true in centers elsewhere in the world such as Asia where the distribution of small bowel pathology tends to be different. Lastly, it does not seem to matter whether BAE is performed in the morning or in the afternoon as the diagnostic and therapeutic rates do not differ [27].

Clinical Outcomes with Long-Term Follow-Up

Most of the small bowel endoscopy literature consists of studies looking at the diagnostic and/ or therapeutic yields of VCE or BAE, with relatively little research defined by outcomes that are truly relevant to patient care such as bleeding cessation, rates of rebleeding, time to rebleeding, improvements in hemoglobin levels and transfusion requirements. Recently, there has been increasing attention paid to these types of clinical outcome studies with long-term follow-up.

VCE

As a purely diagnostic test, VCE cannot alter clinical outcomes but can at best localize bleeding lesions to direct subsequent treatments or can demonstrate the absence of significant pathology that could pose a risk for ongoing or future bleed-

ing. This is perhaps best illustrated by studies reporting outcomes with VCE prior to the local availability of BAE. In a retrospective, single-center study of a prospectively maintained database of 95 patients in Seoul, South Korea who underwent VCE between 2003 and 2010 for predominantly overt OGIB, significant bleeding lesions were identified in 40 % of patients [28]. After a median follow-up of 24 months, the rebleeding rate in patients who had a positive VCE (37 %) was higher than in patients with a negative VCE (23 %), with a median time-to-rebleeding of 10 months. However, only four patients with a positive VCE underwent BAE due to the delayed introduction of BAE at this center, demonstrating the lack of benefit of finding a bleeding source on VCE if nothing is done to address the lesion. This mirrors the findings of other smaller studies that showed that without specific treatments to suspected bleeding sites, rates of rebleeding after long-term follow-up are the same in patients with positive and with negative VCE, but do decrease if therapeutic interventions are performed [29, 30]. In a single center study from Barcelona of 105 patients who underwent VCE for both occult and overt OGIB and who were followed for slightly less than 1 year, rebleeding occurred in 31 % of patients at a median of 157 days [31]. However, once again the rate of rebleeding was lower in patients who had received lesion-directed treatment compared to nonspecific treatment (21 % versus 36 %, respectively). In contrast, a large retrospective analysis of 696 patients who underwent VCE for OGIB at a single center in Rome, Italy between 2002 and 2011 demonstrated substantially lower rebleeding rates in patients with negative VCE studies [32]. After a median follow-up of 24 months, the rate of rebleeding was 16 % after negative VCE compared to 45 % after positive VCE ($p = 0.00001$), with the majority of rebleeding episodes occurring within the first year. However, it is unclear from this study how the patients with abnormal VCE were treated, and in particular, whether they underwent lesion-directed therapy by BAE or other means following their VCE. Two trends seem to emerge from these VCE studies assessing recurrence of bleeding over time:

1. Significant lesions identified on VCE require subsequent targeted treatment by other modalities in order for the performance of VCE to confer clinical benefit.
2. The negative predictive value for rebleeding of a normal VCE study is not as robust as was previously thought, since these more recent studies reveal rebleeding rates after negative VCE of 16–35 % [28–32], much higher than earlier studies that suggested rebleeding rates of only 5–11 % after negative VCE [8–10].

In fact, a large, multicenter study of 305 patients who underwent VCE for overt OGIB at 13 hospitals in South Korea from 2006 to 2009 found no decline in rebleeding rates after positive VCE [33]. Despite a diagnostic yield of 52 % in this study, only 12 % of patients received interventional therapies, perhaps due to the low prevalence of angiodysplasia (only found in 10 %) and relatively high rates of ulcerative lesions (26 %) in this population sample. Perhaps as a result, the overall rebleeding rate of 19 % at a mean follow-up of 39 months did not differ based on the presence of findings on VCE or on having received a therapeutic intervention. The significant predictors of rebleeding were angiodysplasia seen on VCE, duration of bleeding >3 months, and an inability to discontinue antiplatelet or anticoagulation drugs in the subgroup who had been taking these medications at the time of their initial bleeding presentation [33]. Therefore, it appears that finding a presumed bleeding source on VCE had little impact on long-term outcome in the Korean OGIB experience. In fact, a retrospective analysis of 125 patients who received VCE for OGIB at the Asan Medical Center in Seoul, South Korea between 2007 and 2009 showed that after 36-month follow-up, positive VCE leading to a specific treatment resulted in only marginally lower rebleeding rates compared to negative VCE without subsequent therapy (21 % versus 27 % respectively, $p=0.50$) [34].

Similar challenges are highlighted by the outcomes from studies focusing on VCE performed solely for the investigation of iron deficiency anemia. A retrospective review of all VCEs performed for unexplained iron deficiency anemia at a single center in Ireland from 2009 to 2011 found a diagnostic yield of 71 %, with 53 % of patients having a source found within the small bowel and 18 % within the upper GI tract or right colon [35]. At a mean follow-up of 9 months, 42 % of patients had persistent anemia, split evenly between patients who had positive and negative VCE, meaning that a patient was no more likely to have resolution of anemia after having positive VCE findings compared to having a normal VCE. Furthermore, even among the patients in whom a positive VCE led to a specific change in treatment, the majority (61 %) remained anemic at follow-up. Despite this limitation, considerable clinical value may be achieved by performing VCE even if it does not lead to long-term resolution of the anemia, since an important additional goal of small bowel investigations is to exclude the presence of worrisome pathology. This may be particularly true in younger patients. A study from the UK looked at the presence of "sinister pathology," defined as small bowel malignancy, significant Crohn's disease inflammation, strictures, or Celiac disease, which was found on VCE performed for the investigation of iron deficiency anemia, and stratified the findings by age group [36]. They found that the prevalence of "sinister pathology" was 25 % in patients ≤40 years-old, but was only 7.5 % in patients >age 40, and that there was a general trend toward an increasing frequency of angioectasias and decreasing incidence of sinister pathology with increasing age. Therefore, even if the clinical outcome studies with VCE demonstrate that it is challenging to achieve long-term resolution of OGIB, particularly for vascular lesions, VCE is still valuable to identify or to exclude so-called sinister pathology, especially in younger patients.

If patients are no more likely to stop bleeding after receiving specific treatment for a culprit lesion identified on VCE than if no potential bleeding source is found, a cynical argument could be made for questioning the value of performing VCE at all for OGIB. However, such an interpretation would be a misread of the literature that we have just discussed. These studies are all retrospective analyses of prospective cohorts, but in no case were patients randomized to receive endoscopic/surgical treatments or not. In fact, there are substantial selection biases inherent in the retrospective nature of these studies that influence the apparent outcomes. It can almost certainly be assumed that patients with the most concerning lesions seen on VCE were the ones most likely to undergo therapeutic interventions. Therefore, it is a probable assumption that were these patients to have not received specific treatments, their rebleeding rates would have been much higher than that in patients with negative VCE. Indeed, such a pattern was observed in several of the previously discussed studies [28, 30]. What merits further examination is the fact that the rate of rebleeding after negative VCE remains so high, and why the rate of rebleeding after treatment of a likely bleeding lesion remains even higher, even though it may be considerably lower than what it might otherwise have been if it were never treated. To further examine these issues, we will turn our attention to clinical outcome studies with BAE.

BAE

As with most areas in the BAE literature, nearly all of the outcomes studies for OGIB relate to DBE. One of the first studies that looked at long-term follow-up after DBE was a telephone survey administered at Stanford and the University of Chicago [37]. At 12 months follow-up, 23 % of patients reported recurrent overt bleeding while 35 % required blood transfusions or iron therapy, and by 30 months 24 % of patients had overt bleeding and 18 % still needed transfusions or iron. This suggests that over half of patients experience rebleeding, with the majority occurring within the first year after the index DBE. In addition, patients with vascular lesions found on DBE were most likely to have ongoing overt or occult bleeding difficulties. However, only one-third of patients in the study population participated in follow-up, likely resulting in substantial selection and other biases that may have unduly influenced the apparent results. A stronger study is a retrospective analysis by Shinozaki et al. of 151 patients who underwent DBE for predominantly inactive

overt OGIB in Japan [38]. The outcome of interest used in this study was "control of bleeding," which was defined as the absence of overt bleeding, blood transfusions or iron therapy, and hemoglobin less than 10.0 g/dL. Overall, 63 % of patients had control of bleeding at a mean follow-up of 30 months. However, this result hides the large discrepancy in outcomes for patients with vascular small bowel lesions compared to patients with other, nonvascular sources of bleeding. Among patients with vascular lesions, 40 % had a recurrent overt bleed within 1 year of their DBE and only 40 % achieved "control of bleeding" at long-term follow-up. In contrast, 84 % of patients with tumors or polyps and 65 % with ulcers or erosions achieved long-term control of bleeding. The significant predictors of failure to achieve "control of bleeding" among the vascular subgroup were the presence of multiple versus single lesions, increased blood transfusion requirements prior to DBE, and the finding of "suspicious" rather than "definite" lesions on endoscopy, perhaps due to the increased probability that the identified lesion was not the true bleeding source [38]. Further evidence supporting the observation that vascular lesions in the small bowel are the most difficult to treat with long-term success was provided by a retrospective study of 147 consecutive patients who underwent single balloon endoscopy (SBE) for OGIB at Washington University from 2008 to 2010 [39]. More than 90 % of patients had small bowel pathology identified on VCE prior to undergoing enteroscopy, resulting in a diagnostic yield of 65 % on SBE, with 83 % of positive findings being vascular lesions (angioectasias and Dieulafoy lesions). Mean follow-up of 24 months was achieved for 110 patients (37 lost to follow-up), split evenly between those with overt and occult OGIB presentations. Recurrent bleeding was defined as overt bleeding signs; hospitalization for GI bleeding; any endoscopic, surgical or radiologic intervention for bleeding; or need for blood transfusion or iron therapy. The overall rebleeding rate was 45 %, with greater success among patients with positive findings on SBE (41 % rebleeding) compared to patients who had a normal SBE (56 % rebleeding). Interestingly, the rate of rebleeding among patients found to have vascular lesions on SBE did not significantly differ from that among patients without a bleeding source identified (48 % versus 56 %; $p=0.47$), leading the authors to speculate that most patients with OGIB who have no bleeding source found on BAE likely have vascular lesions that have gone undetected. Strikingly, there was no rebleeding in the small group of patients found to have nonvascular bleeding sources. What is clear from these few clinical outcomes studies following BAE is that while a significant proportion of patients achieve long-term success, a considerable number have ongoing or recurrent bleeding problems, particularly those found to have vascular lesions in the small bowel.

Recognizing the challenge of achieving durable long-term success when treating small bowel vascular lesions, several studies have now specifically focused on clinical outcomes with OGIB patients in this category. The first was published by May et al. from Germany who reported long-term follow-up of 50 patients who received argon plasma coagulation (APC) to treat small bowel vascular lesions while undergoing DBE for predominantly overt OGIB [40]. Rebleeding was defined as overt melena or hematochezia or as an occult drop in hemoglobin >1.0 g/dL, and occurred in 46 % of patients after a long clinical follow-up period of 55 months. Despite the high rate of rebleeding in nearly half of patients, treatment with APC (see Video 9.1) made a positive impact on clinical outcomes by significantly improving hemoglobin levels and reducing blood transfusion requirements. The mean hemoglobin level improved from 7.6 g/dL prior to DBE to 11.0 g/dL at follow-up, while 60 % of patients were transfused a median of 9 units of blood prior to DBE and only 16 % were transfused a median of 2 units afterwards. A similar rebleeding rate was seen in a retrospective follow-up study from France that included 98 patients who received successful endoscopic therapy to vascular lesions in the small bowel while undergoing DBE for overt and occult OGIB [41]. At 3 years' follow-up, 46 % of patients experienced recurrent overt bleeding or iron deficiency anemia

with need for blood transfusions or iron therapy, with the majority found to be bleeding from the same type of vascular lesions within the same segment of the small bowel as seen on the index DBE. The significant predictors of rebleeding on multivariate regression were the total number of vascular lesions ($p=0.001$) and the presence of valvular or arrhythmic heart disease ($p=0.007$). An interesting, multicenter prospective follow-up study has recently been published, again from France, that included 183 patients with both overt and occult OGIB who were found to have angiodysplasia on VCE and subsequently went on to receive endoscopic therapy during DBE [42]. The lesions seen on VCE were classified according to the system previously proposed by Saurin et al. [43]: P0=no bleeding potential; P1=uncertain bleeding potential (e.g., mucosal red spots); P2=high bleeding potential (e.g., classic angiodysplasia); P3=actively bleeding lesion (see Table 9.2). The authors then defined P1 lesions as having a low likelihood of bleeding, and P2 and P3 lesions as having a high likelihood of bleeding [42]. Rebleeding was defined as overt bleeding signs, need for blood transfusion, or decline in hemoglobin >2 g/dL after excluding other potential causes. At 1-year follow-up, 35 % of patients had experienced rebleeding, with cardiac disease (hazard ratio 2.04; $p<0.01$) and an overt bleeding presentation (hazard ratio 1.78; $p=0.03$) predictive of rebleeding risk on multivariate regression. Perhaps the most unique finding from this study was the analysis demonstrating that patients who received endoscopic therapy during DBE to P1 lesions considered low likelihood for bleeding when seen on VCE had significantly increased

Table 9.2 Classification of small bowel vascular lesions

Saurin et al. [43] classification for capsule endoscopy	Yano–Yamamoto DBE classification [54]
P0: no bleeding potential	Type 1: angiodysplasias
P1: uncertain bleeding potential (e.g., mucosal red spots)	1a: punctate erythema <1 mm
	1b: patchy erythema >2 mm
P2: high bleeding potential (e.g., classic angiodysplasia)	Type 2: Dieulafoy lesions
	Type 3: arteriovenous malformations
P3: actively bleeding lesion	

rates of rebleeding compared to patients with high likelihood lesions (P2 and P3) treated during DBE (hazard ratio 1.87), with a longer time-to-rebleeding among the patients with high likelihood lesions. What this shows is that minor abnormalities identified on VCE are unlikely to represent the true bleeding source and therefore, the expected benefit of treating such lesions via DBE is likely to be limited. A limitation with this study is that the mean wait time from VCE to DBE was over 4 months. Since we know that the sooner that VCE or DBE is performed after a bleeding episode the greater the likelihood of finding significant bleeding lesions, and since this current study tells us that the benefit of endoscopic therapy during DBE is most realized when applied to higher risk lesions, any delay between bleeding presentation, localization of high likelihood bleeding lesion on VCE, and treatment of that lesion during DBE may be detrimental to clinical outcome.

Repeat Investigations for Recurrent OGIB

The first step when patients have recurrent bleeding episodes after already undergoing thorough small bowel workup is often to repeat EGD and/or colonoscopy, particularly due to the fact that studies of small bowel endoscopy for OGIB have found that as many as one-fourth of bleeding sites are within reach of conventional endoscopes, including lesions such as GAVE, gastric and duodenal ulcers, Dieulafoy's, and colonic angioectasias [44–46]. A recent study from the Netherlands that examined VCE performed for the investigation of OGIB found that 28 % of bleeding sources were within reach of EGD or colonoscopy, with over half of these being vascular lesions [47]. The substantial prevalence of "missed" pathology found within areas reachable by conventional endoscopes demonstrates the potential importance of repeating these tests, but should not necessarily be interpreted as meaning that the initial endoscopist was at fault for "missing" the lesions. By their very nature, vascular lesions such as Dieulafoy's tend to

come and go and often their detection have as much to do with fortuitous timing than with any skill or the completeness of the endoscopic examination. However, once repeat EGD and/or colonoscopy have confirmed that the likely source of recurrent bleeding is indeed the small bowel, repeat small bowel endoscopy should be considered depending on the nature of the bleeding and the results of previous small bowel investigations (see Table 9.1). There is evidence supporting the strategy to repeat VCE in this context despite a previously normal small bowel evaluation, particularly if the presentation changes from occult to overt bleeding and/or if there is a significant decline in hemoglobin >4 g/dL, or if iron deficiency anemia becomes severe enough that the hemoglobin falls below 10 g/dL [48, 49]. If the VCE is negative then there may be a role for performing CT enterography (CTE), which may identify bleeding sources not seen on VCE, particularly small bowel mass lesions that are better detected by radiologic imaging. In a comparative study in which 58 patients with both overt and occult OGIB underwent both VCE and CTE, VCE detected only one-third of the mass lesions seen on CTE [50]. A separate study administered CTE for the investigation of OGIB after patients had a VCE that was not definitively diagnostic [51]. In this cohort, 28 % of patients with a non-diagnostic VCE had a bleeding source confirmed by CTE. However, aside from finding small bowel tumors that result in surgical resection, it is unclear whether the identification of additional pathology such as vascular lesions by CTE that were missed by VCE actually results in any change in clinical outcome. This question has yet to be studied.

In contrast, repeating DBE after recurrent OGIB seems to be most useful among patients in whom prior DBE had identified a bleeding source. A single center retrospective study from Los Angeles examined the endoscopic findings of repeat DBE for recurrent OGIB that were performed at a median of 30 weeks after an index DBE. A bleeding source was found on repeat DBE in 81 % of patients who had a positive initial DBE and in none of the patients who had a negative initial DBE ($p < 0.001$), with bleeding lesions almost entirely comprised of angiodys-plasias [52]. Therefore, proceeding directly to DBE in patients with recurrent OGIB after a pre-viously positive DBE may be a reasonable approach. Furthermore, a recent study from Japan illustrates the clinical benefit of repeating DBE to provide additional endoscopic therapy to small bowel vascular lesions in patients with recurrent bleeding [53]. Patients with overt OGIB who had received endoscopic therapy to small bowel vascular lesions during DBE performed between 2000 and 2010 were selected for long-term follow-up. After excluding 9 patients who died from other causes and 6 patients who were lost to follow-up, 43 patients remained for analy-sis. The rate of recurrent overt bleeding over a mean follow-up of 4.9 years was 37 %. The sig-nificant predictors of recurrent overt bleeding were the presence of multiple rather than single vascular lesions (52 % versus 20 %; $p=0.017$) and the type of vascular lesions identified on the initial DBE. The latter is an interesting finding because this is the first study to show that the type of small bowel vascular lesion, defined according to the Yano–Yamamoto classification (see Table 9.2) [54], predicts risk of subsequent rebleeding. According to this classification, angioectasias are considered type 1 lesions, Dieulafoy lesions are type 2, and arteriovenous malformations are type 3. Type 1 lesions are fur-ther subdivided into type 1a that consist of punc-tate erythema <1 mm with or without oozing, and type 1b that are patchy erythema that may be up to several mm in size. The rates of rebleeding in this study were 50 % for type 1a lesions, 26 % for type 1b lesions, 29 % for type 2 lesions, and 100 % for type 3 lesions (only one patient had a type 3 lesion) [53]. The authors concluded that patients with type 1a lesions treated during their initial DBE may be at increased risk of subse-quent rebleeding. However, when these patients with type 1a lesions underwent repeat DBE for recurrent overt OGIB, nearly all of them were found to have either type 1b or type 2 lesions that were subsequently treated endoscopically. Given the high rate of rebleeding among patients with type 1a lesions and the tendency to find more significant lesions on repeat DBE, a reasonable

conclusion is that type 1a lesions, which essen-tially consist of tiny red spots that are often seen throughout the small bowel when performing VCE and DBE, are not true bleeding sources and that in those cases it is more likely that the real culprit lesion was not found during the initial small bowel workup. This finding provides fur-ther strength to the argument that OGIB patients found only to have low likelihood bleeding lesions on VCE are unlikely to derive much ben-efit from endoscopic therapy to those lesions via DBE. However, what this study also shows is that repeating DBE to perform additional endoscopic therapy in patients with recurrent overt bleeding, even if the initial DBE only identified rather triv-ial vascular lesions, can be expected to improve the long-term clinical outcome [53]. When the patients who underwent repeat DBE after every episode of overt bleeding are compared to those who did not undergo repeat DBE, the incidence of rebleeding beyond the first year of follow-up decreased significantly from 0.5 bleeding episodes/patient/year to 0.1 episodes/patient/year ($p=0.006$), suggesting that a therapeutic gain is achieved by continuing to perform endoscopic therapy to small bowel vascular lesions when patients have recurrent OGIB. Whether such patients who initially had vascular lesions with low likelihood for bleeding should proceed immediately to BAE or whether they should first undergo repeat VCE to find the true bleeding source, or whether they should simply be clini-cally followed until having a recurrent bleeding episode, is a question that remains unanswered and requires further study.

Conclusion

The field of small bowel endoscopy has advanced rapidly over the past decade such that VCE and BAE are now well-established components of most tertiary referral centers around the world. Despite the fact that OGIB is the primary indica-tion for these procedures, clinically meaningful outcome studies with long-term follow-up have only begun to emerge in the past few years. This means that we are only beginning to develop a realistic understanding of the impact that VCE and BAE actually have on the clinical course of patients. This chapter has attempted to summarize the most relevant literature regarding the outcomes of small bowel endoscopy performed for OGIB. It is now increasingly apparent that the risk of recurrent bleeding is substantially greater for small bowel vascular lesions compared to masses or inflammatory lesions. It is also evident that patients who develop OGIB due to vascular lesions in the small bowel may not be "cured" by endoscopic treatment via DBE. In fact, multiple DBE procedures may be necessary to achieve the best long-term outcome when patients experience rebleeding, which at the very least can improve hemoglobin levels and reduce transfusion requirements if not complete resolution of the bleeding tendency.

An unexpected finding that has emerged from the recent literature is the high rates of rebleeding after negative VCE. In the early years of small bowel endoscopy it appeared that a normal VCE provided real reassurance against future risk of bleeding. The more recent data with longer follow-up now indicate that rebleeding rates in patients with negative VCE may be as high as in patients with positive VCE, suggesting that a normal VCE in patients with OGIB has simply been unable to identify the real bleeding source. How to best utilize these technologies to optimize long-term clinical outcomes will need to remain the focus of intensive research efforts in the decade to come, hopefully allowing us to eventually determine the best strategy to manage OGIB patients.

References

1. Liao Z, Gao R, Xu C, Li Z-S. Indications and detection, completion, and retention rates of small-bowel capsule endoscopy: a systematic review. Gastrointest Endosc. 2010;71(2):280–6.
2. Xin L, Liao Z, Jiang Y-P, Li Z-S. Indications, detectability, positive findings, total enteroscopy, and complications of diagnostic double-balloon endoscopy: a systematic review of data over the first decade of use. Gastrointest Endosc. 2011;74(3):563–70.
3. Pasha SF, Leighton JA, Das A, Harrison ME, Decker GA, Fleischer DE, et al. Double-balloon enteroscopy and capsule endoscopy have comparable diagnostic yield in small-bowel disease: a meta-analysis. Clin Gastroenterol Hepatol. 2008;6(6):671–6.
4. Chen X, Ran Z-H, Tong J-L. A meta-analysis of the yield of capsule endoscopy compared to double-balloon enteroscopy in patients with small bowel diseases. World J Gastroenterol. 2007;13(32):4372–8.
5. Teshima CW, Kuipers EJ, van Zanten SV, Mensink PBF. Double balloon enteroscopy and capsule endoscopy for obscure gastrointestinal bleeding: an updated meta-analysis. J Gastroenterol Hepatol. 2011;26(5):796–801.
6. Gay G, Delvaux M, Fassler I. Outcome of capsule endoscopy in determining indication and route for push-and-pull enteroscopy. Endoscopy. 2006;38(1):49–58.
7. Li X, Chen H, Dai J, Gao Y, Ge Z. Predictive role of capsule endoscopy on the insertion route of double-balloon enteroscopy. Endoscopy. 2009;41(9):762–6.
8. Lewis BS, Eisen GM, Friedman S. A pooled analysis to evaluate results of capsule endoscopy trials. Endoscopy. 2005;37(10):960–5.
9. Lai LH, Wong GLH, Chow DKL, Lau JYW, Sung JJY, Leung WK. Long-term follow-up of patients with obscure gastrointestinal bleeding after negative capsule endoscopy. Am J Gastroenterol. 2006;101(6):1224–8.
10. Macdonald J, Porter V, McNamara D. Negative capsule endoscopy in patients with obscure GI bleeding predicts low rebleeding rates. Gastrointest Endosc. 2008;68(6):1122–7.
11. Carey EJ, Leighton JA, Heigh RI, Shiff AD, Sharma VK, Post JK, et al. A single-center experience of 260 consecutive patients undergoing capsule endoscopy for obscure gastrointestinal bleeding. Am J Gastroenterol. 2007;102(1):89–95.
12. Lepileur L, Dray X, Antonietti M, Iwanicki-Caron I, Grigioni S, Chaput U, et al. Factors associated with diagnosis of obscure gastrointestinal bleeding by video capsule enteroscopy. Clin Gastroenterol Hepatol. 2012;10(12):1376–80.
13. Pennazio M, Santucci R, Rondonotti E, Abbiati C, Beccari G, Rossini FP, et al. Outcome of patients with obscure gastrointestinal bleeding after capsule endoscopy: report of 100 consecutive cases. Gastroenterology. 2004;126(3):643–53.
14. Ge Z-Z, Chen H-Y, Gao Y-J, Hu Y-B, Xiao S-D. Best candidates for capsule endoscopy for obscure gastrointestinal bleeding. J Gastroenterol Hepatol. 2007;22(12):2076–80.
15. Tanaka S, Mitsui K, Yamada Y, Ehara A, Kobayashi T, Seo T, et al. Diagnostic yield of double-balloon endoscopy in patients with obscure GI bleeding. Gastrointest Endosc. 2008;68(4):683–91.
16. Bresci G, Parisi G, Bertoni M, Tumino E, Capria A. The role of video capsule endoscopy for evaluating obscure gastrointestinal bleeding: usefulness of early use. J Gastroenterol. 2005;40(3):256–9.
17. Lecleire S, Iwanicki-Caron I, Di-Fiore A, Elie C, Alhameedi R, Ramirez S, et al. Yield and impact of

emergency capsule enteroscopy in severe obscure-overt gastrointestinal bleeding. Endoscopy. 2012; 44(4):337–42.

18. Singh A, Marshall C, Chaudhuri B, Okoli C, Foley A, Person SD, et al. Timing of video capsule endoscopy relative to overt obscure GI bleeding: implications from a retrospective study. Gastrointest Endosc. 2013;77(5):761–6.

19. May A, Wardak A, Nachbar L, Remke S, Ell C. Influence of patient selection on the outcome of capsule endoscopy in patients with chronic gastrointestinal bleeding. J Clin Gastroenterol. 2005;39(8):684–8.

20. Esaki M, Matsumoto T, Yada S, Yanaru-Fujisawa R, Kudo T, Yanai S, et al. Factors associated with the clinical impact of capsule endoscopy in patients with overt obscure gastrointestinal bleeding. Dig Dis Sci. 2010;55(8):2294–301.

21. Parikh DA, Mittal M, Leung FW, Mann SK. Improved diagnostic yield with severity of bleeding. J Dig Dis. 2011;12(5):357–63.

22. Estévez E, González-Conde B, Vázquez-Iglesias JL, de Los Angeles Vázquez-Millán M, Pértega S, Alonso PA, et al. Diagnostic yield and clinical outcomes after capsule endoscopy in 100 consecutive patients with obscure gastrointestinal bleeding. Eur J Gastroenterol Hepatol. 2006;18(8):881–8.

23. Shahidi NC, Ou G, Svarta S, Law JK, Kwok R, Tong J, et al. Factors associated with positive findings from capsule endoscopy in patients with obscure gastrointestinal bleeding. Clin Gastroenterol Hepatol. 2012; 10(12):1381–5.

24. Byeon J, Chung J, Choi K, Choi K, Kim B, Myung S, et al. Clinical features predicting the detection of abnormalities by double balloon endoscopy in patients with suspected small bowel bleeding. J Gastroenterol Hepatol. 2008;23(7 Pt 1):1051–5.

25. Sakai E, Endo H, Taniguchi L, Hata Y, Ezuka A, Nagase H, et al. Factors predicting the presence of small bowel lesions in patients with obscure gastrointestinal bleeding. Dig Endosc. 2013;25(4):412–20.

26. Sanaka MR, Navaneethan U, Kosuru B, Yerneni H, Lopez R, Vargo JJ. Antegrade is more effective than retrograde enteroscopy for evaluation and management of suspected small-bowel disease. Clin Gastroenterol Hepatol. 2012;10(8):910–6.

27. Sanaka MR, Navaneethan U, Upchurch BR, Lopez R, Vannoy S, Dodig M, et al. Diagnostic and therapeutic yield is not influenced by the timing of small-bowel enteroscopy: morning versus afternoon. Gastrointest Endosc. 2013;77(1):62–70.

28. Koh S-J, Im JP, Kim JW, Kim BG, Lee KL, Kim SG, et al. Long-term outcome in patients with obscure gastrointestinal bleeding after negative capsule endoscopy. World J Gastroenterol. 2013;19(10):1632–8.

29. Redondo-Cerezo E, Gómez-Ruiz CJ, Sánchez-Manjavacas N, Viñuelas M, Jimeno C, Pérez-Vigara G, et al. Long-term follow-up of patients with small-bowel angiodysplasia on capsule endoscopy. Determinants of a higher clinical impact and rebleeding rate. Rev Esp Enferm Dig. 2008;100(4):202–7.

30. Park JJ, Cheon JH, Kim HM, Park HS, Moon CM, Lee JH, et al. Negative capsule endoscopy without subsequent enteroscopy does not predict lower long-term rebleeding rates in patients with obscure GI bleeding. Gastrointest Endosc. 2010;71(6):990–7.

31. Cañas-Ventura A, Márquez L, Bessa X, Dedeu JM, Puigvehí M, Delgado-Aros S, et al. Outcome in obscure gastrointestinal bleeding after capsule endoscopy. World J Gastrointest Endosc. 2013;5(11): 551–8.

32. Riccioni ME, Urgesi R, Cianci R, Rizzo G, D'Angelo L, Marmo R, et al. Negative capsule endoscopy in patients with obscure gastrointestinal bleeding reliable: recurrence of bleeding on long-term follow-up. World J Gastroenterol. 2013;19(28):4520–5.

33. Min YW, Kim JS, Jeon SW, Jeen YT, Im JP, Cheung DY, et al. Long-term outcome of capsule endoscopy in obscure gastrointestinal bleeding: a nationwide analysis. Endoscopy. 2014;46(01):59–65.

34. Kim J-B, Ye BD, Song Y, Yang D-H, Jung KW, Kim KJ, et al. Frequency of rebleeding events in obscure gastrointestinal bleeding with negative capsule endoscopy. J Gastroenterol Hepatol. 2013;28(5):834–40.

35. Holleran GE, Barry SA, Thornton OJ, Dobson MJ, McNamara DA. The use of small bowel capsule endoscopy in iron deficiency anaemia: low impact on outcome in the medium term despite high diagnostic yield. Eur J Gastroenterol Hepatol. 2013;25(3): 327–32.

36. Koulaouzidis A, Yung DE, Lam JHP, Smirnidis A, Douglas S, Plevris JN. The use of small-bowel capsule endoscopy in iron-deficiency anemia alone; be aware of the young anemic patient. Scand J Gastroenterol. 2012;47(8–9):1094–100.

37. Gerson L, Batenic M, Ross A, Semrad C. Long-term outcomes after double balloon enteroscopy for obscure gastrointestinal bleeding. Clin Gastroenterol Hepatol. 2009;7(6):664–9.

38. Shinozaki S, Yamamoto H, Yano T, Sunada K, Miyata T, Hayashi Y, et al. Long-term outcome of patients with obscure gastrointestinal bleeding investigated by double balloon endoscopy. Clin Gastroenterol Hepatol. 2010;8(2):151–8.

39. Kushnir VM, Tang M, Goodwin J, Hollander TG, Hovis CE, Murad FM, et al. Long-term outcomes after single-balloon enteroscopy in patients with obscure gastrointestinal bleeding. Dig Dis Sci. 2013;58(9):2572–9.

40. May A, Friesing-Sosnik T, Manner H, Pohl J, Ell C. Long-term outcome after argon plasma coagulation of small-bowel lesions using double-balloon enteroscopy in patients with mid-gastrointestinal bleeding. Endoscopy. 2011;43(9):759–65.

41. Samaha E, Rahmi G, Landi B, Lorenceau-Savale C, Malamut G, Canard J-M, et al. Long-term outcome of patients treated with double balloon enteroscopy for small bowel vascular lesions. Am J Gastroenterol. 2012;107(2):240–6.

42. Rahmi G, Samaha E, Vahedi K, Delvaux M, Gay G, Lamouliatte H, et al. Long-term follow-up of patients

undergoing capsule and double-balloon enteroscopy
for identification and treatment of small-bowel vascular
lesions: a prospective, multicenter study. Endoscopy.
2014;46(7):591–7.
43. Saurin J-C, Delvaux M, Gaudin J-L, Fassler I,
Villarejo J, Vahedi K, et al. Diagnostic value of endoscopic capsule in patients with obscure digestive
bleeding: blinded comparison with video push-
enteroscopy. Endoscopy. 2003;35(7):576–84.
44. Elijah D, Daas A, Brady P. Capsule endoscopy for
obscure GI bleeding yields a high incidence of significant treatable lesions within reach of standard upper
endoscopy. J Clin Gastroenterol. 2008;42(8):962–3.
45. Fry LC, Bellutti M, Neumann H, Malfertheiner P,
Mönkemüller K. Incidence of bleeding lesions within
reach of conventional upper and lower endoscopes in
patients undergoing double-balloon enteroscopy for
obscure gastrointestinal bleeding. Aliment Pharmacol
Ther. 2009;29(3):342–9.
46. Tee H-P, Kaffes AJ. Non-small-bowel lesions encountered during double-balloon enteroscopy performed
for obscure gastrointestinal bleeding. World J
Gastroenterol. 2010;16(15):1885–9.
47. Hoedemaker RA, Westerhof J, Weersma RK,
Koornstra JJ. Non-small-bowel abnormalities identified during small bowel capsule endoscopy. World J
Gastroenterol. 2014;20(14):4025–9.
48. Viazis N, Papaxoinis K, Vlachogiannakos J,
Efthymiou A, Theodoropoulos I, Karamanolis DG. Is
there a role for second-look capsule endoscopy in
patients with obscure GI bleeding after a nondiagnostic first test? Gastrointest Endosc. 2009;69(4):
850–6.
49. Bar-Meir S. Video capsule endoscopy or double-
balloon enteroscopy: are they equivalent? Gastrointest
Endosc. 2009;69(4):875–6.
50. Huprich JE, Fletcher JG, Fidler JL, Alexander JA,
Guimarães LS, Siddiki HA, et al. Prospective blinded
comparison of wireless capsule endoscopy and multiphase CT enterography in obscure gastrointestinal
bleeding. Radiology. 2011;260(3):744–51.
51. Agrawal JR, Travis AC, Mortele KJ, Silverman SG,
Maurer R, Reddy SI, et al. Diagnostic yield of dual-
phase computed tomography enterography in patients
with obscure gastrointestinal bleeding and a non-
diagnostic capsule endoscopy. J Gastroenterol
Hepatol. 2012;27(4):751–9.
52. Byeon JS, Mann NK, Jamil LH, Lo SK. Is a repeat
double balloon endoscopy in the same direction
useful in patients with recurrent obscure gastrointestinal bleeding? J Clin Gastroenterol. 2013;
47(6):496–500.
53. Shinozaki S, Yamamoto H, Yano T, Sunada K,
Hayashi Y, Shinhata H, et al. Favorable long-term outcomes of repeat endotherapy for small-intestine vascular lesions by double-balloon endoscopy.
Gastrointest Endosc. 2014;80(1):112–7.
54. Yano T, Yamamoto H, Sunada K, Miyata T, Iwamoto
M, Hayashi Y, et al. Endoscopic classification of vascular lesions of the small intestine (with videos).
Gastrointest Endosc. 2008;67(1):169–72.

Video Legends

Video 9.1 - Angiodysplasia treated with argon plasma coagulation during DBE.

Inflammatory Bowel Disease

10

Edward J. Despott and Chris Fraser

Introduction

The term idiopathic inflammatory bowel disease (IBD) encompasses inflammatory conditions of the gastrointestinal (GI) tract of undetermined etiology, which are characterized by their chronicity and a tendency to induce significant morbidity through multiple relapses of disease activity [1]. IBD is mainly classified into two major conditions: ulcerative colitis (UC) and Crohn's disease (CD). UC is hallmarked by varying degrees of inflammation mainly confined to the colonic mucosa while CD is a more heterogeneous chronic inflammatory disorder, which may induce transmural inflammation of any part of the GI tract [2, 3]. CD often manifests itself with distal small bowel (SB) involvement with or with-out colonic involvement and its transmural nature may induce stricturing and bowel wall penetration [2, 3]. There is no gold standard test for IBD and the diagnosis is usually made by a thorough corroboration of clinical features and hematological, biochemical, endoscopic, radiological and histopathological findings [2, 3]. In about 5–15 % of patients with colonic IBD, classification of the disease remains a challenge despite investigation findings and in these cases the condition remains unclassified (IBDU) [2, 4, 5].

The SB has a propensity for involvement with CD in up to 66 % of patients at diagnosis [6]; as such, patients with suspected or established CD and IBDU usually require assessment of the SB for the presence of inflammatory lesions (Videos 10.1, 10.2, and 10.3). In patients with UC, assessment of the SB is warranted if suspicion of a potential diagnosis of CD is raised [2]. The remarkable progress in SB imaging technology established over the last decade has greatly facilitated accurate assessment of the nature and extent of SB disease in such patients.

Endoscopic advances in the form of capsule endoscopy (SBCE) and device-assisted enteroscopy (DAE) have revolutionized the assessment of the SB mucosa [2, 7–11]. These two types of endoscopic technologies have now been established to be complementary to each other with SBCE (the less invasive and more patient-friendly of the two), often used as a "scout" for pathology, which may potentially require further characterization and biopsy/endotherapy by DAE [2, 12].

Electronic supplementary material: The online version of this chapter (doi: 10.1007/978-3-319-14415-3_10) contains supplementary material, which is available to authorized users. Videos can also be accessed at http://link.springer.com/chapter/10.1007/978-3-319-14415-3_10.

E.J. Despott, M.R.C.P (Gastro), F.E.B.G.H, M.D. (Res) (✉)
Royal Free Unit for Endoscopy, Institute for Liver and Digestive Health, Royal Free Hospital, University College London, Pond Street, London NW3 2QG, UK
e-mail: edespott@doctors.org.uk

C. Fraser, M.B., Ch.B., M.D., F.R.C.P.
Centre for Liver and Digestive Disorders, Royal Infirmary of Edinburgh, Edinburgh, UK

Wolfson Unit for Endoscopy, St. Mark's Hospital and Academic Institute, Harrow, Middlesex, UK

These innovations in SB endoscopy have also been paralleled by a similarly impressive evolution in diagnostic imaging technologies. Dedicated SB radiological investigation in the form of computed tomographic and magnetic resonance enterography/enteroclysis (CTE and MRE respectively) now also allows a complementary, thorough assessment and staging of SB disease activity and extra-luminal complications in patients with suspected or established CD [2, 12–16].

Small Bowel Capsule Endoscopy (SBCE)

SBCE allows patient-friendly, non-invasive, wireless ambulatory endoscopic assessment of the SB mucosa [2, 9, 12], which has been shown to have a high sensitivity (96–100 %) for mucosal lesions compatible with the presence of active SB CD [2, 12, 17–21]. The lack of a gold standard for the diagnosis of CD, however, has required the use of surrogates and adoption of "diagnostic yield" in clinical studies evaluating this parameter [2, 12, 15, 16, 21–25]. Moreover, mucosal lesions that may be caused by active SB CD are not specific to this condition and may have

alternative underlying etiologies, which include pharmacological agent use (non-steroidal anti-inflammatory drugs [NSAIDs] in particular), infections, vasculitides, and neoplastic disease [25–28]; these SBCE findings should therefore be interpreted within the clinical context in corroboration with findings of other complementary investigations (Fig. 10.1).

Capsule retention (CR)—defined as an SB capsule remaining within the GI tract for at least 2 weeks or requiring urgent medical, endoscopic or surgical intervention for retrieval [29]—is the main potential complication of SBCE. Given the propensity for SB stricture formation in CD, precautionary measures to avoid CR require particular attention in this setting. Although for suspected CD the CR rate is low (of the order of 1.6 % and comparable with other indications for SBCE), the rate of CR in patients with known CD has been reported to be as high as 13 % [30–33]. This highlights the critical requirement for clinicians to actively attempt to exclude the presence of stricturing disease by direct questioning for abdominal pain and other obstructive symptoms and appropriate use of the PillCam™ patency capsule (PC) (Given Imaging, Israel) and "pre-test" cross-sectional imaging where SBCE is indicated [34–36].

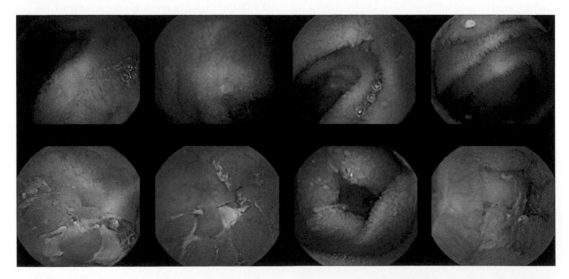

Fig. 10.1 CD SB lesions of varying degrees of severity, SBCE views. These appearances are not specific to CD and may be induced by other etiologies (including other inflammatory conditions and the use of pharmacological agents; e.g., NSAIDs). Images: Prof. O. Epstein, Ms. H. Palmer, Dr. M. I. Hamilton and Dr. E. J. Despott, Royal Free Unit for Endoscopy, Royal Free London NHS Foundation Trust

Comparisons of SBCE with Dedicated SB Radiological Imaging

A meta-analysis by Dionisio et al. compared the diagnostic yield (DY) of SBCE and other diagnostic imaging modalities (including SB follow-through [SBFT], CTE, and MRE) in patients with suspected or known CD [22]. This showed a significant incremental yield (IY) for SBCE as compared with SBFT and CTE in the setting of suspected CD (SBCE versus SBFT IY=32 %, $P<0.0001$ and SBCE versus CTE: IY=47 %, $P<0.00001$). While this meta-analysis has shown a similar performance for SBCE and MRE, a prospective study by Jensen et al. in 93 patients with suspected or known CD comparing SBCE, CTE, and MRE (using ileo-colonoscopy [IC] as the gold standard) showed that SBCE may be more sensitive than MRE for the detection of subtle mucosal lesions and proximal SB pathology [37]. CTE and MRE have been shown to have similar sensitivities and although MRE provides a safer option for patients by the avoidance of ionizing radiation, this technology is more expensive and less widely available [38, 39].

A previous prospective, randomized 4-way comparison of SBCE, CTE, SB follow-through (SBFT) and IC by Solem et al. [16] performed in patients with suspected (or known) CD (using consensus criteria as the reference standard) showed similar sensitivities (83 % for SBCE, 67 % for CTE and IC, and 50 % for SBFT) but lower specificity for SBCE as compared with the other tests (100 %, $P<0.05$). These results underline the importance of interpretation of SBCE findings within the appropriate clinical context [16]. Pre-test patient selection by the use of objective parameters (including clinical manifestations and serological inflammatory markers), as recommended by the International Conference on Capsule Endoscopy (ICCE) [40] and fecal calprotectin may enhance the specificity and positive predictive value of SBCE findings [41–48]. Given that NSAIDs may induce similar SB mucosal lesions to those seen in the presence of active CD, thorough exclusion of recent use of these agents should also be actively sought while investigating patients with SBCE in this setting [28, 49, 50].

Comparisons of SBCE with Flexible Endoscopy

In their meta-analysis, Dionisio et al. showed that when compared with push enteroscopy (PE), SBCE had an overall weighted incremental yield (IYw) of 42 % and within the same comparison, for the sub-groups of patients with suspected and known CD SBCE had an IYw of 18 % and 57 % respectively [22]. This meta-analysis also showed that SBCE had an overall IYw of 39 % when compared with ileo-colonoscopy (IC). Sub-group analysis of patients with suspected and known CD for the latter comparison showed a SBCE IYw of 22 % and 13 % respectively [22]. In their 4-way comparative study, using clinical consensus as the gold standard, Solem et al. showed similar sensitivities for IC and SBCE but higher specificities for IC [16]. Two additional studies [51, 52] compared these two modalities for the assessment of postoperative SB CD recurrence and although the results were at variance, both studies showed that SBCE detected more proximal lesions than IC.

A meta-analysis from the Mayo Clinic [53] demonstrated similar diagnostic yields for SBCE and double-balloon enteroscopy (DBE). In another meta-analysis [54] although SBCE appeared to have significantly higher diagnostic yield than DBE performed via either anterograde or retrograde route alone, the yield of positive findings for these two endoscopic modalities was similar when DBE was performed via both routes combined.

Role of SBCE in the Diagnosis and Management of IBD

Suspected CD

Since up to 90 % of patients with SB CD have terminal ileal involvement [55], IC is considered to be the first choice of endoscopic investigation to help establish a diagnosis of CD [6]. In cases where IC is not attainable or remains inconclusive [56, 57] and there is no clinical evidence to support the presence of obstructive disease,

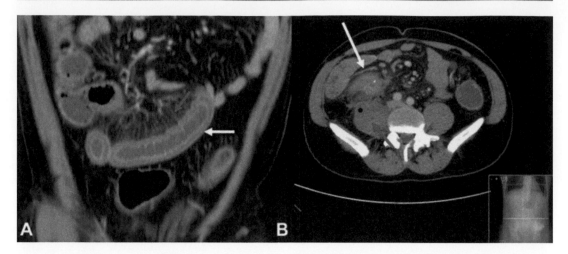

Fig. 10.2 (**a**) Coronal plane CTE image in a patient with active CD demonstrating an inflamed ileal loop with mural thickening and hyper-enhancement (*white arrow*) and prominence of the mesenteric vasa recta (the "comb sign") (*red arrow*). (**b**) Transverse plane CTE image of another patient with active CD demonstrating an inflam-matory mass at the ileo-colic anastomosis (*white arrow*), which has fistulated into the right psoas muscle causing an intra-muscular abscess (*red arrow*). Images: Courtesy of Drs Abdullah Sharif and Katie Planche of the Department of Radiology, Royal Free London NHS Foundation Trust

SBCE may be considered for the assessment of the SB mucosa; otherwise CTE or MRE should be the investigation of choice [2, 12]. The clinical value of any SBCE findings and its cost-effectiveness would be enhanced by careful patient selection with application of pre-test probability criteria [41–48] and avoidance of potential confounding factors e.g. recent NSAID use [12, 28, 49, 50].

Known CD

In the presence of known CD, further assessment of the SB is frequently warranted for staging of disease activity in the presence of symptoms regardless of IC findings [6, 12]. In this setting, cross-sectional radiological imaging in the form of CTE or MRE takes precedence since these would facilitate the identification of stricturing and or transmural/extramural disease activity and associated complications while also allowing enhanced anatomical mapping of disease extent and distribution [2, 6, 12] (Figs. 10.2 and 10.3). The use of SBCE may still be warranted if cross-sectional imaging in patients with known CD remains inconclusive, if there are ongoing symp-toms, and/or if any additional findings may influence patient management [24, 37]. However, clinicians should be mindful of the higher risk of CR in this setting. Ensuring functional SB patency by the use of a PC is considered mandatory if SBCE is to be undertaken in patients with known CD [2, 12].

Assessment of CD severity as a guide to management can usually be undertaken by dedicated SB cross-sectional imaging, however, three retrospective studies have also demonstrated the potential usefulness of SBCE in this regard [58–60]. Another retrospective study of patients with known CD (*n*=108) by Flamant et al. [61] focused on the clinical importance of jejunal disease detected by SBCE. This study from France demonstrated the presence of jejunal lesions in 56 % of patients (17 % of these had solitary jejunal disease) and found that jejunal disease was independently associated with a higher risk of relapse, suggesting the underlying presence of a more aggressive CD phenotype. In another retrospective study from France (*n*=71; 3 month follow-up) lesion severity as assessed by SBCE led to an adjustment of medical management in 54 % of patients. The role of SBCE for the assessment of mucosal healing is also being assessed [62, 63],

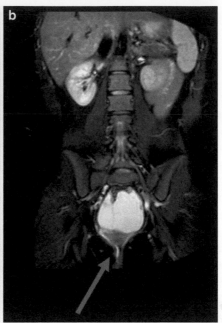

Fig. 10.3 MRE images in a patient with active CD and previous pan-proctocolectomy demonstrating a loculated pelvic fluid collection and perineal fistula (*red arrows*). (**a**) Sagittal plane. (**b**) coronal plane. Images: Courtesy of Drs Abdullah Sharif and Katie Planche of the Department of Radiology, Royal Free London NHS Foundation Trust

albeit this indication has not yet been recommended for use in routine clinical practice. More objective disease activity indices such as the Capsule Endoscopy Crohn's Disease Activity Index (CECDAI) (Niv score) or Lewis score may help to standardize reporting of disease activity identified at SBCE in clinical trials and clinical practice [64, 65].

IBDU and UC

In the setting of IBDU, although the supportive evidence is scant and mainly relates to the findings of one retrospective study ($n = 120$) [66] and three small prospective studies [67–69], mucosal lesions compatible with SB CD have been reported in 17–70 % of patients with previously unclassified disease [66, 67, 69]. Within the appropriate clinical context, SBCE therefore may be a useful modality to assist reclassification and may lead to modification of disease management strategies in patients with this condition [2, 12, 70]. The role of SBCE in UC remains limited but

it may be useful in patients who manifest atypical symptoms and in those with unexplained iron deficiency [2, 12, 71]. Usefulness of SBCE in the preoperative assessment of patients undergoing ileal pouch-anal anastomosis (IPAA) surgery was investigated prospectively by Murrell et al. in a longitudinal study of 68 patients [72]. At 12 months follow-up, the results of this study showed no significant correlation between preoperative SBCE findings and IPAA outcome. Pre-IPAA assessment by SBCE therefore appears to be of limited value and is currently not recommended in day-to-day clinical practice [2, 12].

Flexible Enteroscopy

The development of DAE over the last decade has allowed minimally invasive, flexible endoscopic access to the depths of the SB with far less restriction than ever before. The term DAE is used to collectively describe flexible enteroscopic technologies that use device assistance to apply gentle SB wall traction to minimize SB stretching and looping in order to facilitate advancement of a dedicated enteroscope deep into the SB. DAE comprises balloon-assisted and spiral enteroscopy technologies (BAE and SE, respectively), which all make use of a flexible stabilizing overtube and enteroscope. BAE collectively describes the main types of DAE that employ the use of balloon-assisted SB traction. Double-balloon enteroscopy (DBE) (Fujifilm, Saitama, Japan) incorporates the use of two balloons [11, 73] while single-balloon enteroscopy (SBE) (Olympus, Tokyo, Japan) uses a single traction balloon respectively [8, 10]. SE (Spirus-Medical™, Stoughton, MA, USA) does not incorporate balloon traction but alternatively makes use of a soft-plastic spiral for SB traction [74].

Since DBE was the first type of DAE technology to be introduced into clinical practice [73, 75], most of the evidence is DBE related [76–83], albeit experience with other DAE technologies is also increasing [7, 84–90]. Although DAE is considered complimentary to SBCE and this is often used to guide further evaluation and/or therapy by DAE [91, 92], the potential presence of SB strictures may preclude the use of SBCE in patients with CD and recourse to DAE is often guided by SB cross-sectional imaging findings in this condition [93].

The main advantages of DAE relate to its ability to allow direct assessment of the SB mucosa (via the anterograde or retrograde routes), facilitation of tissue biopsy, and the application of endotherapy. In the setting of CD, DAE therefore may assist with confirmation of diagnosis, evaluation of disease activity and response to medical therapy, facilitation of endoscopic balloon dilatation (EBD) of SB strictures (in appropriately selected cases), and with retrieval of retained SB capsules [2, 12, 76, 79–83, 93–97]. Disadvantages of DAE include its relative invasiveness and procedure duration (often in excess of 60 min) [98]. DAE proficiency requires dedicated training. In addition, there are technical challenges particularly related to the retrograde-route and those patients with prior surgery and extensive adhesions, which may hinder success [99, 100]. DAE has been shown to be safe and complication rates are of the order of about 1 % overall and up to

9 % for procedures involving endotherapy [7, 83, 84, 94, 101–103].

Role of DAE in the Diagnosis and Management of IBD

Diagnosis and Assessment

A key meta-analysis from the Mayo clinic by Pasha et al. (11 studies, including 9 that compared yield of inflammatory lesions) confirmed that DBE and SBCE had similar diagnostic yields [53]. This was also demonstrated by another meta-analysis (including eight studies) [54], which showed that the yields of bi-directional DBE and SBCE were similar. For diagnostic and assessment purposes, DAE is usually reserved for cases where other less-invasive investigations remain inconclusive or where histopathological corroboration (to rule out infection or malignancy) is deemed to be essential [2, 12, 104]. When DAE is clinically indicated, correlation with other imaging modalities allows for "targeting" of suspect lesions and may enhance its diagnostic yield and clinical effectiveness [76, 80, 91, 103]. Direct evaluation of SB mucosal lesions is also useful for the diagnostic process and the presence of mesenteric border SB ulceration has been shown to be highly suggestive of underlying CD [81] (Fig. 10.4). A small pediatric study ($n=20$) from the Netherlands, which compared the findings of SBE with ultrasound (+ Doppler) and MRE, found that SBE facilitated definitive diagnosis of active CD in 14/20 patients (70 %) and suggested that earlier use of DAE may expedite the diagnostic process [85]. DAE may also be useful in the guidance of medical management by direct endoscopic assessment of disease activity [78, 93, 96, 105]. In a retrospective study of 40 patients with established CD, Mensink et al. [96] showed that DBE identified active SB disease in 24 (60 %) patients and as a result, management was altered in 75 % of those with positive findings. These results were confirmed by another prospective longitudinal study performed by the same investigators in another 50 patients with known CD. In this second study, the

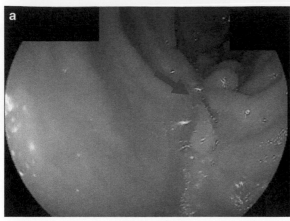 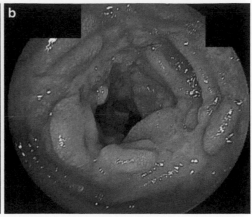

Fig. 10.4 CD SB lesions as seen at DBE in two different patients. (**a**) Healing ulceration at the mesenteric side of the ileum (*blue arrow*). (**b**) Severe ulceration and edema affecting the jejunum, leading to inflammatory stricturing. Images: Dr E. J. Despott, Royal Free Unit for Endoscopy, Royal Free London NHS Foundation Trust

findings at DBE had a direct impact on the medical management of 38 % of patients, 88 % of whom remained in remission with a significantly improved Crohn's disease activity index (CDAI) at 12 months of follow-up [93].

Endotherapy of SB Strictures at DAE

Within the appropriate clinical setting, selected CD-related strictures may be amenable to endoscopic balloon dilation (EBD). This has been shown to be effective and may reduce the need for surgical intervention in some patients [75–77, 79, 82, 94, 97, 106]. In order to reduce the risk of major complications (which may be of the order of 2–11 %) and enhance clinical effectiveness, careful patient selection is mandatory [76, 94, 97]. Prior to consideration for EBD, SB cross-sectional imaging should be used to evaluate stricture anatomy and characteristics, length, number and location [76, 94, 97]. EBD of shorter strictures, less than 5 cm, is associated with better clinical outcomes [76, 79, 94, 106] and the presence of severe, active inflammation and angulated stricture morphology should discourage the use of EBD since this may increase the risk of iatrogenic perforation [76, 79, 94, 97]. In order to further reduce risk, adequate endoscopic views (avoiding tight angulation) and a stable enteroscope position should be obtained before EBD is considered [76, 94, 97]. Intra-procedure fluoroscopy may enhance safety and outcome [94, 97] and is recommended. The most frequently used technique for EBD employs the use of a transparent, wire-guided, through-the-scope (TTS) balloon dilator—e.g., controlled radial expansion (CRE™) (Boston Scientific, USA) or Hercules™ (Cook Medical, Ireland)—which allows EBD to be performed under direct endoscopic vision [76, 94, 97] by water insufflation to the required pressure and balloon diameter for 1–2 min [76] (Fig. 10.5).

Three studies have focused on outcomes of EBD of SB strictures in patients with CD [76, 79, 94]. Pohl et al. attempted EBD of CD-related strictures in a study of 19 patients [79]. EBD was considered suitable in 10/19 and at 10 months follow-up, 6 of these patients remained asymptomatic and without the need for surgery. Despott et al. performed a study in 11 patients with confirmed CD SB strictures who were referred for DBE-facilitated endotherapy [76]. EBD was achieved in 9/11 patients. In the remaining two patients, adhesive disease prevented enteroscopic access to the strictures. One patient with actively inflamed strictures suffered a delayed perforation, warranting surgical resection of the diseased SB. At a mean follow-up period of 20.5 months, the remaining eight patients experienced significant symptomatic relief after EBD as noted by

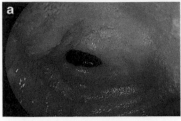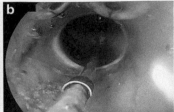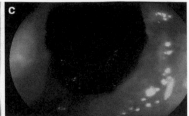

Fig. 10.5 EBD of a short (mainly fibrotic) CD-induced jejunal stricture using a through-the-scope CRE™ (Boston Scientific, USA) transparent, wire-guided balloon dilator under direct endoscopic vision at DBE.

(**a**) Pre-EBD. (**b**) during EBD. (**c**) post-EBD, (**c**) Images: Dr E. J. Despott, Royal Free Unit for Endoscopy, Royal Free London NHS Foundation Trust

improved symptom-related VAS scores. Although two patients required repeat EBD, none of them required surgery. Similar findings were shown by Hirai et al. [94]. In their study of 25 patients, EBD was successful with regard to short-term dilation in 18/25 (72 %). Although two patients suffered major complications (pancreatitis and hemorrhage) cumulative surgery-free rates at 6 and 12 months follow-up were 83 % and 72 %, respectively. The concept of biodegradable SB stents [107] that may be deployed at DAE for potential improvement of longer-term outcomes in this setting merits further study.

Conclusion

The emergence of advanced, complementary endoscopic and radiological technologies over the last decade has greatly refined our ability to assess the SB for pathology in patients with suspected or known/established IBD. Given the absence of a diagnostic gold standard, the interpretation of endoscopic and radiological findings requires corroboration with clinical and other investigation results. Although the relative role of each of these SB imaging technologies in practice shall ultimately be governed by individual clinical scenarios, access to local resources and patient preference, the application of pre-test criteria and consideration of dedicated international consensus guidance may further enhance their clinical and economic effectiveness.

The use of DAE is likely to continue to be reserved for cases where direct endoscopic and histopathological evaluation is required and for selected cases where EBD of SB strictures is indicated. The impact and potential future role of SB endoscopy in the evaluation of mucosal healing and response to medical management strategies warrants further investigation.

Disclosure E. J. Despott has received education and research grants from Aquilant Medical (UK), Fujifilm and Keymed-Olympus.

References

1. Molodecky NA, Soon IS, Rabi DM, Ghali WA, Ferris M, Chernoff G, et al. Increasing incidence and prevalence of the inflammatory bowel diseases with time, based on systematic review. Gastroenterology. 2012;142:46.
2. Bourreille A, Ignjatovic A, Aabakken L, Loftus Jr EV, Eliakim R, Pennazio M, et al. Role of small-bowel endoscopy in the management of patients with inflammatory bowel disease: an international OMED-ECCO consensus. Endoscopy. 2009;41(7):618–37.
3. Cosnes J, Gower-Rousseau C, Seksik P, Cortot A. Epidemiology and natural history of inflammatory bowel diseases. Gastroenterology. 2011;140(6):1785–94.
4. Stewenius J, Adnerhill I, Ekelund G, Floren CH, Fork FT, Janzon L, et al. Ulcerative colitis and indeterminate colitis in the city of Malmo, Sweden. A 25-year incidence study. Scand J Gastroenterol. 1995;30(1):38–43.
5. Zhou N, Chen WX, Chen SH, Xu CF, Li YM. Inflammatory bowel disease unclassified. J Zhejiang Univ Sci B. 2011;12(4):280–6.
6. Van AG, Dignass A, Panes J, Beaugerie L, Karagiannis J, Allez M, et al. The second European evidence-based Consensus on the diagnosis and management of Crohn's disease: definitions and diagnosis. J Crohns Colitis. 2010;4(1):7–27.

7. Akerman PA, Cantero D. Spiral enteroscopy and push enteroscopy. Gastrointest Endosc Clin N Am. 2009;19(3):357–69.

8. Hartmann D, Eickhoff A, Tamm R, Riemann JF. Balloon-assisted enteroscopy using a single-balloon technique. Endoscopy. 2007;39 Suppl 1:E276.

9. Iddan G, Meron G, Glukhovsky A, Swain P. Wireless capsule endoscopy. Nature. 2000;405(6785):417.

10. Tsujikawa T, Saitoh Y, Andoh A, Imaeda H, Hata K, Minematsu H, et al. Novel single-balloon enteroscopy for diagnosis and treatment of the small intestine: preliminary experiences. Endoscopy. 2008;40(1):11–5.

11. Yamamoto H, Sekine Y, Sato Y, Higashizawa T, Miyata T, Iino S, et al. Total enteroscopy with a nonsurgical steerable double-balloon method. Gastrointest Endosc. 2001;53(2):216–20.

12. Annese V, Daperno M, Rutter MD, Amiot A, Bossuyt P, East J, et al. European evidence based consensus for endoscopy in inflammatory bowel disease. J Crohns Colitis. 2013;7(12):982–1018.

13. Dubcenco E, Jeejeebhoy KN, Petroniene R, Tang SJ, Zalev AH, Gardiner GW, et al. Capsule endoscopy findings in patients with established and suspected small-bowel Crohn's disease: correlation with radiologic, endoscopic, and histologic findings. Gastrointest Endosc. 2005;62(4):538–44.

14. Golder SK, Schreyer AG, Endlicher E, Feuerbach S, Scholmerich J, Kullmann F, et al. Comparison of capsule endoscopy and magnetic resonance (MR) enteroclysis in suspected small bowel disease. Int J Colorectal Dis. 2006;21(2):97–104.

15. Hara AK, Leighton JA, Heigh RI, Sharma VK, Silva AC, De PG, et al. Crohn disease of the small bowel: preliminary comparison among CT enterography, capsule endoscopy, small-bowel follow-through, and ileoscopy. Radiology. 2006;238(1):128–34.

16. Solem CA, Loftus Jr EV, Fletcher JG, Baron TH, Gostout CJ, Petersen BT, et al. Small-bowel imaging in Crohn's disease: a prospective, blinded, 4-way comparison trial. Gastrointest Endosc. 2008;68(2):255–66.

17. Koulaouzidis A, Rondonotti E, Karargyris A. Small-bowel capsule endoscopy: a ten-point contemporary review. World J Gastroenterol. 2013;19(24):3726–46.

18. Leighton JA. The role of endoscopic imaging of the small bowel in clinical practice. Am J Gastroenterol. 2011;106(1):27–36.

19. Lewis BS, Eisen GM, Friedman S. A pooled analysis to evaluate results of capsule endoscopy trials. Endoscopy. 2005;37(10):960–5.

20. Mow WS, Lo SK, Targan SR, Dubinsky MC, Treyzon L, Abreu-Martin MT, et al. Initial experience with wireless capsule enteroscopy in the diagnosis and management of inflammatory bowel disease. Clin Gastroenterol Hepatol. 2004;2(1):31–40.

21. Tukey M, Pleskow D, Legnani P, Cheifetz AS, Moss AC. The utility of capsule endoscopy in patients with suspected Crohn's disease. Am J Gastroenterol. 2009;104(11):2734–9.

22. Dionisio PM, Gurudu SR, Leighton JA, Leontiadis GI, Fleischer DE, Hara AK, et al. Capsule endoscopy has a significantly higher diagnostic yield in patients with suspected and established small-bowel Crohn's disease: a meta-analysis. Am J Gastroenterol. 2010;105(6):1240–8.

23. Efthymiou A, Viazis N, Vlachogiannakos J, Georgiadis D, Kalogeropoulos I, Mantzaris G, et al. Wireless capsule endoscopy versus enteroclysis in the diagnosis of small-bowel Crohn's disease. Eur J Gastroenterol Hepatol. 2009;21(8):866–71.

24. Voderholzer WA, Beinhoelzl J, Rogalla P, Murrer S, Schachschal G, Lochs H, et al. Small bowel involvement in Crohn's disease: a prospective comparison of wireless capsule endoscopy and computed tomography enteroclysis. Gut. 2005;54(3):369–73.

25. Levesque BG. Yield to diagnostic accuracy: capsule endoscopy in Crohn's disease. Gastrointest Endosc. 2010;71(1):128–30.

26. Goldstein JL, Eisen GM, Lewis B, Gralnek IM, Zlotnick S, Fort JG. Video capsule endoscopy to prospectively assess small bowel injury with celecoxib, naproxen plus omeprazole, and placebo. Clin Gastroenterol Hepatol. 2005;3(2):133–41.

27. Graham DY, Opekun AR, Willingham FF, Qureshi WA. Visible small-intestinal mucosal injury in chronic NSAID users. Clin Gastroenterol Hepatol. 2005;3(1):55–9.

28. Maiden L, Thjodleifsson B, Theodors A, Gonzalez J, Bjarnason I. A quantitative analysis of NSAID-induced small bowel pathology by capsule enteroscopy. Gastroenterology. 2005;128(5):1172–8.

29. Cave D, Legnani P, de Franchis R, Lewis BS. ICCE consensus for capsule retention. Endoscopy. 2005;37(10):1065–7.

30. Cheifetz AS, Kornbluth AA, Legnani P, Schmelkin I, Brown A, Lichtiger S, et al. The risk of retention of the capsule endoscope in patients with known or suspected Crohn's disease. Am J Gastroenterol. 2006;101(10):2218–22.

31. Hoog CM, Bark LA, Arkani J, Gorsetman J, Brostrom O, Sjoqvist U. Capsule retentions and incomplete capsule endoscopy examinations: an analysis of 2300 examinations. Gastroenterol Res Pract. 2012;2012:518718.

32. Liao Z, Gao R, Xu C, Li ZS. Indications and detection, completion, and retention rates of small-bowel capsule endoscopy: a systematic review. Gastrointest Endosc. 2010;71(2):280–6.

33. Rondonotti E, Herrerias JM, Pennazio M, Caunedo A, Mascarenhas-Saraiva M, de Franchis R. Complications, limitations, and failures of capsule endoscopy: a review of 733 cases. Gastrointest Endosc. 2005;62(5):712–6.

34. Herrerias JM, Leighton JA, Costamagna G, Infantolino A, Eliakim R, Fischer D, et al. Agile patency system eliminates risk of capsule retention in patients with known intestinal strictures who undergo capsule endoscopy. Gastrointest Endosc. 2008;67(6):902–9.

35. Karagiannis S, Faiss S, Mavrogiannis C. Capsule retention: a feared complication of wireless capsule endoscopy. Scand J Gastroenterol. 2009;44(10): 1158–65.
36. Postgate AJ, Burling D, Gupta A, Fitzpatrick A, Fraser C. Safety, reliability and limitations of the given patency capsule in patients at risk of capsule retention: a 3-year technical review. Dig Dis Sci. 2008;53(10):2732–8.
37. Jensen MD, Nathan T, Rafaelsen SR, Kjeldsen J. Diagnostic accuracy of capsule endoscopy for small bowel Crohn's disease is superior to that of MR enterography or CT enterography. Clin Gastroenterol Hepatol. 2011;9(2):124–9.
38. Fiorino G, Bonifacio C, Peyrin-Biroulet L, Minuti F, Repici A, Spinelli A, et al. Prospective comparison of computed tomography enterography and magnetic resonance enterography for assessment of disease activity and complications in ileocolonic Crohn's disease. Inflamm Bowel Dis. 2011;17(5):1073–80.
39. Siddiki HA, Fidler JL, Fletcher JG, Burton SS, Huprich JE, Hough DM, et al. Prospective comparison of state-of-the-art MR enterography and CT enterography in small-bowel Crohn's disease. AJR Am J Roentgenol. 2009;193(1):113–21.
40. Mergener K, Ponchon T, Gralnek I, Pennazio M, Gay G, Selby W, et al. Literature review and recommendations for clinical application of small-bowel capsule endoscopy, based on a panel discussion by international experts. Consensus statements for small-bowel capsule endoscopy, 2006/2007. Endoscopy. 2007;39(10):895–909.
41. Adler SN, Yoav M, Eitan S, Yehuda C, Eliakim R. Does capsule endoscopy have an added value in patients with perianal disease and a negative work up for Crohn's disease? World J Gastrointest Endosc. 2012;4(5):185–8.
42. Bardan E, Nadler M, Chowers Y, Fidder H, Bar-Meir S. Capsule endoscopy for the evaluation of patients with chronic abdominal pain. Endoscopy. 2003; 35(8):688–9.
43. De BM, Bellumat A, Cian E, Valiante F, Moschini A, De BM. Capsule endoscopy findings in patients with suspected Crohn's disease and biochemical markers of inflammation. Dig Liver Dis. 2006;38(5): 331–5.
44. Koulaouzidis A, Douglas S, Rogers MA, Arnott ID, Plevris JN. Fecal calprotectin: a selection tool for small bowel capsule endoscopy in suspected IBD with prior negative bi-directional endoscopy. Scand J Gastroenterol. 2011;46(5):561–6.
45. Koulaouzidis A, Douglas S, Plevris JN. Lewis score correlates more closely with fecal calprotectin than Capsule Endoscopy Crohn's Disease Activity Index. Dig Dis Sci. 2012;57(4):987–93.
46. May A, Manner H, Schneider M, Ipsen A, Ell C. Prospective multicenter trial of capsule endoscopy in patients with chronic abdominal pain, diarrhea and other signs and symptoms (CEDAP-Plus Study). Endoscopy. 2007;39(7):606–12.
47. Sipponen T, Haapamaki J, Savilahti E, Alfthan H, Hamalainen E, Rautiainen H, et al. Fecal calprotectin and S100A12 have low utility in prediction of small bowel Crohn's disease detected by wireless capsule endoscopy. Scand J Gastroenterol. 2012; 47(7):778–84.
48. Valle J, Alcantara M, Perez-Grueso MJ, Navajas J, Munoz-Rosas C, Legaz ML, et al. Clinical features of patients with negative results from traditional diagnostic work-up and Crohn's disease findings from capsule endoscopy. J Clin Gastroenterol. 2006;40(8):692–6.
49. Kalla R, McAlindon ME, Sanders DS, Sidhu R. Subtle mucosal changes at capsule endoscopy in diarrhoea predominant Irritable Bowel Syndrome. Med Hypotheses. 2012;79(3):423.
50. Maiden L, Thjodleifsson B, Seigal A, Bjarnason II, Scott D, Birgisson S, et al. Long-term effects of non-steroidal anti-inflammatory drugs and cyclooxygenase-2 selective agents on the small bowel: a cross-sectional capsule enteroscopy study. Clin Gastroenterol Hepatol. 2007;5(9):1040–5.
51. Bourreille A, Jarry M, D'Halluin PN, Ben-Soussan E, Maunoury V, Bulois P, et al. Wireless capsule endoscopy versus ileocolonoscopy for the diagnosis of postoperative recurrence of Crohn's disease: a prospective study. Gut. 2006;55(7):978–83.
52. Pons Beltrán V, Nos P, Bastida G, Beltran B, Arguello L, Aguas M, et al. Evaluation of postsurgical recurrence in Crohn's disease: a new indication for capsule endoscopy? Gastrointest Endosc. 2007;66(3):533–40.
53. Pasha SF, Leighton JA, Das A, Harrison ME, Decker GA, Fleischer DE, et al. Double-balloon enteroscopy and capsule endoscopy have comparable diagnostic yield in small-bowel disease: a meta-analysis. Clin Gastroenterol Hepatol. 2008;6(6):671–6.
54. Chen X, Ran ZH, Tong JL. A meta-analysis of the yield of capsule endoscopy compared to double-balloon enteroscopy in patients with small bowel diseases. World J Gastroenterol. 2007;13(32):4372–8.
55. Jensen MD, Nathan T, Rafaelsen SR, Kjeldsen J. Ileoscopy reduces the need for small bowel imaging in suspected Crohn's disease. Dan Med J. 2012;59(9):A4491.
56. Marshall JB, Barthel JS. The frequency of total colonoscopy and terminal ileal intubation in the 1990s. Gastrointest Endosc. 1993;39(4):518–20.
57. Samuel S, Bruining DH, Loftus Jr EV, Becker B, Fletcher JG, Mandrekar JN, et al. Endoscopic skipping of the distal terminal ileum in Crohn's disease can lead to negative results from ileocolonoscopy. Clin Gastroenterol Hepatol. 2012;10(11):1253–9.
58. Long MD, Barnes E, Isaacs K, Morgan D, Herfarth HH. Impact of capsule endoscopy on management of inflammatory bowel disease: a single tertiary care center experience. Inflamm Bowel Dis. 2011;17(9):1855–62.
59. Lorenzo-Zuniga V, de Vega VM, Domenech E, Cabre E, Manosa M, Boix J. Impact of capsule

endoscopy findings in the management of Crohn's Disease. Dig Dis Sci. 2010;55(2):411–4.

60. Sidhu R, McAlindon ME, Drew K, Hardcastle S, Cameron IC, Sanders DS. Evaluating the role of small-bowel endoscopy in clinical practice: the largest single-centre experience. Eur J Gastroenterol Hepatol. 2012;24(5):513–9.

61. Flamant M, Trang C, Maillard O, Sacher-Huvelin S, Le RM, Galmiche JP, et al. The prevalence and outcome of jejunal lesions visualized by small bowel capsule endoscopy in Crohn's disease. Inflamm Bowel Dis. 2013;19(7):1390–6.

62. Chevaux JB, Fiorino G, Frederic M, Peyrin-Biroulet L. Capsule endoscopy in Crohn's disease. Curr Drug Targets. 2012;13(10):1261–7.

63. Swaminath A, Legnani P, Kornbluth A. Video capsule endoscopy in inflammatory bowel disease: past, present, and future redux. Inflamm Bowel Dis. 2010;16(7):1254–62.

64. Lewis BS. Expanding role of capsule endoscopy in inflammatory bowel disease. World J Gastroenterol. 2008;14(26):4137–41.

65. Niv Y, Ilani S, Levi Z, Hershkowitz M, Niv E, Fireman Z, et al. Validation of the Capsule Endoscopy Crohn's Disease Activity Index (CECDAI or Niv score): a multicenter prospective study. Endoscopy. 2012;44(1):21–6.

66. Mehdizadeh S, Chen G, Enayati PJ, Cheng DW, Han NJ, Shaye OA, et al. Diagnostic yield of capsule endoscopy in ulcerative colitis and inflammatory bowel disease of unclassified type (IBDU). Endoscopy. 2008;40(1):30–5.

67. Di NG, Oliva S, Ferrari F, Riccioni ME, Staiano A, Lombardi G, et al. Usefulness of wireless capsule endoscopy in paediatric inflammatory bowel disease. Dig Liver Dis. 2011;43(3):220–4.

68. Lopes S, Figueiredo P, Portela F, Freire P, Almeida N, Lerias C, et al. Capsule endoscopy in inflammatory bowel disease type unclassified and indeterminate colitis serologically negative. Inflamm Bowel Dis. 2010;16(10):1663–8.

69. Maunoury V, Savoye G, Bourreille A, Bouhnik Y, Jarry M, Sacher-Huvelin S, et al. Value of wireless capsule endoscopy in patients with indeterminate colitis (inflammatory bowel disease type unclassified). Inflamm Bowel Dis. 2007;13(2):152–5.

70. Kalla R, McAlindon ME, Drew K, Sidhu R. Clinical utility of capsule endoscopy in patients with Crohn's disease and inflammatory bowel disease unclassified. Eur J Gastroenterol Hepatol. 2013;25(6):706–13.

71. Dignass A, Eliakim R, Magro F, Maaser C, Chowers Y, Geboes K, et al. Second European evidence-based consensus on the diagnosis and management of ulcerative colitis part 1: definitions and diagnosis. J Crohns Colitis. 2012;6(10):965–90.

72. Murrell Z, Vasiliauskas E, Melmed G, Lo S, Targan S, Fleshner P. Preoperative wireless capsule endoscopy does not predict outcome after ileal pouch-anal anastomosis. Dis Colon Rectum. 2010;53(3):293–300.

73. Yamamoto H, Yano T, Kita H, Sunada K, Ido K, Sugano K. New system of double-balloon enteroscopy for diagnosis and treatment of small intestinal disorders. Gastroenterology. 2003;125(5):1556–7.

74. Akerman PA, Agrawal D, Cantero D, Pangtay J. Spiral enteroscopy with the new DSB overtube: a novel technique for deep peroral small-bowel intubation. Endoscopy. 2008;40(12):974–8.

75. Yamamoto H, Kita H, Sunada K, Hayashi Y, Sato H, Yano T, et al. Clinical outcomes of double-balloon endoscopy for the diagnosis and treatment of small-intestinal diseases. Clin Gastroenterol Hepatol. 2004;2(11):1010–6.

76. Despott EJ, Gupta A, Burling D, Tripoli E, Konieczko K, Hart A, et al. Effective dilation of small-bowel strictures by double-balloon enteroscopy in patients with symptomatic Crohn's disease (with video). Gastrointest Endosc. 2009;70(5):1030–6.

77. Kondo J, Iijima H, Abe T, Komori M, Hiyama S, Ito T, et al. Roles of double-balloon endoscopy in the diagnosis and treatment of Crohn's disease: a multicenter experience. J Gastroenterol. 2010;45(7):713–20.

78. Oshitani N, Yukawa T, Yamagami H, Inagawa M, Kamata N, Watanabe K, et al. Evaluation of deep small bowel involvement by double-balloon enteroscopy in Crohn's disease. Am J Gastroenterol. 2006;101(7):1484–9.

79. Pohl J, May A, Nachbar L, Ell C. Diagnostic and therapeutic yield of push-and-pull enteroscopy for symptomatic small bowel Crohn's disease strictures. Eur J Gastroenterol Hepatol. 2007;19(7):529–34.

80. Seiderer J, Herrmann K, Diepolder H, Schoenberg SO, Wagner AC, Goke B, et al. Double-balloon enteroscopy versus magnetic resonance enteroclysis in diagnosing suspected small-bowel Crohn's disease: results of a pilot study. Scand J Gastroenterol. 2007;42(11):1376–85.

81. Sunada K, Yamamoto H, Hayashi Y, Sugano K. Clinical importance of the location of lesions with regard to mesenteric or antimesenteric side of the small intestine. Gastrointest Endosc. 2007;66(3 Suppl):S34–8.

82. Sunada K, Yamamoto H, Yano T, Sugano K. Advances in the diagnosis and treatment of small bowel lesions with Crohn's disease using double-balloon endoscopy. Therap Adv Gastroenterol. 2009;2(6):357–66.

83. Xin L, Liao Z, Jiang YP, Li ZS. Indications, detectability, positive findings, total enteroscopy, and complications of diagnostic double-balloon endoscopy: a systematic review of data over the first decade of use. Gastrointest Endosc. 2011;74(3):563–70.

84. Aktas H, de Ridder L, Haringsma J, Kuipers EJ, Mensink PB. Complications of single-balloon enteroscopy: a prospective evaluation of 166 procedures. Endoscopy. 2010;42(5):365–8.

85. de Ridder L, Mensink PB, Lequin MH, Aktas H, de Krijger RR, van der Woude CJ, et al. Single-balloon enteroscopy, magnetic resonance enterography, and

abdominal US useful for evaluation of small-bowel disease in children with (suspected) Crohn's disease. Gastrointest Endosc. 2012;75:87.

86. Despott EJ, Hughes S, Marden P, Fraser C. First cases of spiral enteroscopy in the UK: let's "torque" about it! Endoscopy. 2010;42(6):517.

87. Mensink PB. Spiral enteroscopy: from "new kid on the block" to established deep small-bowel enteroscopy tool. Endoscopy. 2010;42(11):955–6.

88. Pasha SF, Leighton JA. Enteroscopy in the diagnosis and management of Crohn disease. Gastrointest Endosc Clin N Am. 2009;19(3):427–44.

89. Riccioni ME, Urgesi R, Cianci R, Spada C, Nista EC, Costamagna G. Single-balloon push-and-pull enteroscopy system: does it work? A single-center, 3-year experience. Surg Endosc. 2011;25(9):3050–6.

90. Upchurch BR, Sanaka MR, Lopez AR, Vargo JJ. The clinical utility of single-balloon enteroscopy: a single-center experience of 172 procedures. Gastrointest Endosc. 2010;71(7):1218–23.

91. Gay G, Delvaux M, Fassler I. Outcome of capsule endoscopy in determining indication and route for push-and-pull enteroscopy. Endoscopy. 2006;38(1):49–58.

92. Li X, Chen H, Dai J, Gao Y, Ge Z. Predictive role of capsule endoscopy on the insertion route of double-balloon enteroscopy. Endoscopy. 2009;41(9):762–6.

93. Mensink PB, Aktas H, Zelinkova Z, West RL, Kuipers EJ, van der Woude CJ. Impact of double-balloon enteroscopy findings on the management of Crohn's disease. Scand J Gastroenterol. 2010;45(4):483–9.

94. Hirai F, Beppu T, Sou S, Seki T, Yao K, Matsui T. Endoscopic balloon dilatation using double-balloon endoscopy is a useful and safe treatment for small intestinal strictures in Crohn's disease. Dig Endosc. 2010;22(3):200–4.

95. May A, Nachbar L, Ell C. Extraction of entrapped capsules from the small bowel by means of push-and-pull enteroscopy with the double-balloon technique. Endoscopy. 2005;37(6):591–3.

96. Mensink PB, Groenen MJ, van Buuren HR, Kuipers EJ, van der Woude CJ. Double-balloon enteroscopy in Crohn's disease patients suspected of small bowel activity: findings and clinical impact. J Gastroenterol. 2009;44(4):271–6.

97. Sunada K, Yamamoto H, Kita H, Yano T, Sato H, Hayashi Y, et al. Clinical outcomes of enteroscopy using the double-balloon method for strictures of the small intestine. World J Gastroenterol. 2005;11(7):1087–9.

98. May A, Manner H, Aschmoneit I, Ell C. Prospective, cross-over, single-center trial comparing oral double-balloon enteroscopy and oral spiral enteroscopy in patients with suspected small-bowel vascular malformations. Endoscopy. 2011;43(6):477–83.

99. Despott E, Fraser C. Achieving successful ileal intubation during retrograde double balloon enteroscopy: description of a novel, alternative technique (with video). Endoscopy. 2009;41 Suppl 2:E309–10.

100. Despott EJ, Murino A, Fraser C. Management of deep looping when failing to progress at double-balloon enteroscopy. Endoscopy. 2011;43(Suppl 2 UCTN):E275–6.

101. Gerson LB, Tokar J, Chiorean M, Lo S, Decker GA, Cave D, et al. Complications associated with double balloon enteroscopy at nine US centers. Clin Gastroenterol Hepatol. 2009;7(11):1177–82, 1182.

102. Mensink PB, Haringsma J, Kucharzik T, Cellier C, Perez-Cuadrado E, Monkemuller K, et al. Complications of double balloon enteroscopy: a multicenter survey. Endoscopy. 2007;39(7):613–5.

103. Moschler O, May A, Muller MK, Ell C. Complications in and performance of double-balloon enteroscopy (DBE): results from a large prospective DBE database in Germany. Endoscopy. 2011;43(6):484–9.

104. Pohl J, Delvaux M, Ell C, Gay G, May A, Mulder CJ, et al. European Society of Gastrointestinal Endoscopy (ESGE) Guidelines: flexible enteroscopy for diagnosis and treatment of small-bowel diseases. Endoscopy. 2008;40(7):609–18.

105. Manes G, Imbesi V, Ardizzone S, Cassinotti A, Pallotta S, Porro GB. Use of double-balloon enteroscopy in the management of patients with Crohn's disease: feasibility and diagnostic yield in a high-volume centre for inflammatory bowel disease. Surg Endosc. 2009;23:2790.

106. Thienpont C, D'Hoore A, Vermeire S, Demedts I, Bisschops R, Coremans G, et al. Long-term outcome of endoscopic dilatation in patients with Crohn's disease is not affected by disease activity or medical therapy. Gut. 2010;59(3):320–4.

107. Tokar JL, Banerjee S, Barth BA, Desilets DJ, Kaul V, Kethu SR, et al. Drug-eluting/biodegradable stents. Gastrointest Endosc. 2011;74(5):954–8.

Video Legends

Video 10.1 - CD SB lesions of varying severity. Video: Prof. O. Epstein, Ms. H. Palmer, Dr. M. I. Hamilton and Dr. E. J. Despott, Royal Free Unit for Endoscopy, Royal Free London NHS Foundation Trust.

Video 10.2 - CD SB lesions of varying severity. Video: Prof. O. Epstein, Ms. H. Palmer, Dr. M. I. Hamilton and Dr. E. J. Despott, Royal Free Unit for Endoscopy, Royal Free London NHS Foundation Trust.

Video 10.3 - CD SB lesions of varying severity. Video: Prof. O. Epstein, Ms. H. Palmer, Dr. M. I. Hamilton and Dr. E. J. Despott, Royal Free Unit for Endoscopy, Royal Free London NHS Foundation Trust.

Celiac Disease and Other Malabsorption States

Maximilien Barret, Gabriel Rahmi, Georgia Malamut, Elia Samaha, and Christophe Cellier

Introduction

Celiac disease (CD) is induced by the ingestion of gluten—a major storage protein of wheat, barley, and rye—resulting in small bowel mucosal lesions in genetically predisposed persons who are positive for HLA DQ2 or DQ8 haplotypes. The typical presentation of CD is chronic diarrhea, emaciation, anemia, malabsorption, and abdominal pain, which resolves with a gluten-free dict. However, isolated chronic abdominal pain, constipation, weight loss, neurologic symptoms, dermatitis herpetiformis, autoimmune thyropathy, or hypofertility may also be the initial presentation. In addition, silent forms exist and may present with iron-deficiency anemia, hypoproteinemia, hypocalcemia, elevated liver enzymes, osteoporosis, or there may be incidental recognition at endoscopy performed for other reasons [1].

An inflammatory reaction mediated by CD4+ T cells is triggered and leads to villous atrophy and intraepithelial lymphocytic infiltration. Both are the key histological markers of CD. The main histological classification later revised by Oberhuber [2] was reported by Marsh [3] and defines stage 1 CD by the presence of an isolated increase in intraepithelial lymphocytes (>40 intraepithelial lymphocytes per 100 enterocytes); stage 2 is characterized by crypt hyperplasia; and stage 3 is associated with villous atrophy, classified from 3A to 3C depending on its degree (either partial, subtotal, or total). The diagnosis of CD requires the combination of elevated IgA antitissue transglutaminase antibodies and histological analysis of duodenal biopsies. In cases where there is a high-clinical probability of CD, both tests are usually performed at the same time. In cases of low- clinical probability, recent American College of Gastroenterology (ACG) guidelines suggest starting with serologic testing, including a total IgA measurement, in order to rule out IgA deficiency. If IgA deficiency is present, then IgG antitissue transglutaminase and IgG antideamidated gliadin measurements should be performed. Endoscopy should then be limited to patients with positive serological markers [4].

Electronic supplementary material: The online version of this chapter (doi: 10.1007/978-3-319-14415-3_11) contains supplementary material, which is available to authorized users. Videos can also be accessed at http://link.springer.com/chapter/10.1007/978-3-319-14415-3_11.

M. Barret, M.D., M.Sc. • G. Malamut, M.D., Ph.D.
C. Cellier, M.D., Ph.D. (✉)
Sorbonne Paris Centre, Université Paris Descartes, Paris, France

Department of Gastroenterology and Digestive Endoscopy, Georges Pompidou European Hospital, 20-40, rue Leblanc, Paris Cedex 15 75908, France
e-mail: maximilien.barret@egp.aphp.fr; christophe.cellier@egp.aphp.fr

G. Rahmi, M.D. • E. Samaha, M.D.
Department of Gastroenterology and Digestive Endoscopy, Georges Pompidou European Hospital, 20-40, rue Leblanc, Paris Cedex 15 75908, France

Except in the case of children with restrictive diagnostic criteria (clinical features suggestive of CD, IgA antitissue transglutaminase >10 times the normal values, positive antiendomysial serology, and confirmed HLA DQ2 haplotype), all CD diagnoses require upper gastrointestinal endoscopy with duodenal biopsies [4, 5]. Furthermore, endoscopy is of paramount importance in the follow-up and the diagnosis of complications of CD.

Assessment of Villous Atrophy Through Upper Endoscopy

White Light Endoscopy

The recognition of villous atrophy at endoscopic examination of the duodenal mucosa may be of help in two situations. First, in order to choose the sites where biopsies should be performed to obtain histological confirmation of a suspected CD, and second, in patients investigated for nonspecific digestive symptoms, such as dyspepsia or epigastric pain for example [6]. The following endoscopic features have been described as endoscopic markers of CD (Figs. 11.1 and 11.2, Video 11.1):

- Reduction or loss of duodenal folds, with a sensitivity of 47–88 % and a specificity of 83–97 % [7, 8].
- Scalloping of the mucosa, described as a notched and nodular appearance of the duodenal folds,

with a sensitivity varying from 6 to 44 % [8, 9] and a specificity of 94–100 % [8, 10].
- Mosaic pattern or cobblestone appearance of the duodenal surface, with a sensitivity of 12 % and a specificity of 100 % for CD [8].
- Nodularity, also described in the duodenal bulb [11], has a sensitivity of 6 % and a specificity of 95 % for the diagnosis of CD [8].
- Evidence of submucosal vasculature [12]. Mucosal fissures, crevices, or grooves [10, 12, 13].

The presence of any endoscopic marker of CD has a sensitivity of 37–94 % [14, 15] and a specificity of 92–100 % [15, 16]. The most reliable endoscopic marker in terms of sensitivity appears to be the loss of the duodenal folds, however, with very heterogeneous values among published studies [17]. The specificity of these endoscopic markers of CD is good, with numbers ranging from 92 to 100 % [17]. Among differential diagnoses, nonceliac causes of villous atrophy, such as Whipple's disease, enteropathy associated with primary hypogammaglobulinemia, autoimmune enteropathy, drug-induced toxic enteropathies (angiotensin II receptor blokers, mycophenolate mofetil), and tropical sprue should be considered [4, 18].

These specific endoscopic markers left aside, the judgment of the endoscopist on possible villous atrophy seems to be quite reliable. Although conducted without high-resolution videoendoscopes in most studies, white light endoscopic

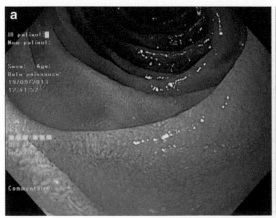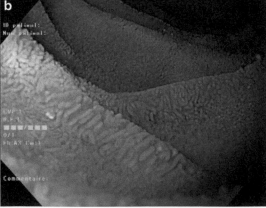

Fig. 11.1 Normal duodenal villi after (**a**) air insufflation and (**b**) water immersion

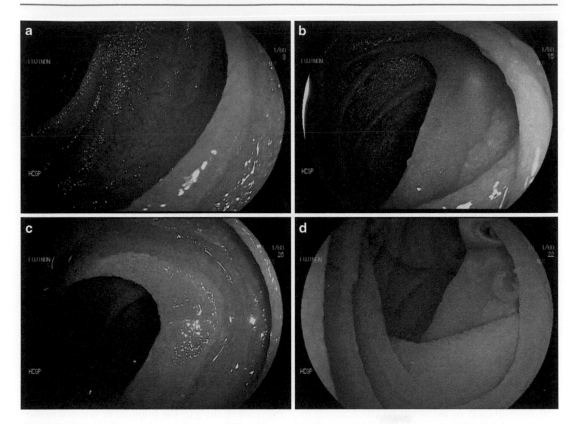

Fig. 11.2 Endoscopic features suggestive of celiac disease. (**a**) Mucosal fissures, grooves, and scalloping of the duodenal mucosa. Focal villous atrophy with (**b**, **c**) air insufflation and (**d**) after water immersion

examination alone could predict the diagnosis of villous atrophy in more than 50 % of cases [10]. A study including 87 patients in an expert endoscopy center even reported sensitivity, specificity, and positive and negative predictive values of 94 %, 100 %, 100 %, and 96 %, respectively [12]. The ability of white light endoscopic examination alone to predict villous atrophy is, however, uncertain, since villous atrophy may be patchy, and early stages of villous atrophy are not easily identified by endoscopy [18, 19]. Hence, mucosal biopsies should be performed even in an endoscopically normal duodenal mucosa.

Advanced Endoscopic Imaging Techniques

Numerous techniques have been assessed to improve the visualization of the mucosal pattern in the duodenum. First and foremost, Cammarota et al. have demonstrated the interest of the "immersion technique"; i.e., the observation of duodenal mucosa after air exsufflation and instillation of 90–150 mL of water in the duodenal lumen. As presented in Figs. 11.1 and 11.2, and confirmed by several studies from this group, the water immersion technique could improve the sensitivity of upper endoscopy for the diagnosis of villous atrophy to more than 90 % [20]. However, these promising results have not been confirmed by other teams.

Chromoendoscopy appears to enhance the borders of flat lesions in the colon, stomach, and duodenum, but there is little data in the literature to suggest a benefit of dye spraying in the duodenum to increase the detection of villous atrophy. Methylene blue chromoendoscopy, even in expert hands, did not bring any improvement in the diagnosis of villous atrophy [12]. Indigo carmine in combination with magnification endoscopy showed greater than 90 % sensitivity for villous atrophy, including partial villous atrophy [13]. A second work confirmed the interest of indigo carmine dye spraying, with or without magnification endoscopy, to improve the detection of villous atrophy, especially in the duodenal bulb [21].

Magnification endoscopy may improve the sensitivity of endoscopy for the diagnosis of villous atrophy, with numbers ranging from 90 to 100 %, either alone [22–24], associated with acetic acid [14] or indigo carmine dye spraying [13]. Cammarota et al. even reported a 100 % sensibility of magnification endoscopy coupled with the water immersion technique [23].

Optical coherence tomography (OCT), an imaging technique similar to the B mode ultrasonography, used by ophthalmologists to assess retinal disorders, has recently been applied to digestive endoscopy. Masci et al. have reported in two studies an acceptable concordance between villous atrophy diagnosed by OCT and pathological examination of duodenal biopsies, resulting in a sensitivity of 82 % and a specificity of 100 % [25, 26].

Endocytoscopy is a novel diagnostic technique allowing for in vivo real-time visualization of the mucosa under 450× magnification. This noninvasive technique has been shown to be useful in in vivo and real-time and can adequately characterize the villous architecture of the duodenal mucosa in patients with celiac disease. Moreover, endocytoscopy accurately identifies mucosal histopathology of advanced CD [27, 28].

The potential contribution of confocal endomicroscopy to the diagnosis of celiac disease has been evaluated of course, with the promising capability of assessing both the degree of villous atrophy and the density of intraepithelial lymphocytes. Three studies have been published to date, all using a device from Pentax® which is currently unavailable [29–31]. Despite an 80–100 % overall specificity, sensitivity values for villous atrophy, crypt hyperplasia, and intraepithelial lymphocyte infiltration were 70–74 %, 52 %, and 81 %, respectively.

In conclusion, advanced endoscopic imaging techniques have not changed much over time in the endoscopic evaluation of a patient with suspected CD. The evidence thus far for clinical practice suggests that high-definition white light upper videoendoscopy and careful examination of the mucosa for patchy lesions are the most effective methods and remain the standard protocol for diagnosing CD. Recent studies suggest that water immersion and/or indigo carmine dye spraying preceding mucosal biopsies may also be helpful.

Intestinal Biopsy Technique

Intestinal mucosal biopsies remain the cornerstone of the diagnosis of CD. They should be repeated after 6–12 months on a gluten-free diet, in order to assess the healing of duodenal mucosa and the new growth of duodenal villi. Complete mucosal healing is variable in adults, and usually requires 2–3 years [32]. However, complete mucosal healing of the duodenum has been associated with a good prognosis, because of a lower rate of T cell lymphoma [33]. Hence, the American College of Gastroenterology clinical guidelines recommend that the first assessment of villous architecture recovery of duodenal histology should wait until 2 years on a gluten-free diet (even in case of symptom regression and normalization of antibody levels), or 6–12 months in case of nonresponsive CD [4].

The current guidelines recommend that the endoscopist should obtain at least four biopsies from the second portion of the duodenum and one or two biopsies in the duodenal bulb [4]. Indeed, villous atrophy, along with other histological abnormalities, can be patchy in the small intestine [34], and the number of 4 is a cutoff above which the sensitivity of biopsies rises significantly [35]. About 10 % of patients with CD have a villous atrophy restricted to the duodenal bulb [36]: hence, one or two biopsies, ideally in the 9 and 12 o'clock positions, should be added to the four biopsies from the second portion of the duodenum [4]. However, gastroenterologists should be aware of potential pitfalls in the interpretation of these duodenal bulb biopsies, due to peptic duodenitis or the epithelial changes in the immediate vicinity of Brünner's glands.

Jumbo biopsy forceps have not been proven superior to standard biopsy forceps [37]. Expert opinion suggests that only a single biopsy specimen should be obtained with each pass of the biopsy forceps, in order to collect relatively large biopsy specimens [4].

Other Endoscopic Findings in Celiac Disease Patients

Villous atrophy left aside, gastroesophageal reflux disease is the most prevalent endoscopic finding in celiac patients, and interestingly, dyspeptic symptoms typically regress under a gluten-free diet. Celiac disease is associated with a decrease in the basal pressure of the lower esophageal sphincter and peptic esophagitis is twice as frequent in CD patients as in nonceliac dyspeptic controls [38]. Along with this finding, the prevalence of Barrett's esophagus may be twice as high in CD patients as in controls [39]. Nonerosive gastric mucosal lesions, typically varioliform, have also been reported to be associated with CD. Histologically, they present as lymphocytic gastritis, of which the significance is still under debate [18].

Ulcers, strictures, or protruding lesions can be observed in any part of the small bowel in CD patients. These lesions are highly suspicious of a malignant T cell proliferation or, more seldom, of an adenocarcinoma, and should be biopsied. Strong consideration should be given for sending the patient to an expert center.

Intraepithelial lymphocytic infiltrate of the terminal ileum has been reported in association with CD, and this finding should lead the endoscopist to perform duodenal biopsies to rule out villous atrophy [40]. Finally, CD is more frequently associated with other digestive conditions, such as microscopic colitis (either lymphocytic or collagenous colitis) or inflammatory bowel disease. These conditions should be searched for in case of persistent diarrhea or abdominal pain on a strict gluten-free diet [18].

Small Bowel Capsule Endoscopy in Celiac Disease

Small bowel capsule endoscopy (CE) is a promising technique in the field of CD because of its ability to image the entire small bowel mucosa with high-quality pictures. Of note, the presence of fluid enhances the visualization of intestinal villi. Furthermore, it is less invasive than upper endoscopy, and thus more acceptable for patients. The main limitation of CE in CD is the risk of capsule retention proximal to a stricture, but this is relatively rare in this setting. However, radiological imaging of the small bowel using magnetic resonance (MR) or computed tomography (CT) enterography or the patency capsule should always precede CE in the presence of abdominal pain compatible with obstruction and/or a small bowel stricture.

The sensitivity of CE for the diagnosis of CD ranges from 77 to 92 %, with a specificity of 91–100 % [41, 42]. These diagnostic performances may be even better than those of optical endoscopy. However, histological assessment of the duodenal mucosa remains mandatory to establish the diagnosis of CD, and CE remains restricted to patients with a high clinical and biological suspicion of CD and who either refuse upper endoscopy, or have normal or indefinite biopsies for CD [41]. The endoscopic markers of CD are the same as in optical endoscopy: reduced duodenal folds, scalloping of folds, mucosal fissures, crevices or grooves, mosaic pattern, and visible submucosal vessels. These signs should draw the attention of the gastroenterologist interpreting a small bowel capsule study and typical features can be seen (Fig. 11.3 and Video 11.2).

The biggest impact of CE in CD is the diagnostic workup of nonresponsive or complicated CD. In nonresponsive CD, after 6–12 months of a well-conducted gluten-free diet, the patient should undergo further diagnostic investigations, searching for causes of refractory celiac disease. Once radiological imaging of the small bowel has excluded a digestive stricture, CE should be considered to search for small bowel ulcers, especially located beyond the distal duodenum. The results of the capsule study can aid the endoscopist in

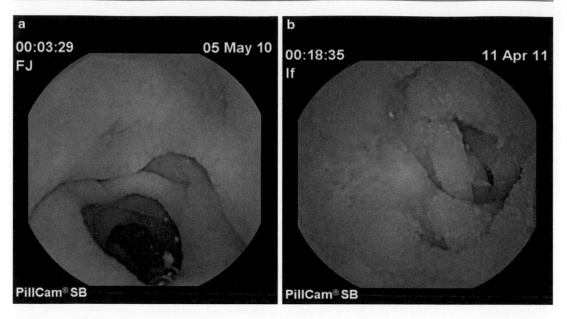

Fig. 11.3 Endoscopic features of celiac disease on capsule endoscopy. (**a**) Villous atrophy and scalloping, and (**b**) jejunal ulcer in the setting of ulcerative jejunitis

choosing between standard esogastroduodenoscopy, push enteroscopy, or deep enteroscopy [43, 44]. It should be noted that there are currently no national or international guidelines to support this management, given the relatively high prevalence of small bowel mucosal ulcers (generally attributable to nonsteroidal anti-inflammatory drug [NSAID] intake) in CE procedures performed in uncomplicated CD patients [45]. CE could also play a role in the annual follow-up of patients with refractory celiac disease, by searching for jejunal or ileal mucosal ulcers suggesting ulcerative jejunitis or malignant transformation of CD.

Role of Enteroscopy in Celiac Disease

Push enteroscopy, balloon-assisted enteroscopy, and/or spiral enteroscopy have very few indications in CD, especially since the development of small bowel capsule endoscopy. It is a time-consuming and invasive procedure, carrying a risk of perforation in patients with diseased small bowel. Rarely, does enteroscopy add much in the evaluation of CD. Since mucosal lesions are known to be patchy in CD, some physicians have

advocated for enteroscopy in order to obtain jejunal mucosal samples, particularly when duodenal biopsies are normal. However, several studies have shown that the diagnostic yield of jejunal biopsies in this setting is insignificant. Cellier et al. demonstrated that enteroscopy did not change the management of responsive CD patients [46]. In another study including more than 140 patients, Thijs et al. found a 2 % rate of pathological jejunal biopsies when duodenal biopsies were normal [47]. Meijer et al. reported a 6 % clinically significant discrepancy between duodenal and jejunal biopsies in more than 100 celiac patients [48]. Given the 96 % sensitivity of the duodenal biopsies (including duodenal bulb biopsies) for the diagnosis of CD, there is little data to support routine upper enteroscopy in the diagnosis of CD for patients with positive serology and negative duodenal biopsies [4].

In contrast, for nonresponsive or complicated CD, enteroscopy remains a useful diagnostic tool. Refractory celiac disease is defined by the persistence of villous atrophy after at least 6 months on a strict gluten-free diet, in the absence of another cause of villous atrophy [1]. Type I disease, in which the phenotype of intraepithelial lymphocytes is normal, should be distinguished from type

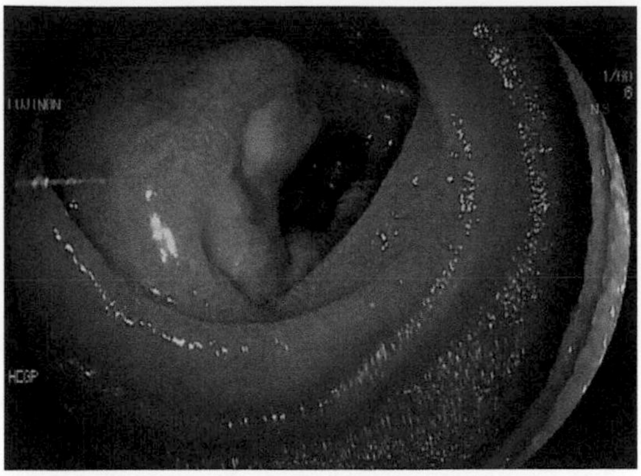

Fig. 11.4 Enteropathy-associated T cell lymphoma, presenting as an ulcerated jejunal stricture diagnosed by push enteroscopy

II, in which clonal expansion of abnormal intraepithelial lymphocytes is observed. This latter form is actually a low-grade T-cell lymphoma and carries a more ominous prognosis. In this setting, enteroscopy allows for the histological follow-up of the duodenal and jejunal mucosa through systematic and targeted mucosal biopsies [43, 49]. Unlike uncomplicated CD, mucosal abnormalities with ulcerative jejunitis can be limited to the jejunum, without any ulcers seen in the duodenum (Fig. 11.3, Video 11.3) [39].

The choice between upper and lower enteroscopy is guided by a preliminary noninvasive workup, including MR or CT enterography, followed by small bowel CE. If abnormalities are detected, then enteroscopy can facilitate the evaluation for a T cell malignant proliferation among jejunal ulcers, or perform histological follow-up of type I refractory celiac disease. Biopsies can aid in the detection of a clonal expansion or an abnormal phenotype of intraepithelial lymphocytes, suggesting the evolution toward type II refractory celiac disease or a T cell lymphoma. This surveillance is conducted yearly in refractory patients, and the choice between esophagogastroduodenoscopy, push enteroscopy, and deep enteroscopy is based primarily on the findings of small bowel capsule endoscopy [43]. Finally, upper enteroscopy allows one to obtain biopsy samples of suspicious lesions of the jejunum, such as deep ulcers or strictures, to rule out adenocarcinoma or T cell lymphoma (Fig. 11.4, Video 11.4).

Contribution of Endoscopy in Other Malabsorption States

In addition to CD, other malabsorptive states can be evaluated with small bowel imaging. The causes of malabsorption can by roughly classified in three groups: (1) maldigestion, mainly linked to gastric and/or small bowel resection or pancreatic exocrine insufficiency; (2) mucosal noninfectious diseases, such as autoimmune enteropathy, common variable immunodeficiency, tropical sprue, and the recently described angiotensin II inhibitor-induced sprue; and (3) microbial causes, including a vast array of bacterial, viral, parasitic, or fungal infections occurring in immunocompetent or immunocompromised hosts, as well as small bowel bacterial overgrowth and Whipple's disease.

The initial diagnostic workup of suspected malabsorption syndrome requires a good history and physical exam followed by laboratory testing and noninvasive imaging where appropriate. Once a small bowel malabsorptive process involving the small bowel has been identified, then esophagogastroduodenoscopy with duodenal biopsies and ileocolonoscopy with systematic biopsies may be warranted and is usually sufficient for a diagnosis.

However, with the development of capsule endoscopy and deep enteroscopy techniques, direct endoscopic imaging and tissue sampling of the entire small bowel is now possible. However, the exact indication for CE in the evaluation of chronic diarrhea or malabsorption states is not mentioned in the last international consensus statement on CE indications [41]. The value of push enteroscopy in the diagnostic workup of malabsorptive states is also not entirely clear. Cuillerier et al. reported that push enteroscopy was of diagnostic value in only 12 % of patients with malabsorption of unclear origin [50]. However, the contribution of jejunal biopsies was limited to patients with inconclusive duodenal histology, and enteroscopy was again of no benefit in patients with normal duodenal mucosa. In contrast, Landi et al. found push enteroscopy to be of help in establishing the diagnosis of malabsorption in 22 % of patients. However, the results of duodenal biopsies were not available in this work [51]. Rarely should deep enteroscopy be needed in the evaluation of these patients.

In terms of specific diseases, the diagnosis of Whipple's disease may as well be made on duodenal and/or jejunal biopsies [52], and usually does not require an extensive small bowel investigation. In the case of primary or secondary intestinal lymphangiectasia, this disease has been diagnosed by CE and histologically assessed by enteroscopy-guided biopsies in some case reports [53]. In one report the diagnostic yield was higher with upper enteroscopy than with capsule endoscopy [54]. Enteroscopic investigation of jejunal ulcers associated with chronic ischemic enteritis has been reported by some authors, and may be of particular benefit in those patients with a high rate of small bowel strictures and capsule retention [55]. Deep enteroscopy may also be used for balloon dilation of ischemic strictures involving the small bowel [56]. Finally, common variable immunodeficiency associated with small bowel lesions (such as nodular lymphoid hyperplasia) is frequently associated with a malabsorption syndrome [57]. Intestinal hyperlymphocytosis and villous atrophy are found in 75 % and 50 % of these patients with gastrointestinal symptoms. CE and deep enteroscopy may be useful in this condition depending on how much of the small bowel is involved [57].

Conclusion

There is no doubt that small bowel imaging techniques are important in the evaluation of CD and other small bowel malabsorptive syndromes. Although serological testing has greatly improved our ability to identify patients with CD, the diagnosis still depends on the histological assessment of duodenal mucosal biopsies. In most cases, upper endoscopy with duodenal biopsies will be sufficient to make the diagnosis.

The use of high-definition endoscopes and complementary endoscopic techniques, such as water immersion, magnification endoscopy, or dye spraying, can help to identify endoscopic markers of CD, and facilitate the performance of targeted biopsies. However, these markers are more specific than they are sensitive, and a normal duodenal endoscopic examination does not exclude the diagnosis of CD. As such, in those suspected of having CD with normal-appearing mucosa, one should perform at least five biopsies, one to two in the duodenal bulb and four in the second portion of the duodenum.

The contribution of CE, push enteroscopy, and deep enteroscopy techniques is most useful for the diagnosis and follow-up of nonresponsive or complicated forms of celiac disease. In patients with other malabsorption states, as in patients with celiac disease, the vast majority of pathological findings can be detected in the duodenum. As such, the indication for CE and deep enteroscopy in the diagnostic workup of these patients is limited.

References

1. Green PH, Cellier C. Celiac disease. N Engl J Med. 2007;357(17):1731–43.
2. Oberhuber G. Histopathology of celiac disease. Biomed Pharmacother. 2000;54:368–72.
3. Marsh MN. Gluten, major histocompatibility complex, and the small intestine. A molecular and immunobiologic approach to the spectrum of gluten sensitivity ('celiac sprue'). Gastroenterology. 1992; 102:330–54.
4. Rubio-Tapia A, Hill ID, Kelly CP, Calderwood AH, Murray JA, American College of Gastroenterology. ACG clinical guidelines: diagnosis and management of celiac disease. Am J Gastroenterol. 2013;108(5): 656–76.
5. Husby S, Koletzko S, Korponay-Szabó IR, Mearin ML, Phillips A, Shamir R, Troncone R, Giersiepen K, Branski D, Catassi C, Lelgeman M, Mäki M, Ribes-Koninckx C, Ventura A, Zimmer KP, ESPGHAN Working Group on Coeliac Disease Diagnosis, ESPGHAN Gastroenterology Committee, European Society for Pediatric Gastroenterology, Hepatology, and Nutrition. European Society for Pediatric Gastroenterology, Hepatology, and Nutrition guidelines for the diagnosis of coeliac disease. J Pediatr Gastroenterol Nutr. 2012;54(1):136–60.
6. Talley NJ, Vakil NB, Moayyedi P. American gastroenterological association technical review on the evaluation of dyspepsia. Gastroenterology. 2005;129(5): 1756–80.
7. Brocchi E, Corazza GR, Caletti G, Treggiari EA, Barbara L, Gasbarrini G. Endoscopic demonstration of loss of duodenal folds in the diagnosis of celiac disease. N Engl J Med. 1988;319(12):741–4.

8. Oxentenko AS, Grisolano SW, Murray JA, et al. The insensitivity of endoscopic markers in celiac disease. Am J Gastroenterol. 2002;97:933–8.

9. Shah VH, Rotterdam H, Kotler DP, Fasano A, Green PH. All that scallops is not celiac disease. Gastrointest Endosc. 2000;51:717–20.

10. Smith AD, Graham I, Rose JD. A prospective endoscopic study of scalloped folds and grooves in the mucosa of the duodenum as signs of villous atrophy. Gastrointest Endosc. 1998;47(6):461–5.

11. Brocchi E, Corazza GR, Brusco G, Mangia L, Gasbarrini G. Unsuspected celiac disease diagnosed by endoscopic visualization of duodenal bulb micronodules. Gastrointest Endosc. 1996;44(5):610–1.

12. Niveloni S, Fiorini A, Dezi R, Pedreira S, Smecuol E, Vazquez H, Cabanne A, Boerr LA, Valero J, Kogan Z, Mauriño E, Bai JC. Usefulness of videoduodenoscopy and vital dye staining as indicators of mucosal atrophy of celiac disease: assessment of interobserver agreement. Gastrointest Endosc. 1998;47(3):223–9.

13. Siegel LM, Stevens PD, Lightdale CJ, Green PH, Goodman S, Garcia-Carrasquillo RJ, Rotterdam H. Combined magnification endoscopy with chromoendoscopy in the evaluation of patients with suspected malabsorption. Gastrointest Endosc. 1997;46(3):226–30.

14. Lo A, Guelrud M, Essenfeld H, Bonis P. Classification of villous atrophy with enhanced magnification endoscopy in patients with celiac disease and tropical sprue. Gastrointest Endosc. 2007;66(2):377–82.

15. Maurino E, Bai JC. Endoscopic markers of celiac disease. Am J Gastroenterol. 2002;97:760–1.

16. Dickcy W, Hughes D. Disappointing sensitivity of endoscopic markers for villous atrophy in a high-risk population: implications for celiac disease diagnosis during routine endoscopy. Am J Gastroenterol. 2001;96:2126–8.

17. Cammarota G, Fedeli P, Gasbarrini A. Emerging technologies in upper gastrointestinal endoscopy and celiac disease. Nat Clin Pract Gastroenterol Hepatol. 2009;6(1):47–56.

18. Lee SK, Green PH. Endoscopy in celiac disease. Curr Opin Gastroenterol. 2005;21(5):589–94.

19. Tursi A, Brandimarte G, Giorgetti GM, Gigliobianco A. Endoscopic features of celiac disease in adults and their correlation with age, histological damage, and clinical form of the disease. Endoscopy. 2002;34(10): 787–92.

20. Cammarota G, Cesaro P, Cazzato A, Cianci R, Fedeli P, Ojetti V, Certo M, Sparano L, Giovannini S, Larocca LM, Vecchio FM, Gasbarrini G. The water immersion technique is easy to learn for routine use during EGD for duodenal villous evaluation: a single-center 2-year experience. J Clin Gastroenterol. 2009; 43(3):244–8.

21. Kiesslich R, Mergener K, Naumann C, Hahn M, Jung M, Koehler HH, Nafe B, Kanzler S, Galle PR. Value of chromoendoscopy and magnification endoscopy in the evaluation of duodenal abnormalities: a prospective, randomized comparison. Endoscopy. 2003;35(7): 559–63.

22. Badreldin R, Barrett P, Wooff DA, Mansfield J, Yiannakou Y. How good is zoom endoscopy for assessment of villous atrophy in coeliac disease? Endoscopy. 2005;37(10):994–8.

23. Cammarota G, Martino A, Pirozzi GA, Cianci R, Cremonini F, Zuccalà G, Cuoco L, Ojetti V, Montalto M, Vecchio FM, Gasbarrini A, Gasbarrini G. Direct visualization of intestinal villi by high-resolution magnifying upper endoscopy: a validation study. Gastrointest Endosc. 2004;60(5):732–8.

24. Banerjee R, Shekharan A, Ramji C, Puli SR, Kalapala R, Ramachandani M, Gupta R, Lakhtakia S, Tandan M, Rao GV, Reddy DN. Role of magnification endoscopy in the diagnosis and evaluation of suspected celiac disease: correlation with histology. Indian J Gastroenterol. 2007;26(2):67–9.

25. Masci E, Mangiavillano B, Albarello L, Mariani A, Doglioni C, Testoni PA. Pilot study on the correlation of optical coherence tomography with histology in celiac disease and normal subjects. J Gastroenterol Hepatol. 2007;22(12):2256–60.

26. Masci E, Mangiavillano B, Barera G, Parma B, Albarello L, Mariani A, Doglioni C, Testoni PA. Optical coherence tomography in pediatric patients: a feasible technique for diagnosing celiac disease in children with villous atrophy. Dig Liver Dis. 2009;41(9):639–43.

27. Matysiak-Budnik T, Coron E, Mosnier JF, Le Rhun M, Inoue H, Galmiche JP. In vivo real-time imaging of human duodenal mucosal structures in celiac disease using endocytoscopy. Endoscopy. 2010;42(3):191–6.

28. Pohl H, Rösch T, Tanczos BT, Rudolph B, Schlüns K, Baumgart DC. Endocytoscopy for the detection of microstructural features in adult patients with celiac sprue: a prospective, blinded endocytoscopy-conventional histology correlation study. Gastrointest Endosc. 2009;70(5):933–41.

29. Günther U, Daum S, Heller F, Schumann M, Loddenkemper C, Grünbaum M, et al. Diagnostic value of confocal endomicroscopy in celiac disease. Endoscopy. 2010;42(3):197–202.

30. Leong RW, Nguyen NQ, Meredith CG, Al-Sohaily S, Kukic D, Delaney PM, et al. In vivo confocal endomicroscopy in the diagnosis and evaluation of celiac disease. Gastroenterology. 2008;135(6):1870–6.

31. Venkatesh K, Abou-Taleb A, Cohen M, Evans C, Thomas S, Oliver P, Taylor C, Thomson M. Role of confocal endomicroscopy in the diagnosis of celiac disease. J Pediatr Gastroenterol Nutr. 2010;51(3):274–9.

32. Rubio-Tapia A, Rahim MW, See JA, Lahr BD, Wu TT, Murray JA. Mucosal recovery and mortality in adults with celiac disease after treatment with a gluten-free diet. Am J Gastroenterol. 2010;105(6):1412–20.

33. Elfström P, Granath F, Ekström Smedby K, Montgomery SM, Askling J, Ekbom A, et al. Risk of lymphoproliferative malignancy in relation to small intestinal histopathology among patients with celiac disease. J Natl Cancer Inst. 2011;103(5):436–44.

34. Ravelli A, Villanacci V, Monfredini C, Martinazzi S, Grassi V, Manenti S. How patchy is patchy villous atrophy ? Distribution pattern of histological lesions in the duodenum of children with celiac disease. Am J Gastroenterol. 2010;105(9):2103–10.

35. Lebwohl B, Kapel RC, Neugut AI, Green PH, Genta RM. Adherence to biopsy guidelines increases celiac disease diagnosis. Gastrointest Endosc. 2011;74(1): 103–9.

36. Evans KE, Aziz I, Cross SS, Sahota GR, Hopper AD, Hadjivassiliou M, et al. A prospective study of duodenal bulb biopsy in newly diagnosed and established adult celiac disease. Am J Gastroenterol 2011; 106:1837–42.

37. Dandalides SM, Carey WD, Petras R, Achkar E. Endoscopic small bowel mucosal biopsy: a controlled trial evaluating forceps size and biopsy location in the diagnosis of normal and abnormal mucosal architecture. Gastrointest Endosc. 1989;35(3): 197–200.

38. Cuomo A, Romano M, Rocco A, Budillon G, Del Vecchio BC, Nardone G. Reflux oesophagitis in adult coeliac disease: beneficial effect of a gluten free diet. Gut. 2003;52(4):514–7.

39. Maieron R, Elli L, Marino M, Floriani I, Minerva F, Avellini C, et al. Celiac disease and intestinal metaplasia of the esophagus (Barrett's esophagus). Dig Dis Sci. 2005;50(1):126–9.

40. Dickey W, Hughes DF. Histology of the terminal ileum in coeliac disease. Scand J Gastroenterol. 2004; 39:665–7.

41. Mergener K, Ponchon T, Gralnek I, Pennazio M, Gay G, Selby W, et al. Literature review and recommendations for clinical application of small-bowel capsule endoscopy, based on a panel discussion by international experts. Consensus statements for small-bowel capsule endoscopy, 2006/2007. Endoscopy. 2007; 39(10):895–909.

42. Murray JA, Rubio-Tapia A, Van Dyke CT, Brogan DL, Knipschield MA, Lahr B, et al. Mucosal atrophy in celiac disease: extent of involvement, correlation with clinical presentation, and response to treatment. Clin Gastroenterol Hepatol. 2008;6(2): 186–93.

43. Barret M, Malamut G, Rahmi G, Samaha E, Edery J, Verkarre V, et al. Diagnostic yield of capsule endoscopy in refractory celiac disease. Am J Gastroenterol. 2012;107(10):1546–53.

44. Culliford A, Daly J, Diamond B, Rubin M, Green PH. The value of wireless capsule endoscopy in patients with complicated celiac disease. Gastrointest Endosc. 2005;62(1):55–61.

45. Atlas DS, Rubio-Tapia A, Van Dyke CT, Lahr BD, Murray JA. Capsule endoscopy in nonresponsive celiac disease. Gastrointest Endosc. 2011;74(6): 1315–22.

46. Cellier C, Cuillerier E, Patey-Mariaud de Serre N, Marteau P, Verkarre V, Brière J, et al. Push enteroscopy in celiac sprue and refractory sprue. Gastrointest Endosc. 1999;50(5):613–7.

47. Thijs WJ, van Baarlen J, Kleibeuker JH, Kolkman JJ. Duodenal versus jejunal biopsies in suspected celiac disease. Endoscopy. 2004;36(11):993–6.

48. Meijer JW, Wahab PJ, Mulder CJ. Small intestinal biopsies in celiac disease: duodenal or jejunal? Virchows Arch. 2003;442(2):124–8.

49. Hadithi M, Al-toma A, Oudejans J, van Bodegraven AA, Mulder CJ, Jacobs M. The value of double-balloon enteroscopy in patients with refractory celiac disease. Am J Gastroenterol. 2007;102(5):987–96.

50. Cuillerier E, Landi B, Cellier C. Is push enteroscopy useful in patients with malabsorption of unclear origin? Am J Gastroenterol. 2001;96(7):2103–6.

51. Landi B, Tkoub M, Gaudric M, Guimbaud R, Cervoni JP, Chaussade S, Couturier D, Barbier JP, Cellier C. Diagnostic yield of push-type enteroscopy in relation to indication. Gut. 1998;42(3):421–5.

52. Fenollar F, Puéchal X, Raoult D. Whipple's disease. N Engl J Med. 2007;356(1):55–66.

53. Oh TG, Chung JW, Kim HM, Han SJ, Lee JS, Park JY, Song SY. Primary intestinal lymphangiectasia diagnosed by capsule endoscopy and double balloon enteroscopy. World J Gastrointest Endosc. 2011; 3(11):235–40.

54. Takenaka H, Ohmiya N, Hirooka Y, Nakamura M, Ohno E, Miyahara R, Kawashima H, Itoh A, Watanabe O, Ando T, Goto H. Endoscopic and imaging findings in protein-losing enteropathy. J Clin Gastroenterol. 2012;46(7):575–80.

55. Van De Winkel N, Cheragwandi A, Nieboer K, van Tussenbroek F, De Vogelaere K, Delvaux G. Superior mesenteric arterial branch occlusion causing partial jejunal ischemia: a case report. J Med Case Rep. 2012;6:48.

56. Nishimura N, Yamamoto H, Yano T, Hayashi Y, Sato H, Miura Y, Shinhata H, Sunada K, Sugano K. Balloon dilation when using double-balloon enteroscopy for small-bowel strictures associated with ischemic enteritis. Gastrointest Endosc. 2011;74(5):1157–61.

57. Malamut G, Verkarre V, Suarez F, Viallard JF, Lascaux AS, Cosnes J, Bouhnik Y, Lambotte O, Béchade D, Ziol M, Lavergne A, Hermine O, Cerf-Bensussan N, Cellier C. The enteropathy associated with common variable immunodeficiency: the delineated frontiers with celiac disease. Am J Gastroenterol. 2010; 105(10):2262–75.

Video Legends

Video 11.1 - Typical mucosal findings in a patient with celiac disease: reduction of intestinal folds and scalloping of the mucosa in the jejunum.

Video 11.2 - Intestinal ulceration with bleeding on capsule endoscopy (given SB2) in a patient with celiac disease.

Video 11.3 - Ulcerative jejunitis associated with a jejunal stricture.

Video 11.4 - Biopsies performed with double balloon enteroscopy showed a T cell lymphoma.

Small-Bowel Strictures Dilation and Stent Placement

12

Todd H. Baron

Introduction

Endoscopic dilation of strictures can be achieved with the use of upper endoscopes, colonoscopes, push enteroscopes, and balloon-assisted enteroscopes. Placement of self-expandable stents in the small bowel is most commonly used for palliation of malignant duodenal obstruction from pancreatic cancer but can be placed more distally in select patients. This chapter will review balloon dilation and stent placement in the small bowel.

Small-Bowel Strictures

There are diverse causes of small-bowel strictures due to benign and malignant diseases (Table 12.1). Those in the duodenum are usually due to peptic ulcer disease and pancreatic cancer, respectively. Strictures found more distally are

Electronic supplementary material: The online version of this chapter (doi: 10.1007/978-3-319-14415-3_12) contains supplementary material, which is available to authorized users. Videos can also be accessed at http://link.springer.com/chapter/10.1007/978-3-319-14415-3_12.

T.H. Baron, M.D., F.A.S.G.E. (✉)
Division of Gastroenterology & Hepatology,
University of North Carolina, Chapel Hill,
130 Mason Farm Road, CB 7080, Chapel Hill, NC
27599, USA
e-mail: todd_baron@med.unc.edu

usually due to nonsteroidal anti-inflammatory drugs (NSAIDs) and Crohn's disease. The natural history and response to dilation therapy for benign strictures vary depending on disease process and concomitant medical therapy.

Balloon Dilation

The use of dilation will be discussed principally for management of benign diseases. In patients with prior abdominal and pelvic surgery it is particularly important to distinguish between adhesive disease and stricture disease since the former does not respond to dilation and dilation may result in perforation (Figs. 12.1, 12.2, 12.3, and 12.4).

Whether the endoscope is passed transorally or transrectally or via a stoma [1] depends on location of the stricture and any prior surgery. For example, most strictures in the duodenum will be within reach of an upper endoscope. On the other hand, reaching the second duodenum in patients with markedly distended stomachs from chronic obstruction may be difficult and a colonoscope may be useful. For passage of dilating balloons, the diameter of the working channel does not need to be large and thus standard upper endoscopes and pediatric colonoscopes as well as enteroscopes can be used. However, if one anticipates a large quantity of retained food then a large diameter may be more effective for suction. Accessories to remove food (e.g., Roth nets) should be readily available.

Table 12.1 Causes of small-bowel strictures

Benign
Peptic ulcer
NSAIDs (diaphragm disease)
Crohn's disease
Radiation
Postinfectious (viral)
Ischemic
Radiation
Eosinophilic enteritis
Trauma
Anastomotic
Stenosing enteritis
Malignant
Pancreatic adenocarcinoma (primary or recurrent)
Metastatic disease
Lymphoma
Miscellaneous
Pouch strictures

Moderate sedation or monitored anesthesia care (MAC) may be used, but airway protection with general anesthesia should be considered in patients with anticipated retained gastric contents and for prolonged procedures.

Fluoroscopy should be readily available and used for anticipated complex strictures in cases where the endoscope cannot be passed across the lesion and with angulated stenoses. Accessories for pancreaticobiliary endoscopy (catheters, stone extraction balloons, guidewires) and water-soluble contrast are helpful to traverse and define the anatomy of complex strictures.

Dilating balloons are available in a variety of sizes and lengths [2]. In addition, multisize balloons that inflate sequentially are also available as are balloons that accept a guidewire. Some balloons (CRE™, Boston Scientific, Marlborough, MA) come prepackaged with a "guidewire," which is approximately 15 cm longer than the length of the balloon and can be adjusted and locked. Prior to the procedure, one should also be certain that the balloon catheter is long enough to pass through the chosen endoscope (colonoscope, enteroscope).

The endoscope is advanced to the site of the lesion. If the lesion can be easily traversed with the endoscope this should be attempted and obviates the need for a guidewire. If the endoscope cannot be passed, one should always consider use of fluoroscopy to be certain that the balloon is passing across the stricture. Additionally, the use of a guidewire allows passage of the balloon distal to the stricture and prevents impaction of the tip against the opposite bowel wall, which could result in perforation. Inflation of contrast in the balloon is helpful to be certain the balloon has crossed the entire stricture and whether the waist has effaced with dilation.

When long-length endoscopes are used for strictures in the jejunum it is helpful to use a clear cap attached to the tip, which can help negotiate tight corners and to assess the stricture at angulations [3]. Use of a lubricant (silicone or vegetable oil) within the endoscope channel also facilitates passage of the balloon within the working channel, which can be difficult when the endoscope is looped and/or when the tip is angulated.

The diameter of the balloon chosen is based upon disease process, prior therapy, and diameter of the stricture. For example, in patients with short, membranous strictures the risk of perforation is less and response is more likely than for a long-fibrotic stricture due to Crohn's or radiation therapy. In the former, larger diameter balloons can be used more safely. In general, one should not dilate very tight, pinhole strictures to a diameter larger than 10–12 mm in one session. Additionally, slower dilation times and staged dilations are believed to be safer.

Outcomes Following Balloon Dilation

As previously mentioned, the response to balloon dilation is variable based upon the disease process, associated inflammation, and concomitant medical therapy. More than one dilation may be needed, and the optimal diameter to be reached and maintained as well as the interval between planned dilations are unknown.

There are many series on the outcomes following balloon dilation for Crohn's disease strictures [4–11]. Short-term and long-term success (3 years) are approximately 80 % and 70 %, respectively [4].

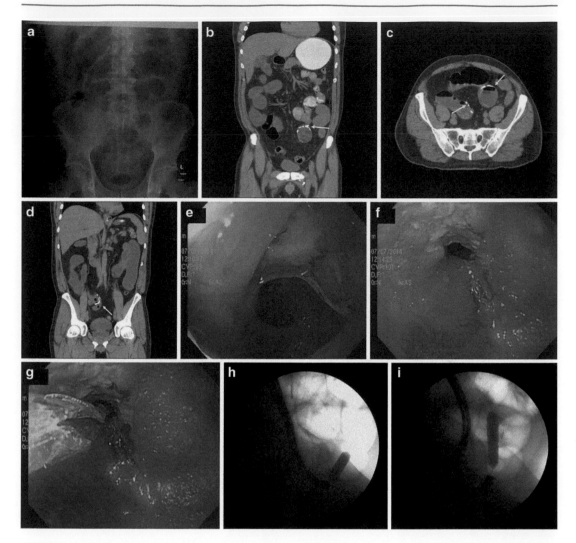

Fig. 12.1 A 60-year-old patient with multiple small-bowel resections for "adhesional strictures." Prior to referral he had >30 hospitalizations for small-bowel obstruction. (**a**) Flat film demonstrates diffuse small-bowel dilation. (**b–d**) *Arrows* demonstrate multiple anastomoses with diffuse upstream small-bowel dilation. Endoscopy demonstrates (**e, f**) ulcerated ileal stenoses treated with (**g–i**) balloon dilation

Adverse events following endoscopic balloon dilation include sedation issues, perforation, and bleeding. Perforation is considered the most common, serious, and likely adverse event to result in need for surgery.

Miscellaneous Treatments

Injection of corticosteroids (Fig. 12.2d) or biologic agents (such as infliximab) into strictures during the same session as balloon dilation may improve long-term outcome of dilation, although this remains unproven. Indeed in one study the outcome was worse with steroid injection compared to placebo [12].

The use of a needle-knife to electroincise webs [13] and strictures [14, 15] has been used (Fig. 12.5); although it is likely best reserved for use by experienced endoscopists since it is performed freehand and may result in inadvertent perforation. Impacted small-bowel capsules can be removed, often concomitantly with web incision or balloon dilation of small-bowel strictures (Fig. 12.6).

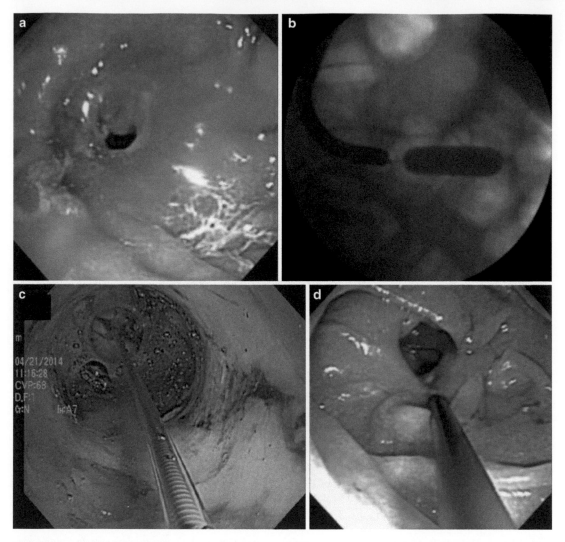

Fig. 12.2 (**a**) High-grade duodenal stricture in Crohn's patient treated with (**b, c**) balloon dilation and (**d**) steroid injection

Stent Placement

Most stents used for small bowel use are self-expandable metal stents (SEMS) (Fig. 12.7, Videos 12.1, 12.2, and 12.3). They are composed of a variety of metal alloys [16], although almost all are now composed of nitinol. SEMS are preloaded in a collapsed (constrained) position, mounted on a small-diameter delivery catheter. A central lumen within the delivery system allows for passage over a guidewire. Once the guidewire has been advanced beyond the site of pathology, the predeployed stent is passed over the guidewire and positioned across the stricture. The constraint system is released or withdrawn, which results in subsequent radial expansion of the stent and of the stenosed lumen (if present) during deployment. The radial expansile forces and degree of shortening differ between stent types [17]. SEMS may also have a covering membrane

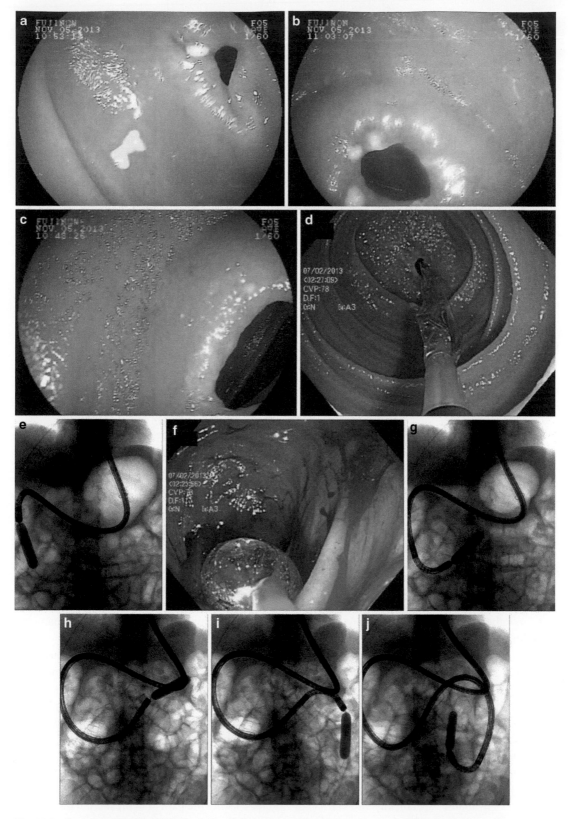

Fig. 12.3 (a–c) Multiple NSAID webs in duodenum and jejunum treated with (d–j) balloon dilation. Patient was taking ibuprofen for rheumatoid arthritis. Eight webs were dilated over two endoscopy sessions using both the single balloon and double balloon enteroscopes

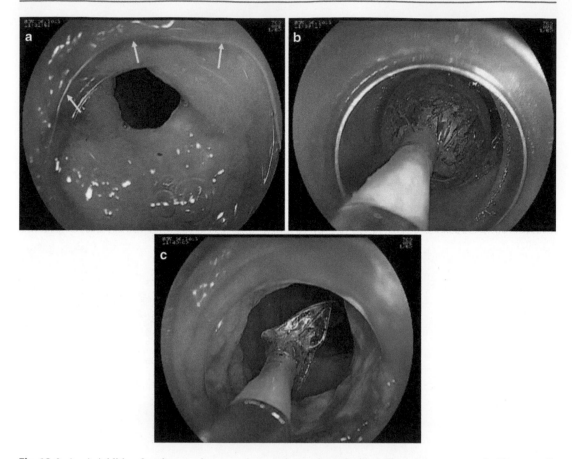

Fig. 12.4 (**a–c**) Additional endoscopy images using cap (*arrows*) on double balloon enteroscope to facilitate small-bowel web dilation (Images courtesy of Louis Wong Kee Song, Rochester, MN.)

(covered or coated stents) to close fistulae and to prevent tumor ingrowth (and subsequent re-obstruction) through the mesh wall.

The uncovered portion of SEMS becomes deeply imbedded into both the tumor and surrounding tissue [18, 19]. This prevents migration. Covering of the SEMS prevents imbedding and promotes stent migration; fully covered metal stents do not imbed and can be removed but are prone to migration [20]. In general, uncovered SEMS should not be used for treatment of benign strictures since they are usually not removable and can result in long-term problems such as tissue hyperplasia, obstruction, and ulceration.

Only three stents from two different manufacturers are available specifically for relief of enteral obstruction and all are uncovered (Table 12.2). These stents pass directly through the working channel of the endoscope (through-the-scope, TTS). Non-TTS stent placement (esophageal or colonic) into the duodenum with native anatomy is difficult, but possible. Additionally, one can also use smaller diameter (10 mm) TTS biliary stents alone or in side-by-side fashion (the latter allows a diameter of up to 20 mm to be achieved). A final option in the U.S. if a covered and removable stent is desired is the use of a covered TTS esophageal stent. Currently, the only such prosthesis available is the Niti-S (Taewoong Medical, Seoul, South Korea).

Optimal endoscopic stent placement may be impaired by the presence of retained gastric contents. Placing the patient in the left lateral decubitus position prevents aspiration, but often results in a suboptimal fluoroscopic image. Placing the

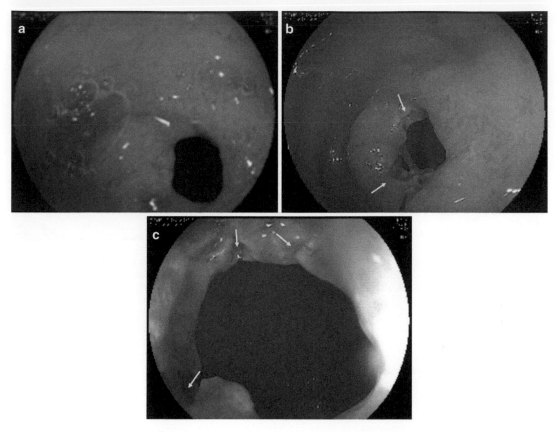

Fig. 12.5 (**a**) Short-stricture/small-bowel web re-treated with (**b, c**) endoscopic electrosection (Images courtesy of Louis Wong Kee Song, Rochester, MN.)

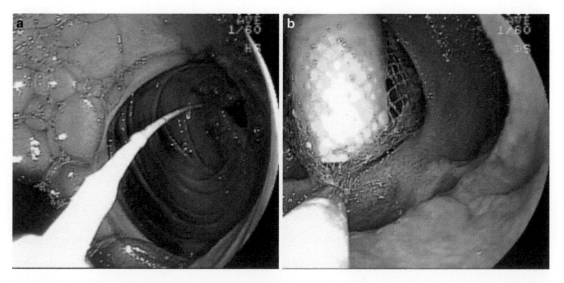

Fig. 12.6 (**a**) Distal jejunal anastomotic Crohn's stricture with impacted small-bowel endoscopy capsule. (**b**) Following balloon dilation, the capsule was removed with a Roth net

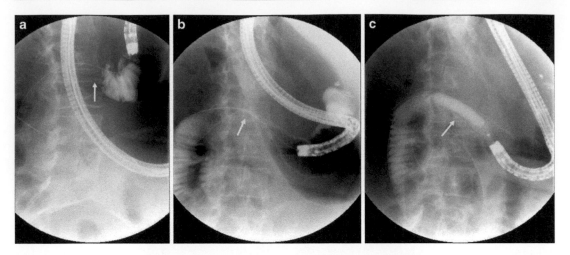

Fig. 12.7 Palliation of duodenal obstruction due to pancreatic cancer. (**a**) Injection of contrast through a biliary catheter outlines stricture in the duodenum (*arrow*). (**b**) Radiograph taken immediately after deployment of duo-denal SEMS. Note proximal end is in the gastric antrum. Stent remains tightly contracted (*arrow*) and (**c**) is dilated with 10–12 mm CRE balloon (*arrow*)

Table 12.2 Expandable duodenal stents

	Materials	Deployed diameters	Deployed lengths (cm)	Features
Boston Scientific				
Wallstent Enteral®a	Elgiloy® (Cobalt-Chromium-Nickel)	20 mm 22 mm	6, 9	TTS delivery; reconstrainable; 39–49 % foreshortening during expansion
Wallflex Enteral Duodenala	Nitinol	22 mm body, 27 mm proximal flare	6, 9, 12	TTS delivery; reconstrainable; 30–38 % foreshortening during expansion
Cook Endoscopy				
Evolution Duodenal Stenta	Nitinol	22 mm (proximal and distal flares 27 mm)	6, 9, 12	TTS delivery; reconstrainable; 45 % foreshortening during expansion
MI Tech				
Hanarostent pyloroduodenal	Nitinol Uncovered Partially covered	18 mm	8, 11, 14 6, 9, 11, 13	TTS delivery (uncovered), reconstrainable
Taewoong Medical				
Pyloric	Nitinol Uncovered Covered	18, 20 (proximal and distal flares 24 and 28 mm)	6, 8, 10, 12	TTS delivery
CS Ella				
SX-ELLA pyloroduodenal	Nitinol Uncovered	20, 22, 25	8, 9, 11, 13.5	TTS delivery

aFDA-approved

patient in the prone or supine position is preferred for fluoroscopic visualization, but if the latter is chosen the patient should be carefully monitored and suctioned, and any gastric contents removed, if possible, as soon as the stomach is entered. Endotracheal intubation should be strongly considered to prevent aspiration.

Before undertaking gastroduodenal stent placement it is important to assess the status of the biliary tree first, since placement of an expandable stent across the papilla may make subsequent endoscopic access to the papilla difficult, if not impossible. In addition, in patients with proximal duodenal strictures, the stent may not need to cross the papilla to achieve palliation. Thus, a stent should be chosen that is adequate to cross the lesion, but not excessively long so as to prevent access to the papilla. Large-caliber therapeutic channel endoscopes (working channel ≥3.8 mm) are needed to place TTS stents and thus, it is frequently not possible to pass the endoscope across the stricture; this is not necessary to achieve placement, and aggressive dilation of the stricture should be avoided to prevent perforation.

The stricture is traversed using biliary endoscopic techniques and accessories using fluoroscopic guidance. Sphincterotomes are also useful since they can be bowed to change the direction of orientation, especially those that can be rotated. In addition, changing from a forward-viewing endoscope to a side-viewing endoscope may improve access to lumen of the stricture. Once the stricture is traversed with the guidewire, catheter contrast can be injected to define stricture length. The stent chosen should be about 4 cm longer than the measured stricture.

Enteral stents foreshorten up to 40 % during deployment and all deploy from the distal end. Thus, in order to prevent malpositioning of the stent it is important to maintain the endoscope in a position about 3–4 cm proximally from the proximal end of the stricture while continuously monitoring the proximal end. The stent will appear to move away from the tip of the endoscope as it is delivered and while it expands and shortens; thus, the endoscopist almost always needs to pull back on the delivery system during deployment to maintain proper position.

For strictures in the second duodenum there is some debate about whether or not the proximal end of the stent should remain in the proximal duodenum or in the gastric antrum because of the potential difference in functional result. Stent-induced perforation has been reported with stents that possess sharp ends when the proximal end remains in the duodenum [21]. However, newer stents with rounded edges may reduce this adverse event.

Placement of stents beyond the duodenum can be achieved using TTS stents that pass through the working channel of a colonoscope. To reach lesions far from the mouth or anus, balloon enteroscopes can be used. Commercially available stents are not long enough to pass through standard balloon enteroscopes, but can be achieved by passing the delivery system through "short" double balloon enteroscopes or by passing them through the overtube of standard length balloon enteroscopes [22–25], or use of a spiral enteroscope [26].

Outcome Following Small-Bowel Stent

There are many publications describing the efficacy of SEMS for palliating gastric outlet obstruction (GOO) due to pancreatic cancer. In a systematic review of 32 case series, including 10 prospective series of gastric and pancreaticobiliary malignancies [27], 606 patients underwent attempted stent placement. Technical success, defined as successful stent placement and deployment, was achieved in 589 (97 %). Technical failure was attributed to severe obstruction, difficult anatomy, malpositioning, and one failed delivery. Clinical success, defined as relief of symptoms and improved oral intake, occurred in 89 % of the technical successes. Clinical failures were due to early stent migration (20 %) and disease progression (61 %), and procedural adverse events (AEs) (15 %) such as malpositioned stent or partially expanded stent. Severe complications included bleeding (1 %). There were no procedure-related deaths. Nonsevere AEs occurred in 27 % of attempted stent placements. The most commonly

Table 12.3 Adverse events following small-bowel stent placement

Perforation: immediate/delayed
Obstruction: tumor ingrowth, overgrowth, and tissue hyperplasia
Bleeding
Migration

reported nonsevere AE was stent occlusion (17 %) primarily due to tumor growth or obstruction away from the stent. Migration occurred in 5 % of patients, generally managed with additional stent placement. Pain was reported in 2 % of subjects. The mean survival was 12.1 weeks. The majority of nonsevere AEs were related to stent obstruction. Adverse events following small-bowel stent placement are seen in Table 12.3.

Surgical gastroenterostomy has been compared to endoscopic SEMS for palliation of unresectable malignant GOO stenosis. Time to ingestion of both liquids and light consistency diet and post-procedure length of hospital stay are significantly shorter in the endoscopic stent group compared to surgical groups. Initial postprocedural and procedural costs are higher in the gastrojejunostomy groups [28]. However, recurrent obstruction occurs more often in the stent group. In a systematic review endoscopic SEMS placement is the preferred strategy over open or laparoscopic gastrojejunostomy for palliation of malignant gastric outlet obstruction in patients with a short life expectancy on the basis of effectiveness, fewer complications, reduced cost, and earlier resumption of per oral intake [29]. No difference in morbidity mortality is seen in these studies.

References

1. Chen M, Shen B. Ileoscopic balloon dilation of Crohn's disease strictures via stoma. Gastrointest Endosc. 2014;79:688–93.
2. ASGE Technology Committee, Siddiqui UD, Banerjee S, Barth B, Chauhan SS, Gottlieb KT, et al. Tools for endoscopic stricture dilation. Gastrointest Endosc. 2013;78:391–404.
3. Hayashi Y, Yamamoto H, Yano T, Kitamura A, Takezawa T, Ino Y, et al. A calibrated, small-caliber tip, transparent hood to aid endoscopic balloon dilation of intestinal strictures in Crohn's disease: successful use of prototype. Endoscopy. 2013; 45(Suppl 2 UCTN):E373–4.
4. Hirai F, Beppu T, Takatsu N, Yano Y, Ninomiya K, Ono Y, et al. Long-term outcome of endoscopic balloon dilation for small bowel strictures in patients with Crohn's disease. Dig Endosc. 2014;26:545–51.
5. Hirai F, Beppu T, Sou S, Seki T, Yao K, Matsui T. Endoscopic balloon dilatation using double-balloon endoscopy is a useful and safe treatment for small intestinal strictures in Crohn's disease. Dig Endosc. 2010;22:200–4.
6. Manes G, Imbesi V, Ardizzone S, Cassinotti A, Pallotta S, Porro GB. Use of double-balloon enteroscopy in the management of patients with Crohn's disease: feasibility and diagnostic yield in a high-volume centre for inflammatory bowel disease. Surg Endosc. 2009;23:2790–5.
7. Stienecker K, Gleichmann D, Neumayer U, Glaser HJ, Tonus C. Long-term results of endoscopic balloon dilatation of lower gastrointestinal tract strictures in Crohn's disease: a prospective study. World J Gastroenterol. 2009;15:2623–7.
8. Despott EJ, Gupta A, Burling D, Tripoli E, Konieczko K, Hart A, et al. Effective dilation of small-bowel strictures by double-balloon enteroscopy in patients with symptomatic Crohn's disease (with video). Gastrointest Endosc. 2009;70:1030–6.
9. Foster EN, Quiros JA, Prindiville TP. Long-term follow-up of the endoscopic treatment of strictures in pediatric and adult patients with inflammatory bowel disease. J Clin Gastroenterol. 2008;42:880–5.
10. Pohl J, May A, Nachbar L, Ell C. Diagnostic and therapeutic yield of push-and-pull enteroscopy for symptomatic small bowel Crohn's disease strictures. Eur J Gastroenterol Hepatol. 2007;19:529–34.
11. Singh VV, Draganov P, Valentine J. Efficacy and safety of endoscopic balloon dilation of symptomatic upper and lower gastrointestinal Crohn's disease strictures. J Clin Gastroenterol. 2005;39:284–9.
12. East JE, Brooker JC, Rutter MD, Saunders BP. A pilot study of intrastricture steroid versus placebo injection after balloon dilatation of Crohn's strictures. Clin Gastroenterol Hepatol. 2007;5:1065–9.
13. Blanco-Rodríguez G, Penchyna-Grub J, Porras-Hernández JD, Trujillo-Ponce A. Transluminal endoscopic electrosurgical incision of fenestrated duodenal membranes. Pediatr Surg Int. 2008;24:711–4.
14. Kerkhof M, Dewint P, Koch AD, van der Woude CJ. Endoscopic needle-knife treatment of refractory ileo-ascending anastomotic stricture. Endoscopy. 2013;45(Suppl 2 UCTN):E57–8. doi:10.1055/s-0032-1325973.
15. Paine E, Shen B. Endoscopic therapy in inflammatory bowel diseases (with videos). Gastrointest Endosc. 2013;78:819–35.
16. Baron TH. Expandable gastrointestinal stents. Gastroenterology. 2007;133:1407–11.
17. Chan AC, Shin FG, Lam YH, et al. A comparison study on physical properties of self-expandable

esophageal metal stents. Gastrointest Endosc. 1999;49:462–5.

18. Silvis SE, Sievert Jr CE, Vennes JA, Abeyta BK, Brennecke LH. Comparison of covered versus uncovered wire mesh stents in the canine biliary tract. Gastrointest Endosc. 1994;40:17–21.

19. Bethge N, Sommer A, Gross U, von Kleist D, Vakil N. Human tissue responses to metal stents implanted in vivo for the palliation of malignant stenoses. Gastrointest Endosc. 1996;43:596–602.

20. Eloubeidi MA, Lopes TL. Novel removable internally fully covered self-expanding metal esophageal stent: feasibility, technique of removal, and tissue response in humans. Am J Gastroenterol. 2009; 104:1374–81.

21. Small AJ, Petersen BT, Baron TH. Closure of a duodenal stent-induced perforation by endoscopic stent removal and covered self-expandable metal stent placement (with video). Gastrointest Endosc. 2007;66:1063–5.

22. Popa D, Ramesh J, Peter S, Wilcox CM, Mönkemüller K. Small bowel stent-in-stent placement for malignant small bowel obstruction using a balloon-assisted overtube technique. Clin Endosc. 2014;47:108–11.

23. Pérez-Cuadrado E, Carballo F, Latorre R, Soria F, López-Albors O. An endoscopic technique for treating symptomatic distal jejunum obstruction by leaving the overtube in place. Rev Esp Enferm Dig. 2013;105:107–9.

24. Espinel J, Pinedo E. A simplified method for stent placement in the distal duodenum: enteroscopy overtube. World J Gastrointest Endosc. 2011;3:225–7.

25. Ross AS, Semrad C, Waxman I, Dye C. Enteral stent placement by double balloon enteroscopy for palliation of malignant small bowel obstruction. Gastrointest Endosc. 2006;64:835–7.

26. Lennon AM, Chandrasekhara V, Shin EJ, Okolo 3rd PI. Spiral-enteroscopy-assisted enteral stent placement for palliation of malignant small-bowel obstruction (with video). Gastrointest Endosc. 2010;71:422–5.

27. Dormann A, Meisner S, Verin N, Wenk LA. Self-expanding metal stents for gastroduodenal malignancies: systematic review of their clinical effectiveness. Endoscopy. 2004;36:543–50.

28. Mittal A, Windsor J, Woodfield J, Casey P, Lane M. Matched study of three methods for palliation of malignant pyloroduodenal obstruction. Br J Surg. 2004;91:205–9.

29. Jeurnink SM, van Eijck CH, Steyerberg EW, Kuipers EJ, Siersema PD. Stent versus gastrojejunostomy for the palliation of gastric outlet obstruction: a systematic review. BMC Gastroenterol. 2007;7:18.

Video Legends

Video 12.1 - Placement of expandable metal stent in a patient with prior pyloric sparing Whipple and biliary obstruction. There is downstream obstruction due to recurrent tumor in the afferent limb. The stricture could not be traversed with biliary accessories using an adult colonoscope. The single balloon endoscope was advanced to the lesion and allowed an en face view of the stricture. It was then traversed. A guidewire and catheter were left in place. The adult colonoscope was then loaded over the wire and an enteral stent placed.

Video 12.2 - Placement of a WallFlex stent to open an ileal obstruction. Video courtesy of Louis M. Wong Kee Song, MD, at Mayo, Rochester.

Video 12.3 - Placement of a WallFlex stent to open a gastric outlet obstruction at the ligament of Treitz. Video courtesy of Louis M. Wong Kee Song, MD, at Mayo, Rochester.

Small-Bowel Tumors, Polyps, and Polyposis Syndromes

13

Alessandra Bizzotto, Maria Elena Riccioni,
Rosario Landi, Clelia Marmo, Brunella Barbaro,
and Guido Costamagna

Small-Bowel Tumors

Epidemiology, Pathology, Clinical Presentation, and Prognosis

The small bowel accounts for almost 75 % of the anatomical length and 90 % of the absorptive surface of the alimentary tract. Despite this, small-bowel tumors (SBTs) are remarkably rare entities, accounting for approximately 3–6 % of all primary gastrointestinal tumors and 1–3 % of all gastrointestinal malignancies [1, 2]. Owing to their rarity, coupled with the limited access to the small intestine, due to its mobility and tortuosity, SBTs pose unique diagnostic and management challenges. According to autopsy data, approximately 40 different histological subtypes of

Electronic supplementary material: The online version of this chapter (doi: 10.1007/978-3-319-14415-3_13) contains supplementary material, which is available to authorized users. Videos can also be accessed at http://link.springer.com/chapter/10.1007/978-3-319-14415-3_13.

A. Bizzotto, M.D. • M.E. Riccioni, M.D. (✉) • R. Landi
C. Marmo, M.S. • G. Costamagna, M.D., F.A.C.G.
Digestive Endoscopy Unit, Università Cattolica del Sacro Cuore, Largo A. Gemelli, Rome 00168, Italy
e-mail: melena.riccioni@rm.unicatt.it;
gcostamagna@rm.unicatt.it

B. Barbaro, M.D.
Department of Bioimaging and Radiological Sciences, Università Cattolica del Sacro Cuore,
Largo A. Gemelli, Rome 00168, Italy
e-mail: brunella.barbaro@rm.unicatt.it

tumors arise in the small bowel, with the four most common being carcinoids (35–42 %), adenocarcinomas (30–40 %), mesenchymal tumors—mainly gastrointestinal stromal tumors (GISTs) (10–15 %) (Fig. 13.1)—and lymphomas (15–20 %). The sites at higher risk are the duodenum and duodenal/jejunal junction for adenocarcinomas (Fig. 13.2) and the ileum for carcinoids (Fig. 13.3), whereas lymphomas (Fig. 13.4) occur most commonly in the jejunum or ileum [2, 3].

SBTs typically present in middle-aged adults and elderly people, especially during the sixth and seventh decades, with a slight male predominance. There is a geographical variation with SBTs being more frequent in Western countries, as well as a racial/ethnic difference, with a higher incidence of adenocarcinomas and malignant carcinoids among black populations [2–4]. Although a complete understanding of the pathogenesis of SBTs has not yet been reached, it is generally postulated that the small bowel has some protection against cancer that the adjacent organs lack [4]. In particular protective factors may be rapid cell turnover, rapid transit times, low-bacterial load, alkaline environment, low levels of activating enzymes or precarcinogens, high levels of lymphoid aggregates, and IgA. Environmental and behavioral factors may certainly also play a role. Finally, some medical or genetic cancerous and noncancerous bowel conditions, such as celiac disease, inflammatory bowel disease, inherited polyposis (discussed later in this chapter) and nonpolyposis syndromes, confer an increased risk

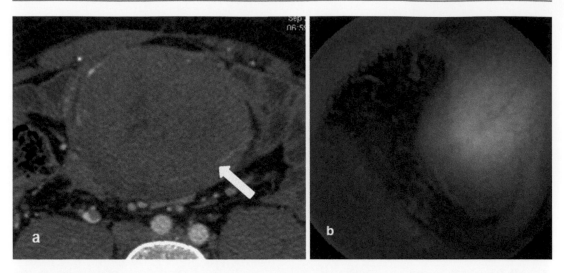

Fig. 13.1 An ileal GIST: at abdominal CT in the axial scans (**a**) and at CE (**b**)

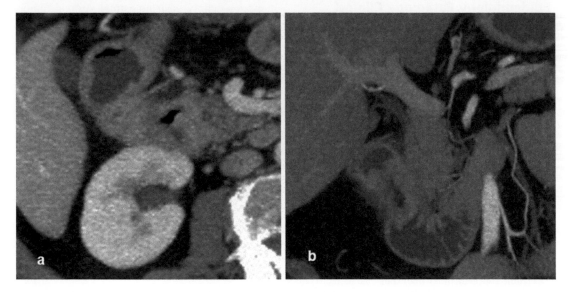

Fig. 13.2 CTE showing, in axial scan, a duodenal lesion (**a**) and, in coronal scan, neoplastic stenosis with thickening of the wall (**b**)

for developing SBTs [3, 4]. Hence, patients presenting with SBTs should always be assessed for one of these underlying conditions [5].

As for secondary small-bowel cancers, they can occur either by direct invasion or as a result of distant metastasis spread. Metastatic SBTs derive from melanomas, prostate, lung, kidney, breast, and testes. Melanoma is the most common metastatic tumor to the small bowel. Intestinal melanomas can be primary tumors but

more commonly are metastases, affecting the jejunum and ileum [6] (Fig. 13.5, Video 13.1).

The rising incidence rates of primary SBTs [2] partially reflect both a better understanding and increased awareness of the disease, with a higher index of clinical suspicion and a lower threshold to order further investigations. It is also related to the improvements in diagnostic capabilities with the advent of novel endoscopic devices and high-performance radiological techniques for a

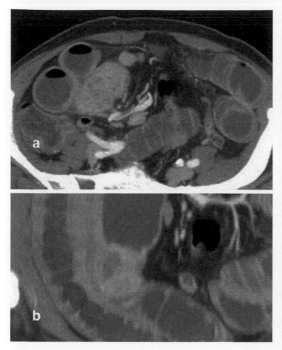

Fig. 13.3 Ileal carcinoid, in CTE axial (**a**) and coronal (**b**) scan, appearing like a solid formation with inhomogeneous enhancement

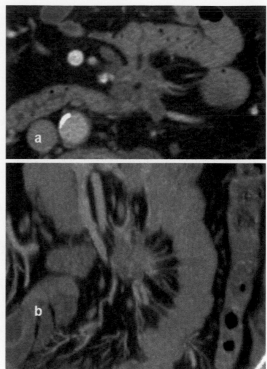

Fig. 13.4 Intestinal lymphoma in patient with HIV at the abdomen CT in axial (**a**) and coronal (**b**) scan

thorough small-bowel evaluation. Due to their rarity and nonspecific clinical presentation, SBTs are indeed difficult to diagnose and quite often detected in advanced stages. Physical examination is usually unrevealing. Symptoms and signs associated to SBTs are vague, nonspecific, indistinct, or inconclusive. They may include any of the following: dyspepsia, minor anemia, vague or cramping abdominal pain, bloating, fatigue, nausea and vomiting related to partial, intermittent, or complete bowel obstruction, weight loss, anorexia, diarrhea, perforation, palpable abdominal mass, jaundice in case of periampullary lesions, frank bleeding, and chronic obscure-occult bleeding. All of these clinical signs and symptoms show poor sensitivity and specificity. Even the serotonine activity-related visible signs and symptoms of carcinoid syndrome (flushing, diarrhea, wheezing) correlate with a tumor that has already progressed [6–9].

Malignant tumors arising from the small bowel have a poor prognosis, with an overall 5-year relative survival rate of 54 % (83 % for carcinoids, 25 % for adenocarcinomas, 62 % for lymphomas, and 45 % for sarcomas) [10]. Many SBTs can remain clinically silent for years. The available literature reports approximately a 10- to 20-month mean delay in diagnosis from first symptoms. Delayed diagnosis contributes to the poor survival prognosis. Diagnosis at an early stage would be desirable, because the mainstay of treatment for adenocarcinomas, GISTs, and carcinoids is complete curative resection. Cancer-directed surgery, early stage disease, and lymph node involvement ratio are key prognostic factors significantly associated with overall survival. On the other hand the diagnosis of a lymphoproliferative disorder may change the management from surgical to medical [11–14]. All of these factors support the need to have a high index of suspicion for small-intestinal neoplasms and to perform a more aggressive diagnostic work-up in patients with vague gastrointestinal symptoms (Video 13.2).

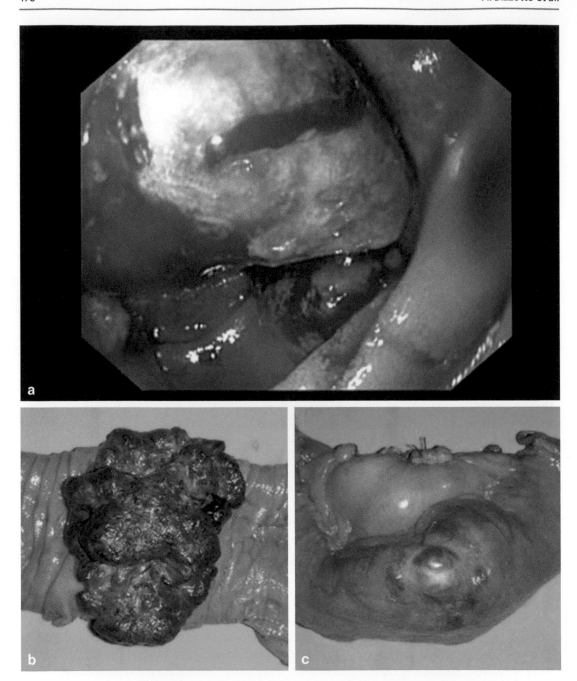

Fig. 13.5 Melanoma of the small bowel, at endoscopic diagnosis (**a**) and surgical specimen after resection (**b, c**)

SBTs in the *Old* Era

Until the advent of capsule endoscopy and device-assisted enteroscopy coupled with the advances in radiology, physicians had to deal with limited diagnostic capabilities for investigating the small bowel. Accurate and early preoperative diagnosis of SBTs proved difficult. Intraoperative enteroscopy (diagnostic yield ranging from 70 to 100 % in patients with obscure-gastrointestinal bleeding) and surgery were the sole, rather invasive, procedures providing definite evidence

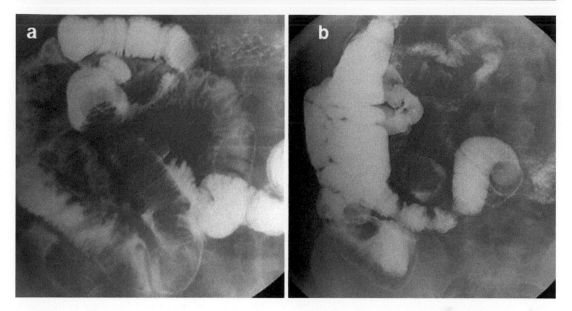

Fig. 13.6 Ileal lipoma with intussusception at SBFT: filling defect with spiral morphology in ileal loop

of lesions, polyps, or masses deeply located in the small intestine and allowing their treatment [15]. Leaving the obsolete sonde enteroscopy out of any consideration, diagnosis of SBTs was mainly based on barium-contrast radiology, such as small-bowel follow-through (SBFT) (Fig. 13.6) or enteroclysis, push enteroscopy, or in selected cases angiography. Although abnormalities may be seen in up to 83 % of patients with SBTs, upper gastrointestinal series with a SBFT deserves limited utility given its low sensitivity for SBTs of 30–44 % [16, 17]. Owing to their partial evaluation of the small bowel and overall low-diagnostic yield, these techniques are gradually being phased out in favor of more efficient and effective endoscopic and radiological techniques.

Regardless of clinical indications, sensitivity at enteroclysis is superior to sensitivity at SBFT: 87–96 % reported by most authors [18]. In particular, enteroclysis is a good technique to identify folds, masses, and large protruding proximally located or obstructive small-bowel lesions. In a series of 71 patients diagnosed with primary mesenteric malignant tumors of the small intestine over a 21-year period, the tumor detection rate of standard enteroclysis was 90 %

as compared to 33 % of SBFT [19]. However, surface coating is suboptimal due to barium dilution and enteroclysis is ineffective in visualizing the luminal surface directly, small sized and flat lesions, and/or lesions of the terminal ileum. Moreover, patient's discomfort, high-radiation dose, and complexity have limited its use [20].

Conventional computed tomography (CT) scan and magnetic resonance (MR) imaging are reliable methods for detection of small-bowel masses, for localization, for assessment of their relationship to adjacent structures, and for staging of metastatic spread and lymph nodes involvement. However, it is important to note that they might miss small intraluminal and mucosal lesions and lack the capacity to distinguish subtypes of SBTs [18, 21]. Over the past years, conventional CT scan and MR imaging have substantially been improved with the adjunct of oral or small-bowel contrasts allowing a more accurate bowel filling and distension, and demonstrating high accuracy for the detection and location of small-bowel lesions [22, 23].

Push enteroscopy is limited to the proximal jejunum, allowing an average of 50–100 cm of the small intestine to be intubated. It is still useful for the identification and sampling of proximal tumors, but is inferior to CE and push-and-pull enteroscopy with regard to the length of the small bowel visualized, as well as the diagnostic yield [24, 25]. In patients referred for obscure-gastrointestinal bleeding (OGIB) and positive radiologic findings, the diagnostic yield of push enteroscopy for SBTs is about 5–6 % [26]. Standard esophagogastroduodenoscopy plays a primary role in the assessment of lesions located in the duodenum. The terminal ileum is success-fully investigated through colonoscopy with ile-oscopy up to 45 cm [27].

SBTs: Outcome and Results in the *New* Era

Since the advent of capsule endoscopy (CE) there has been a growing body of evidence showing its superiority over the traditional small intestine diagnostic tests. CE proved superior to SBFT and push enteroscopy for the diagnosis of small-bowel diseases. CE effectively identifies lesions beyond the reach of push enteroscopy, including SBTs undetected by conventional radiological studies with a diagnostic yield of 52.6–65.2 % [25, 28, 29]. As such, CE has become the front-line diagnostic tool in case of suspected small-bowel diseases, after negative upper GI endoscopy and colonoscopy [30]. However, it is important to emphasize that CE, though providing a complete evaluation of the small bowel, has limitations. In particular, CE is not very good at evaluating the duodenal sweep and the periampullary area. Standard endoscopy methods are still important here [31, 32]. A possible explanation is the rapid capsule transit time across the duodenal sweep.

Clinical studies on CE have reported a fre-quency of SBTs differently ranging between 4 and 10 %. The majority (approximately 60 %) are malignant. Occasionally, small-bowel malig-nancies are secondary tumors, mainly originating from skin melanomas [29, 33–38]. The great variation in the reported frequency of SBTs is likely multifactorial and related to the retrospec-tive design of the studies, the analysis of preva-lence only in patients with OGIB, the absence of

a standardized approach, the inclusion of both benign and malignant tumors [37], and the inclu-sion of hereditary polyposis syndromes. In any case, it appears that CE has increased the rate of diagnosing SBTs and a detection rate even up to 13.7 % has been reported in the recent literature [39]. This might be the result of a selection bias in tertiary referral centers. This is supported by the fact that a recent multicenter European study [40] including 5,129 patients undergoing CE showed a 2.4 % frequency of SBTs. This surpris-ingly low result seems consistent with the 1.6 % detection rate of SBTs reported in another large study based on 1,000 CE examinations [41]. The low frequency of tumors detected might be related to the high number of capsule studies per-formed, as the authors themselves suggest [40].

Chronic occult or overt bleeding is the most common presentation of SBTs [15] and the usual clinical indication for CE in 80 % of cases [29, 35, 37, 40]. Whenever CE is performed for OGIB, SBTs are detected in 6–12 % of cases, the incidence being higher in adults <50 years of age [6, 15, 42]. In descending order of incidence, SBTs reside in the jejunum in 40–60 % of cases, in the ileum in 25–40 % of cases, and less fre-quently in the duodenum (15–20 % of cases) [29, 33, 35–37, 41]. The preponderance of the lesions in the mid-gut may account for the extensive work-up that patients usually have undergone prior to CE. The literature suggests that patients undergo between 3.6 and 5 negative procedures, including SBFT, enteroclysis, push enteroscopy, and abdominal CT scan [33, 37, 43]. As for the endoscopic appearance of SBTs at capsule imaging, many descriptors have been used to describe the findings [39]. The heterogeneous terminology used for capsule images has prompted an expert panel to establish a structured common terminology, which includes nodule, polyp, submucosal, ulcerated, fungating, frond-like or villous, bleeding or nonbleeding mass, or tumor [44, 45]. SBTs generally appear at CE as masses or polyps in 70–80 % of cases and as ulcers or strictures in 20–30 % of cases [46].

Based only on capsule images, it is not pos-sible to distinguish the tumor type or whether a lesion is malignant or benign [46, 47]. Therefore, in case of a suspected SBT—for example, as a result of cross-sectional imaging techniques—the European Society of Gastrointestinal Endoscopy (ESGE) guidelines on flexible enteroscopy recommend balloon-assisted enteroscopy as the first choice, given its potential for histopathological diagnosis through tissue sampling [47]. A novel index aiming to overcome the potential CE false-positive findings and aiming to discriminate a mucosal bulge from a mass was recently developed: the Smooth Protruding Index on Capsule Endoscopy (SPICE) score [48]. A SPICE score higher than 2 had an 83 % sensitivity and 89 % specificity for tumors. Other attempts to differentiate tumors on CE include an automated scale using multiscale wavelet-based analysis in capsule endoscopy images that is reported to have 93 % sensitivity and specificity [49].

CE allows noninvasive evaluation of the entire small bowel in 79–90 % of patients, with a high-diagnostic yield and positive and negative predictive values approaching respectively 83, 97, and 100 % in the evaluation of OGIB [50]. The performance of CE for tumor detection was very good with sensitivity, specificity, NPV, and PPV values reaching 83.3, 100, 97.6, and 100 %, respectively [51]. In the setting of SBTs, the influence of CE on the final diagnosis and management may be as high as 77 % [43]. With regard to therapeutic impact, in one series including 443 CE examinations with a SBT detection rate of 2.5 %, CE had an impact on therapy in 6 out of 11 patients (55 %) [37]. In a large-multicenter study on 1,132 patients, where 4.3 % (57) of SBTs were diagnosed with CE, capsule critically changed the therapeutic course in 12.3 % of patients (7/57) leading to surgical intervention [28]. In the study by Bailey et al., curative resection was performed in 52 % of patients with SBTs and they remained recurrencefree at a mean follow-up of 38 months, most likely because of an earlier stage at diagnosis [29]. Further long-term studies are needed to clarify the impact of CE on outcomes and its role in surveillance of SBTs.

Capsule endoscopy can also play a role in surveillance of small-bowel lesions. CE has been shown to be useful in the surveillance of small-bowel lymphomas and to assess response to treatment, including lymphomas in type II refractory celiac disease [52, 53]. The ESGE guidelines indicate, in these cases too, the importance of balloon-assisted enteroscopy as for the ability to take biopsies [47].

CE is actually a mere visual diagnostic tool. Its major drawbacks include the inability to perform tissue sampling, the absence of therapeutic capabilities, the inability to control its movement through the gastrointestinal tract, and poor localization and sizing of lesions. Another important disadvantage is the misdiagnosis due to false-negative CE examinations [54]. Poor bowel preparation, rapid passage, random movements of the capsule, inadequate bowel distension, or incomplete small-bowel examinations may hamper or prevent diagnosis. The highest miss rate refers to solitary small-bowel mass lesions. In a pooled analysis of 24 trials representing 530 patients, the authors recorded an 18.9 % CE miss-rate for small neoplasms [55]. Recent comparative studies reported on SBTs missed at CE but identified with CT enterography [56, 57] or balloon-assisted enteroscopy (BAE) [58], with two-thirds of the overlooked SBTs involving the duodenum/proximal jejunum [51, 57]. When stratified according to the site of tumor, the diagnostic yield for SBTs in the distal duodenum/proximal jejunum is lower (73 %) than for those located more distally (90 %) [57]. Though a negative CE may be reassuring in many cases, when there is a high index of suspicion, as in the case of persistent or alarm symptoms, the clinician should have a low threshold to further investigate with complementary endoscopic and/or radiologic tests [56–59].

This must also be balanced by the fact that CE can identify nonspecific lesions that are, in fact, false positives. Incidental findings, such as erosions and angiodysplasias, are common and may be mistaken as a source of bleeding [46, 50, 56]. Another limitation of CE is the possible risk of retention. The risk of CE retention due to a stricture or mass, in the setting of a definite or suspected SBT, may be as high as 10 % [40]. A pooled analysis of 227 papers including 22,840 CE procedures found an overall CE retention rate of 1.4 % [60]. A low-retention rate was associated with OGIB, whereas a relatively high retention rate was associated with neoplasms. In many of these cases, however, CE retention may be regarded as a therapeutic adverse event, leading to a diagnosis and ultimately to surgical resection of the lesion and CE retrieval. The use of a dissolvable patency capsule to test for small-bowel patency is a viable method to reduce retention risk in patients at higher risk for obstruction [46].

Following the development of the capsule, the advent of device-assisted enteroscopy (DAE) is a further major breakthrough in the diagnosis and therapy of small-bowel cancerous lesions. DAE encompasses double-balloon enteroscopy (DBE), single-balloon enteroscopy (SBE), and spiral enteroscopy (SE). All of these techniques allow a deep and theoretically total enteroscopy with the assistance of an overtube that facilitates the pleating of the small bowel over the scope and overtube assembly by means of push-pull anchoring movements or rotational movements. Using these techniques, the depth of intubation of the small bowel (240–360 cm on oral approach and 102–140 cm with the retrograde route) is much greater compared to push enteroscopy and ileoscopy [61]. The rate of total enteroscopy has been reported to range from 5 to 86 % and is very operator dependent [62]. Patients having undergone extensive abdominal surgery may be poor candidates for DAE because of adhesions or altered anatomy, which may prevent the endoscope from advancing. The subtypes of DAE share the same indications, drawbacks (invasive nature, prolonged duration, requirement for additional personnel), and complications (pancreatitis, perforation, bleeding, paralytic ileus) without significant differences in technical and clinical success rates [61]. The choice of one or the other technique depends on local expertise and availability. DAE is invasive and labor intensive, but holds the potential for histological diagnosis with tissue sampling. Moreover, it has the ability for therapeutic interventional procedures including polypectomy, hemostasis, palliative dilation, stent placement, tattoos for SBT detection at minimally invasive surgery (Video 13.3), and retrieval of retained capsules [61, 63]. In the setting of SBTs, DAE provides the ability to diagnose, apply therapy, and precisely localize the lesion. Therapeutic maneuvers, however, do raise the complication rate from 1 to 4–5 % [64, 65].

As for CE, the main indication for DAE is OGIB [66–68]. However, DAE is increasingly used to confirm abnormal CE or cross-sectional imaging findings, to evaluate patients with celiac disease for the presence of enteropathy-associated T-cell lymphoma, or to screen or survey patients with intestinal polyposis syndromes (discussed later) [66, 68]. Since the advent of DBE in 2001 many papers addressing the diagnosis and management of SBTs have been published. In the largest series from a Japanese multicenter study (a retrospective analysis of 1,035 patients undergoing DBE for various indications), 13.9 % of patients were found to have SBTs, with 7.3 % primary cancers detected in nonpolyposis patients [68]. In most of the cases the diagnosis was made through DBE and in some cases a therapeutic procedure was directly performed. The most common indication for DBE was OGIB (44 %), followed by obstructive symptoms inclusive of abdominal pain (12 %), evaluation or treatment of diseases such as inherited polyposis syndromes (12 %), the suspected presence of a SBT (9 %), and other indications (23 %) [68]. In this study, as in other studies [67, 69, 70], the incidence of SBTs in patients undergoing DAE is significantly higher than reported in CE studies. The current literature, mostly based on retrospective series, shows heterogeneous results in SBT detection rates by DAE, ranging from 3.6 to 17.4 % [58, 66–71].

The reasons for a high variation in detection rates for SBTs is probably multifactorial, including selection bias. The diagnostic yield of DBE appears to be highest in patients who have positive findings on previous radiologic studies, CE, or octroescan [72]. Many series include benign tumors or patients known to have genetic disorders (Familial Adenomatous Polyposis or Peutz-Jeghers syndrome) where the incidence of SBTs

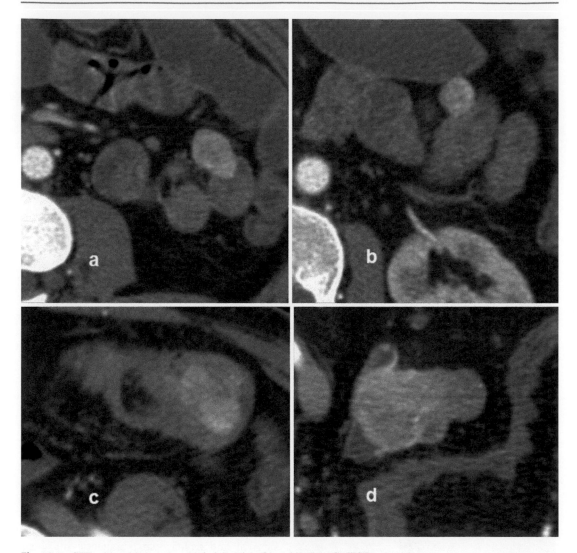

Fig. 13.7 CTE with evidence of multiple jejunal (**a**, **b**) and ileal (**c**, **d**) GISTs

may be expected to be higher or patients may be specifically referred to evaluate and treat specific lesions, as in Peutz-Jeghers syndrome. Smaller studies where inherited polyposis and benign tumors were excluded have indeed reported a surprisingly low (3.6 %) SBT incidence in patients examined by DBE [66]. Finally, the differences may partially reflect a dissimilar referral practice to tertiary referral centers or a true geographic or ethnic patient population difference in the incidence of the various types of SBTs. In the Japanese series [68], lymphomas and GISTs (Figs. 13.7, 13.8, and 13.9) were found more

commonly. Neuroendocrine tumors (NETs) were rarely diagnosed (2.8 %), whereas in the West, based on a 5-year experience at a US referral center, there was a higher incidence of NETs (40 %) [66]. Carcinoid tumor was also reported to be the most common small-bowel cancer identified by DBE in the US study by Cangemi et al. [69]. This geographic variation needs to be further investigated.

There is some information on the comparable diagnostic yield between CE and DAE. A meta-analysis by Pasha et al. found the diagnostic yield for small-bowel lesions to be equal between DBE

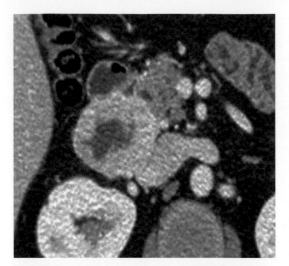

Fig. 13.8 CTE with evidence of duodenal GIST

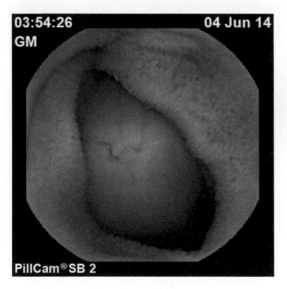

Fig. 13.9 CE finding of jejunal GIST

(57 %) and CE (60 %) [73]. However, as already pointed out, DBE may identify small-bowel mass lesion undetected on CE [58]. Some studies demonstrated DBE to be superior to CE, and CE achieving comparable diagnostic yield compared to DBE only when combined with contrast-enhanced CT (91 % versus 99 %) [59]. On the other hand, tumors may be missed on DBE as well after a positive CE result [74, 75], usually because of their location in an area of the small bowel not examined by DBE.

CE and DAE have to be viewed as complementary tests for the evaluation of patients with suspected SBTs and CE is considered the preferred initial test of choice [76]. CE is a noninvasive test, while DAE is time consuming and more invasive. If no lesions are found on CE, one may avoid the need for an invasive procedure. However, if a lesion is detected, CE can direct the route for a "targeted DAE" and guide the selection of the intubation approach. For deep intubation, according to findings and transit times, the oral approach is preferred when the lesion is suspected to be within the proximal 75 % of the small bowel, whereas a retrograde route is used for more distal lesions [76–78]. If CE is negative but there is a high index of suspicion, further investigations with DAE or cross-sectional imaging should be pursued [56–59]. It should also be mentioned that repeat CE may also identify additional findings in up to 75 % of patients with OGIB, leading to a change in management in 62 % of cases [79]. In some cases, there is a role for deep enteroscopy as the first-diagnostic test without a prior CE, especially when there is a high index of suspicion [63] and/or there is a risk of obstruction and capsule retention [68].

The clinical impact of DAE on the management of small-bowel cancers is illustrated by the high percentage of patients who undergo surgery based upon the findings at DAE [66]. In the series of Lee et al. [67] the results of DBE affected the surgical and endoscopic therapeutic plans and short-term clinical results among patients with SBTs in 64 % of cases. The therapeutic plans were changed more frequently in patients with SBTs than patients with other conditions. Based upon the surgical results, DAE also proved extremely accurate for locating small-bowel neoplasms and for histological diagnosis [69, 70]. DBE was very effective for enteroscopy-guided self-expandable metal stents placement for rescue palliation of malignant small-bowel obstruction with a technical success rate of 94.7 % [80]. Novel areas of innovation and potential application include the use of endoscopic ultrasound for evaluation of SBTs. DAE-guided endoscopic ultrasonography offers adequate imaging and useful information on the wall structure and

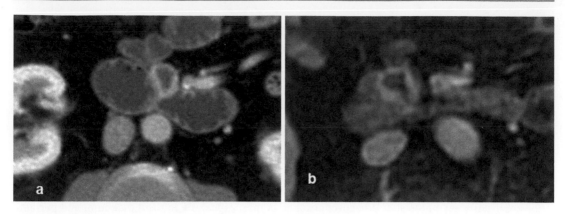

Fig. 13.10 NET at CTE (**a**) and at a MRE (**b**) showing soft tissue contrast

nature of the detected abnormalities in the deep parts of the small bowel. These high-resolution cross-sectional images of SBTs may be helpful in the differential diagnosis of these submucosal tumors [81, 82]. However, further large-scale patient population studies and prospective studies are needed to assess the impact of DAE on long-term outcomes in patients diagnosed with SBTs and to further define its role in the diagnosis, management, and surveillance of treated tumors. In the majority of the studies, complete follow-up was not obtained as the patients following DAE were returned to the primary referring institution or physician [66, 69].

What is the contribution of radiology in this renewed and revolutionized panorama of small-bowel endoscopy? Barium enteroclysis has demonstrated reasonable accuracy in the detection of SBTs and has until recently been the radiological option of choice. However, it is unable to assess the mural and extramural extent of the disease. Despite improvements in multidetector CT, conventional CT scans detect only large-sized intestinal tumors greater than 1.0 cm in diameter. On the other hand, CT enteroclysis/enterography (CTE) provides not only excellent images of the luminal side but also information about mesentery, perienteric fat, lymph node status, and adjacent organs with 100 % sensitivity and 95 % specificity. CTE can detect tumors that are only 5 mm in diameter and the negative and positive predictive values for carcinoid tumor in patients with carcinoid symptoms were 100 and 94.7 %,

respectively. CTE allows for the assessment of extraluminal disease and potential metastatic spread, and helps in preoperative staging [83, 84]. MR enteroclysis/enterography (MRE) offers the advantage of soft tissue contrast and multiplanar imaging without radiation exposure. MRE is able to identify small-intestinal strictures, especially in tumors with intestinal obstruction, based on the signal difference generated by the intestinal wall and luminal contrast agents, and shows very high overall diagnostic accuracy of 95 % for SBTs [85] (Fig. 13.10).

Small-Bowel Polyps and Polyposis Syndromes

Sporadic Duodenal Adenomas, Familial Adenomatous Polyposis (FAP), Peutz-Jeghers Syndrome (PJS), and Hamartomatous Polyps: Basic Outlines

Polyps of the small bowel are a rare entity compared to polyps of the colon. They can be sessile or pedunculated and, according to histology, divided into inflammatory, hyperplastic, hamartomatous, and adenomatous polyps. Hamartomatous polyps and adenomas may arise sporadically or be associated with polyposis syndromes. Small-bowel polyps need to be correctly recognized and histopathologically defined for adequate management, treatment, and follow-up [86].

The duodenum can easily be investigated with conventional upper GI endoscopy. Brunner gland hyperplasia is commonly seen in the context of peptic duodenitis, appearing as nodular duodenitis. In most cases no intervention is necessary but it may deserve treatment when causing problems such as hemorrhage, intestinal obstruction, intussusceptions, or is associated with suspicious lesions [87]. Sporadic duodenal adenomas are an uncommon incidental finding during upper GI endoscopy and are found in up to 5 % [88]. They are usually asymptomatic. Whenever possible, sporadic adenomas should be removed with endoscopic resection, which is preferred over surgical intervention [89]. There is no evidence to support surveillance endoscopy or regular follow-up of these lesions, especially in elderly patients or patients with relevant comorbidity [90]. However, there is accumulating data based on retrospective cohort or case-control studies, suggesting a clinically important association with colorectal neoplasia [91]. Colonoscopic assessment is thus advisable in all patients diagnosed with sporadic duodenal adenomas [92]. The broad category of intestinal polyposis syndromes embraces familial adenomatous polyposis (FAP), as well as hamartomatous polyposis syndromes. The hamartomatous polyposis syndromes consist mainly of Peutz-Jeghers syndrome (PJS), PTEN-associated hamartomatous syndromes (including Cowden syndrome and Bannayan-Riley-Ruvalcaba syndrome [BRRS]), juvenile polyposis, Cronkhite-Canada syndrome, and hereditary-mixed polyposis syndrome (HMPS). The two most common inherited intestinal polyposis syndromes are FAP and PJS [92]. As already mentioned, the clinically most relevant classification of polyposis syndromes relies on the histological typing of polyps, which is crucial for their diagnostic work-up and further management.

FAP and its phenotypic variants are an autosomal dominant inherited disorder caused by germline mutations in the oncosuppressor adenomatous polyposis coli (APC) gene, located on chromosome 5 (segment 5q21-q22). Classic FAP is characterized by the growth of hundreds to thousands of synchronous adenomatous polyps throughout the large bowel during childhood

and adolescence. There is virtually a 100 % lifetime risk of colorectal cancer (CRC) by the age of 40, requiring early prophylactic colectomy before the age of 25. Attenuated FAP (AFAP) is characterized by fewer polyps at presentation, with a tropism to the proximal colon, lower penetration of cancer, and later onset of CRC [92]. Most polyposis syndromes share intestinal extracolonic and extraintestinal features. Besides colon cancer, FAP patients exhibit a higher risk of developing small-bowel adenomas and carcinomas, especially in the duodenum, and periampullary region. Adenomas in the duodenum can be found in 50–90 % of cases, with a lifetime risk of duodenal cancer up to 5 %, as highlighted by three prospective studies on duodenum surveillance [93–95]. Not unusual is the development of ileal pouch adenomas and even cancer after proctocolectomy, correlating with duodenal polyposis and with mutations involving exon 15 of the APC gene [96].

The polyposis associated with the mutation of the gene MUTYH (MUTYH-associated polyposis [MAP]), located on chromosome 1, is a recessive autosomal condition. The clinical presentation is usually similar to AFAP, but the condition can also mimic classic FAP. Data regarding intestinal extracolonic tumors are scarce: duodenal polyposis seems to be less frequent (reported in up to 17 % of patients) and the risk of developing a duodenal cancer is unknown [97]. To date, given the predominant descriptive and retrospective studies, guidelines for the management of FAP and MAP patients are mainly based on expert opinion recommendations [98] in which the clinical usefulness of a systematic small-bowel screening and surveillance program has yet to be determined. Current guidelines recommend scheduled standard upper endoscopic surveillance in relation to the Spigelman classification to investigate the duodenal polyposis, though there is no consensus at which age to start. Based on expert opinion it is advisable to start between the ages of 25 and 30 [98]. Furthermore, current guidelines suggest endoscopic follow-up of the remnant rectum after colectomy with ileorectal anastomosis and of the pouch after proctocolectomy with ileal pouch-anal anastomosis respectively at 3- to 6-month and 6- to 12-month intervals [98].

Peutz-Jeghers is an autosomal dominant inherited polyposis disorder most frequently (80–90 % of cases) arising from a germline mutation of the serine/threonine kinases gene (STK11), located on chromosome 19 (segment 19p13.3). This disorder is characterized by characteristic hamartomatous gastrointestinal polyps, mainly involving the small bowel (60–90 %), in association with mucocutaneous pigmentation. The natural history of the disease is associated with repeated polyp-related complications, consisting of intussusception, obstruction, or bleeding, often requiring endoscopic polypectomy or surgical resection [99, 100]. The overall risk of developing a cancer at any site is significantly high, with an estimated 15-fold increased risk compared to the general population, as reported by Giardiello et al. in a meta-analysis involving 210 patients from 79 families with PJS [101]. Specifically, PJS patients are at risk of developing stomach, small bowel, colon, pancreas, and breast cancer, due the hamartomatous polyps harboring adenomatous dysplastic foci, as observed in 3–6 % of the removed hamartomas. Lifetime incidence for small-bowel cancer reaches 13 %. The increased risk for cancer is age dependent and moreover the risk exponentially increases after the age of 50 [101–103]. The small-bowel tropism of Peutz-Jeghers polyps makes their detection and treatment a challenging issue. Current guidelines recommend scheduled small-bowel surveillance with CE or MR imaging, and endoscopic clearance of sizeable polyps given their potential for development of cancer and intestinal obstruction [104]. Surveillance should be initiated at 8 years of age or earlier if the patient is symptomatic and continued every 3 years if polyps are detected at the index examination. If few or no polyps are found at the initial examination, screening should start again at the age of 18.

Among the disorders predisposing to small-bowel cancer, Lynch syndrome must also be mentioned, due to germline mutations in one of the mismatch repair genes. The lifetime risk of developing small-bowel cancer is estimated to be around 4 %. However, little is known about prev-alence and natural history of these tumors and surveillance in this subset of patients is not yet recommended [105]. In a recent prospective series of 35 patients with Lynch syndrome undergoing CE and CTE, CE diagnosed a histologically confirmed cancer in 8.6 % of cases, compared to CTE that missed all but one neoplasia [106]. Despite these promising results, to date the usefulness and cost-effectiveness of small-bowel screening has not been confirmed.

Outcome and Results in the *Old* and *New* Era of Endoscopy and Radiology

Familial Adenomatous Polyposis

Prophylactic colectomy has greatly improved life expectancy for FAP patients and disease-related morbidity and mortality causes shifted from CRC to duodenal and ampullary adenocarcinomas and to extraintestinal manifestations such as desmoid tumors [107]. Lifetime risk to develop duodenal adenomatosis (Fig. 13.11) is 100 %, with an increasing severity with aging [93]. The severity of duodenal polyposis is rated according to the classification derived by Spigelman and describes five stages from 0 to IV, based on polyp number, size, histology, and degree of dysplasia [95, 108]. Aging of subjects is a determinant factor for progression of duodenal adenomatosis. On the other

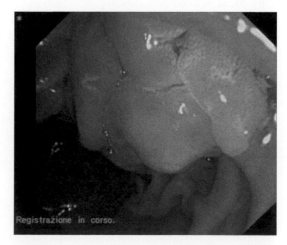

Fig. 13.11 Large duodenal adenomatous polyp in FAP

hand, technical improvements in endoscopic imaging as well contribute to explaining the progression in Spigelman stages, from low to high stages, that has been recorded over the past years [109]. However, the progressive duodenal and periampullary polyposis with advancing age remains a relatively slow process [109–111], as is the progression to cancer. The lifetime risk of developing duodenal cancer is estimated to be approximately 5 % in most series. The current guidelines recommend surveillance of the duodenum with a side-viewing endoscope, to allow detailed inspection of the papilla, and a forward-viewing instrument, at intervals dictated by the Spigelman stage [98]. It has been demonstrated that the higher the Spigelman stage, the higher the risk of small-bowel adenocarcinomas, with a lifetime risk up to 7–36 % in patients with Spigelman stage III and IV, over follow-up periods of 7–10 years [93, 94].

Endoscopic treatment of duodenal and ampullary adenomas is a crucial aspect of the care of FAP patients. With regard to their endoscopic appearance, small-bowel FAP adenomas appear like nonpolypoid, crackled, whitish plaques, or flat lesions, at times coalescing to produce a carpet-like change of the mucosal surface. Even normal-appearing duodenal mucosa may harbor adenomatous dysplastic tissue. High-definition, high-resolution white light imaging, combined with dye spraying or virtual chromoendoscopy, such as NBI or FICE, may help to better demarcate these lesions and improve detection [112, 113]. The main current therapeutic option is endoscopic snare resection, when polyps are amenable to endoscopic treatment. Often duodenal FAP adenomas are numerous (Fig. 13.12), and not all polyps can be removed. On the basis of expert opinion, patients with few small adenomas may undergo follow-up without endoscopic treatment, whereas patients with Spigelman stage III and IV should undergo endoscopic treatment with removal of significant polyps larger than 1 cm or those with high-grade dysplasia. Intensive surveillance and early treatment may delay the need for major duodenal-pancreatic surgery and its potential detrimental effects as well as lead to a reduction in duodenal cancer mortality [98].

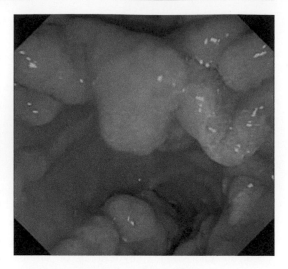

Fig. 13.12 Duodenal polyposis in FAP

Endoscopic treatment of these adenomas is feasible, but challenging, given their flat morphology and associated high overall complication rates (17 %) consisting of bleeding, perforation, and pancreatitis [114]. Moreover, long-term outcome results show a high-recurrence rate. According to the available data on outcome following endoscopic treatment, recurrence rates exceeding 50 % are not unusual [114]. Similarly, a high rate of recurrent adenomas after duodenectomy of 78 % at a mean follow-up period of 46 months has been recently reported [115]. These data support the argument for an intensive surveillance program even after endoscopic or surgical treatment. Trying to reach the neopapilla after duodenectomy might be difficult but the use of a balloon enteroscope may facilitate this.

With regard to adenomas occurring in the pouch, afferent loop, or rectal cuff/anal transitional zone, endoscopic surveillance using indigo-carmine chromoendoscopy is recommended [113, 116] and endoscopic resection of polyps larger than 1 cm or those with high-grade dysplasia is recommended [117]. Pediatric colonoscopes or gastroscopes may be used for this purpose as well. In patients with extensive pouch polyposis not amenable to endoscopic clearance, or where endoscopic surveillance is not practical, pouch excision and terminal ileostomy should

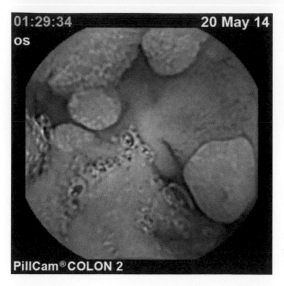

01:29:34   20 May 14
OS

PillCam®COLON 2

Fig. 13.13 CE finding of multiple ileal polyps in FAP

seriously be considered [113]. The advent of CE has changed the approach to small-bowel diseases and has expanded the armamentarium of small-bowel investigation tools. CE, however, cannot replace standard endoscopy in the surveillance of the duodenum. CE is diagnostically inferior to standard endoscopy with regard to the ampullary region [118] and the second part of the duodenum, revealing a 92 % rate of sensitivity for duodenal polyps when compared to conventional upper GI endoscopy and duodenoscopy [31, 32]. Moreover reaching the ligament of Treitz with a forward-viewing endoscope is feasible.

Little is known about the incidence and clinical significance of adenomatous polyps of the jejunum and ileum in FAP patients (Fig. 13.13). Studies using CE [31, 96, 119], push enteroscopy [118], balloon-assisted enteroscopy [120], and radiological imaging [121–123] have revealed that jejunal and ileal polyps frequently occur in FAP patients, especially in those with extensive duodenal polyposis. Recent reports show a prevalence of small-bowel adenomas distal to the duodenum of 75 % [124] and furthermore corroborate the postulated segregation of mutations at exon 15 of the APC gene with a jejunal polyposis phenotype [112, 124]. Adenomas usually do not occur alone. Isolated distal jejunal or ileal polyps are extremely rare (3 %) [31]. A prospective

study by Schulmann et al. [31] of 29 FAP patients demonstrated jejunum and/or ileal adenomas in 59 % (17/29) of patients investigated with both CE and push enteroscopy. The incidence of jejunal and ileal polyps was higher in patients having established duodenal adenomas (16/21 = 76 %) in contrast with patients without duodenal polyposis (1/8 = 12 %). All but one patient with distal jejunum/ileal polyps had proximal polyps as well. Proximal polyps were visualized by PE as well as CE, and were significantly associated with the presence and severity of duodenal polyposis, while distal jejunal and ileal polyps, being beyond the accessibility of push enteroscopy, were detected only by CE. This study showed that CE was as effective as PE in detecting proximal jejunum polyps, in contrast with the analysis of Wong et al. [118] where the authors found PE more accurate than CE in detecting adenomas and determining their size. Furthermore, Schulz et al. [96] proved the simultaneous occurrence of adenomas in the pouch and small intestine after proctocolectomy. On the basis of these findings, the authors recommend CE or even DAE for follow-up examinations when pouch adenomas occur. As for their endoscopic appearance, deep small-bowel polyps exhibit all the same macroscopic features as duodenal or pouch polyps. Nevertheless, the clinical relevance of small-bowel polyps beyond the duodenum is to date not clearly understood. The current evidence does not warrant a generalized screening examination of the deep small bowel. Jejunal cancers have been reported but are rare [125]. This suggests that clinically significant jejunal or ileal polyps are extremely rare [126], even in high-risk patients with advanced duodenal disease, as corroborated by a recent prospective DAE evaluation of jejunal polyposis in a Dutch series [120]. Perhaps, patients with Spigelman stage III–IV duodenal polyposis [119] or patients with specific mutations (mutations in exon 15 of the APC gene) [71] might benefit from a more thorough small-bowel investigation. Some authors, in fact, suggest CE or DAE to be performed in these settings [119, 127]. Genetic testing might be of help to select patients for a small-bowel investigation [71, 127]. Finally, patients who are candidates for duodenectomy might benefit from a preoperative small-bowel endoscopic screening examination, to ensure subsequent surgical reconstruction with a "polyp free" jejunal loop [120], as well as after duodenectomy to screen for recurrence of adenomatous polyps [115].

CE is a safe procedure in polyposis patients. Prior abdominal surgery is not an absolute contraindication to CE [116]. Though CE fails to precisely localize the polyps, and polyp size is generally poorly estimated on CE, comparative studies demonstrated the superiority of CE compared to MR imaging and SBFT in patients with intestinal polyposis [121–123]. CE has shown to be more accurate than MR imaging in detecting small polyps, while for polyps larger than 15 mm, detection rates are similar [122]. One small study using DBE and intraoperative enteroscopy (IOE) to evaluate 41 patients with FAP suggested that DBE is of equivalent value for evaluation of the small-bowel adenomas [124]. Successful and safe deep intubation with DAE, as well as polypectomy and argon plasma coagulation have been described in FAP patients [71, 112, 128]. CE and DAE should play a complementary role in any diagnostic algorithm where CE is used to detect the polyps and to further guide future management, allowing DAE to safely achieve targeted interventional maneuvers. To our knowledge, no studies have assessed long-term outcomes or directly compared CE with DAE in FAP patients.

In an ongoing prospective Italian multicenter research trial, the diagnostic and prognostic values of CE compared to DAE are being assessed in patients with both FAP and PJS [129]. To date 16 patients (10 patients with FAP and 6 with PJS) have been enrolled; 14 patients have previously undergone intestinal surgery. CE was performed in all patients. DAE was performed within 6 months after CE. All patients had antegrade DAE except for two. The maximum mean insertion depth was 300 cm for the oral route and 68 cm from the anal/ileostomy insertion route. Based on the available data, it suggests that CE and DAE share a comparable detection capability for small-bowel lesions, including polyps. The kappa

agreement on lesion detection seems to be good between the two techniques—k: 0.54 p: 0.01 for duodenum, k: 0.58 p: 0.009 for ileum and k (adjusted for prevalence), 0.63 p: 0.6 for jejunum. However, it is important to note that in this subset of patients, postsurgical anatomic status considerably restricts the potential to achieve total deep enteroscopy, even though the majority of the lesions appear to be very proximally or very distally located, within the reach of DAE for therapeutic interventions.

Though radiology has a minor role in FAP as compared to PJS, CT scanning and moreover MR imaging still play an important role in these patients, with regard to detection and surveillance of desmoid tumors, a benign proliferative disease of fibrous tissue origin. Abdominal desmoid tumors are the third major cause of mortality and morbidity in FAP, their incidence ranging between 7 and 17 % during a lifetime. In FAP patients suspected or known to have abdominal desmoid tumors, abdominal CT and MR imaging are performed to detect the tumor, to measure its extent and to rule out significant small-bowel obstruction [107, 130, 131]. MR imaging provides additional information on tumor activity [130, 131]. Desmoid tumors are histologically benign and nonmetastasizing but locally aggressive and infiltrative and may lead to death when invading vital structures. Mesenteric desmoid tumors may cause small-bowel obstruction or other life-threatening complications such as ischemia, hydronephrosis, or the formation of fistulas. In this setting, given the risk of entrapment, CE has to be performed with caution, only after significant small-bowel obstruction has been ruled out. Surgical trauma is a trigger in the development of desmoid tumors and the approach should be conservative with surgery limited to life-threatening complications, since recurrence rates after debulking are reported as high as 75–85 % [107, 131]. Follow-up MR imaging of desmoids indicates more aggressive behavior of recurrences [132]. Early radiological detection of these desmoids with CT and MR imaging may facilitate a conservative medical approach, avoiding surgery [31, 107].

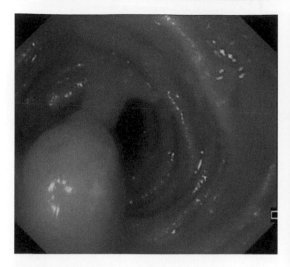

Fig. 13.14 Enteroscopic image of polyp with stalk in PJS

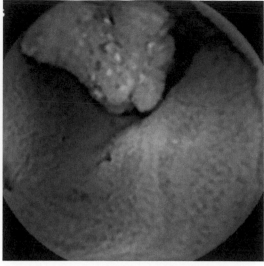

Fig. 13.15 CE finding of a stalked polyp in PJS

Peutz-Jeghers Syndrome

Polyps in PJS are often pedunculated (Fig. 13.14), with a characteristic histological pattern of smooth muscle arborisation [100], and become clinically significant at young ages. The risk of intussusception at the age of 20 is 50 % [133]. A survey of adults with PJS found that by the age of 10 years, 30 % had undergone laparotomy and 68 % of adults had required laparotomy by the age of 18—70 % in an emergency setting [133]. In light of this, the primary goal of small-bowel surveillance is the detection of significant polyps and performing polypectomy before symptoms develop (Video 13.4). Such an approach will help prevent bleeding from ulcerated or infarcted polyps, intussusceptions, obviate the need for urgent laparotomy, and hopefully lengthen the disease-free interval [134]. All symptomatic or significant polyps (>10–15 mm) should be removed [135]. This avoids the risk of multiple enterotomies or small-bowel resections leading to short-bowel syndrome. In addition, given the increased risk for small-bowel cancer (13 % lifetime risk, corresponding to a relative risk 520 times that of the general population) [101], surveillance programs and polyp removal with advancing age should lead to early detection of precancerous lesions and cancer [136]. Before the introduction of the recently developed advanced endoscopy techniques, these deep small-bowel polyps required surgical removal, except for the more proximal that could be removed by PE and IOE [135, 137, 138]. In fact, diagnosis and surveillance mainly relied on small-bowel barium radiographs [137].

PJS is a disease where CE and DAE best exhibit their diagnostic and/or therapeutic strength. Since the first reports following its advent, CE showed its usefulness in the management of these patients. CE immediately proved more effective than barium radiograph in detecting these polyps, with an 80 % detection rate and a positive impact in changing the management in 40 % of patients, leading to IOE with surgical and endoscopic polypectomy [135]. This confirmed its role as a diagnostic strategic tool for the investigation of symptoms and the surveillance of the small bowel in PJS. Significant polyps are commonly detected by CE in PJS (Figs. 13.15 and 13.16), with higher accuracy than SBFT, enteroclysis, and PE [119, 121, 139] and lead to change in management in up to 50 % of subjects [131, 135]. PE is limited to the proximal jejunum, whereas these polyps are distributed throughout the entire small bowel. The evidence suggests that CE is comparable to MR imaging for the detection of large (>15 mm) polyps, while smaller, flatter polyps are seen more often with the capsule [122]. The limitation to CE seems to be that it is less reliable for accurately sizing and locating the detected polyps

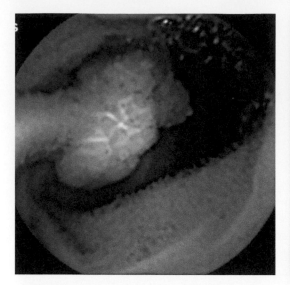

Fig. 13.16 CE finding of a stalked polyp in PJS

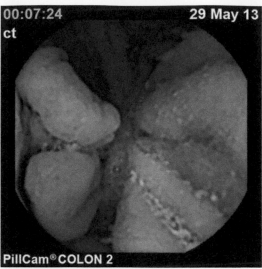

Fig. 13.17 CE finding of multiple polyps in PJS

[122, 139]. Examples of CE for polyp surveillance in PJS are shown in Figs. 13.17 and 13.18. Schulmann et al. [31] reported on 11 patients and an immediate impact on further clinical management according to CE findings. They suggested CE as the first-line surveillance procedure.

Current guidelines propose routine small-bowel surveillance using CE or MR enterography (or still SBFT, except for children) as reasonable techniques, followed by endoscopic clearance of sizeable polyps to prevent polyp-related complications [104]. DAE allows endoscopic treatment using standard snare polypectomy, whilst its use as a method of small-bowel surveillance in PJS is not supported by the current evidence [104]. However, in specific cases (i.e., in symptomatic patients in whom the diagnostic yield of significant polyps appears to be high) balloon-assisted enteroscopy may be considered as the first-diagnostic modality, as stated in the ESGE guidelines on flexible enteroscopy for small-bowel diseases [47].

DAE has been shown to be effective and safe for therapeutic purposes in adults [140–145] as well as in children [146], even in patients with a history of extensive abdominal surgery. Endoscopic resection of polyps is feasible even in cases of numerous or large polyps ≥3 cm, with success rates reaching 96 % [140–145].

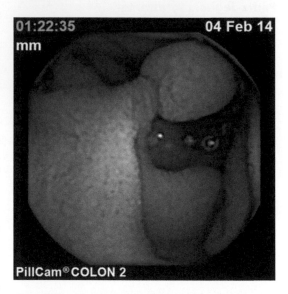

Fig. 13.18 CE finding of multiple polyps in PJS

Complications—including bleeding, perforation, acute pancreatitis, and postpolypectomy syndrome—may occur but rates in the reported series range from 0 % [142, 144] to 7 % [141, 143, 145]. The overall complication rate of endoscopic therapeutic interventions in the small bowel using the DBE device is approximately 3 %. It appears that polypectomy of large polyps ≥3 cm is associated with the highest risk (up to 10 %) and requires significant technical skills and specific precautions, such as prior injection and lift of diluted epinephrine-saline solution with piecemeal resection [147]. Polypectomy should ideally be performed when PJS polyps are relatively small, thereby avoiding the technically more difficult endoscopic resection of large polyps at a later stage [140]. There are studies to show that PJS polyps as large as 5–6 cm have been successfully treated during DAE [141, 144, 145]. If large polyps are endoscopically resected, surgical backup is advisable. Given the high risk of perforation, polyps that are bulky, locally concentrated in large numbers, invaginated, and thick-stalked with serosal retraction into the stalk should not be addressed by polypectomy, even if performed during surgery, but should be surgically removed [148]. Though, some authors recommend DAE for simultaneous diagnosis and treatment of small-bowel polyps in PJS [144] the majority of centers use CE and/or MR enterography as the first-diagnostic tool, followed by a targeted DAE procedure for therapeutic purposes.

References

1. Ubaiah O, Devesa SS, Platz CE, et al. Small intestinal cancer: a population-based study of incidence and survival patterns in the United States, 1992 to 2006. Cancer Epidemiol Biomarkers Prev. 2010; 19(8):1908–18.
2. Bilimoria KY, Bentrem DJ, Wayne JD, et al. Small bowel cancer in the United States: changes in epidemiology, treatment, and survival over the last 20 years. Ann Surg. 2009;249(1):63–71.
3. Pan SY, Morrison H. Epidemiology of cancer of the small intestine. World J Gastrointest Oncol. 2011; 3(3):33–42. 15.
4. Neugut AI, Jacobson JS, Suh S, et al. The epidemiology of cancer of the small bowel. Cancer Epidemiol Biomarkers Prev. 1998;7(3):243–51.
5. Raghav K, Overman MJ. Small bowel adenocarcinomas – existing evidence and evolving paradigms. Nat Rev Clin Oncol. 2009;10(9):534–44.
6. Cheung DY, Choi MG. Current advance in small bowel tumors. Clin Endosc. 2011;44(1):13–21.
7. Dabaja BS, Suki D, Pro B, et al. Adenocarcinoma of the small bowel: presentation, prognostic factors, and outcome of 217 patients. Cancer. 2004;101(3): 518–26.
8. Farhat MH, Shamseddine AI, Barada KA. Small bowel tumors: clinical presentation, prognosis, and outcome in 33 patients in a tertiary care center. J

Oncol. 2008. doi:10.1155/2008/212067. Epub 2008 Dec 2.
9. Talamonti MS, Goetz LH, Rao S, Joehl RJ. Primary cancers of the small bowel: analysis of prognostic factors and results of surgical management. Arch Surg. 2002;137(5):564–70. discussion 570-1.
10. DiSario JA, Burt RW, Vargas H, McWhorter WP. Small bowel cancer: epidemiological and clinical characteristics from a population-based registry. Am J Gastroenterol. 1994;89(5):699–701.
11. Naef M, Bühlmann M, Baer HU. Small bowel tumors: diagnosis, therapy and prognostic factors. Langenbecks Arch Surg. 1999;384(2):176–80.
12. Aparicio T, Zaanan A, Svrcek M, et al. Small bowel adenocarcinoma: epidemiology, risk factors, diagnosis and treatment. Dig Liver Dis. 2014;46(2):97–104.
13. Cananzi FC, Lorenzi B, Belgaumkar A, et al. Prognostic factors for primary gastrointestinal stromal tumors: are they the same in the multidisciplinary treatment era? Langenbecks Arch Surg. 2014;399(3):323–32.
14. Tabrizian P, Sweeney RE, Uhr JH, et al. Laparoscopic resection of gastric and small bowel gastrointestinal stromal tumors: 10-year experience at a single center. J Am Coll Surg. 2014;218(3):367–73.
15. Zuckerman GR, Prakash C, Askin MP, Lewis BS. AGA technical review on the evaluation and management of occult and obscure gastrointestinal bleeding. Gastroenterology. 2000;118(1):201–21.
16. Ekberg O, Ekholm S. Radiography in primary tumors of the small bowel. Acta Radiol Diagn (Stockh). 1980;21(1):79–84.
17. Zollinger Jr RM. Primary neoplasms of the small intestine. Am J Surg. 1986;151(6):654–8.
18. Orjollet-Lecoanet C, Ménard Y, Martins A, et al. CT enteroclysis for detection of small bowel tumors. J Radiol. 2000;81(6):618–27.
19. Bessette JR, Maglinte DD, Kelvin FM, Chernish SM. Primary malignant tumors in the small bowel: a comparison of the small-bowel enema and conventional follow-through examination. AJR Am J Roentgenol. 1989;153(4):741–4.
20. Thoeni RF, Gould RG. Enteroclysis and small bowel series: comaprison of radiation dose and examination time. Radiology. 1991;178:659–62.
21. Gill SS, Heuman DM, Mihas AA. Small intestinal neoplasms. J Clin Gastroenterol. 2001;33:267–82.
22. Soyer P, Boudiaf M, Fishman EK, et al. Imaging of malignant neoplasms of the mesenteric small bowel: new trends and perspectives. Crit Rev Oncol Hematol. 2011;80(1):10–30.
23. Hoeffel C, Mule S, Romaniuk B, et al. Advances in radiological imaging of gastrointestinal tumors. Crit Rev Oncol Hematol. 2009;69(2):153–67.
24. May A, Nachbar L, Schneider M, Ell C. Prospective comparison of push enteroscopy and push-and-pull enteroscopy in patients with suspected small-bowel bleeding. Am J Gastroenterol. 2006;101(9):2016–24.
25. Marmo R, Rotondano G, Piscopo R, et al. Meta-analysis: capsule enteroscopy vs. conventional

modalities in diagnosis of small bowel diseases. Aliment Pharmacol Ther. 2005;22(7):595–604.

26. Berner JS, Mauer K, Lewis BS. Push and sonde enteroscopy for the diagnosis of obscure gastrointestinal bleeding. Am J Gastroenterol. 1994;89(12): 2139–42.

27. Iacopini G, Frontespezi S, Vitale MA, et al. Routine ileoscopy at colonoscopy: a prospective evaluation of learning curve and skill-keeping line. Gastrointest Endosc. 2006;63(2):250–6.

28. Cheung DY, Lee IS, Chang DK, et al. for the Korean Gut Images Study Group. Capsule endoscopy in small bowel tumors: a multicenter Korean study. J Gastroenterol Hepatol. 2010;25(6):1079–86.

29. Bailey AA, Debinski HS, Appleyard MN, et al. Diagnosis and outcome of small bowel tumors found by capsule endoscopy: a three-center Australian experience. Am J Gastroenterol. 2006; 101(10):2237–43.

30. Maieron A, Hubner D, Blaha B, et al. Multicenter retrospective evaluation of capsule endoscopy in clinical routine. Endoscopy. 2004;36(10):864–8.

31. Schulmann K, Hollerbach S, Kraus K, et al. Feasibility and diagnostic utility of video capsule endoscopy for the detection of small bowel polyps in patients with hereditary polyposis syndromes. Am J Gastroenterol. 2005;100(1):27–37.

32. Iaquinto G, Fornasarig M, Quaia M, et al. Capsule endoscopy is useful and safe for small-bowel surveillance in familial adenomatous polyposis. Gastrointest Endosc. 2008;67(1):61–7.

33. Schwartz GD, Barkin JS. Small-bowel tumors detected by wireless capsule endoscopy. Dig Dis Sci. 2007;52:1026–30.

34. de Franchis R, Rondonotti E, Abbiati C, et al. Small bowel malignancy. Gastrointest Endosc Clin N Am. 2004;14(1):139–48.

35. Cobrin GM, Pittman RH, Lewis BS. Increased diagnostic yield of small bowel tumors with capsule endoscopy. Cancer. 2006;107(1):22–7.

36. Estevez E, Gonzalez-Conde B, Vazquez-Iglesias JL, et al. Incidence of tumoral pathology according to study using capsule endoscopy for patients with obscure gastrointestinal bleeding. Surg Endosc. 2007;21:1776–80.

37. Urbain D, De Looze D, Demedts I, et al. Video capsule endoscopy in small-bowel malignancy: a multicenter Belgian study. Endoscopy. 2006;38(4):408–11.

38. Urgesi R, Riccioni ME, Bizzotto A, et al. Increased diagnostic yield of small bowel tumors with PillCam: the role of capsule endoscopy in the diagnosis and treatment of gastrointestinal stromal tumors (GISTs). Italian single-center experience. Tumori. 2012;98(3):357–63.

39. Achour J, Serraj I, Amrani L, Amrani N. Small bowel tumors: what is the contribution of video capsule endoscopy? Clin Res Hepatol Gastroenterol. 2012;36(3):222–6.

40. Rondonotti E, Pennazio M, Toth E, on behalf of the European Capsule Endoscopy Group, the Italian Club for Capsule Endoscopy (CICE) and the Iberian Group for Capsule Endoscopy, et al. Small-bowel neoplasms in patients undergoing video capsule endoscopy: a multicenter European study. Endoscopy. 2008;40(6):488–95.

41. Pasha SF, Sharma VK, Carey EJ, et al. Utility of video capsule endoscopy in the detection of small bowel tumors – a single center experience of 1000 consecutive patients. Presented at ICCE, Madrid, Spain, 8–9 June 2007. Abstract 45. 2007.

42. Leighton JA. The role of endoscopic imaging of the small bowel in clinical practice. Am J Gastroenterol. 2011;106(1):27–36.

43. Spada C, Riccioni ME, Familiari P, et al. Video capsule endoscopy in small-bowel tumors: a single centre experience. Scand J Gastroenterol. 2008;43(4):497–505.

44. Delvaux M, Friedman S, Keuchel M, et al. Structured terminology for capsule endoscopy: results of retrospective testing and validation in 766 small-bowel investigations. Endoscopy. 2005;37(10):945–50.

45. Korman LY, Delvaux M, Gay G, et al. Capsule endoscopy structured terminology (CEST): proposal of a standardized and structured terminology for reporting capsule endoscopy procedures. Endoscopy. 2005;37(10):951–9.

46. Pennazio M, Rondonotti E, de Franchis R. Capsule endoscopy in neoplastic diseases. World J Gastroenterol. 2008;14(34):5245–53.

47. Pohl J, Delvaux M, Ell C, the ESGE Clinical Guidelines Committee, et al. European Society of Gastrointestinal Endoscopy (ESGE) guidelines: flexible enteroscopy for diagnosis and treatment of small-bowel diseases. Endoscopy. 2008;40(7):609–18.

48. Girelli CM, Porta P, Colombo E, et al. Development of a novel index to discriminate bulge from mass on small-bowel capsule endoscopy. Gastrointest Endosc. 2011;74(5):1067–74.

49. Barbosa DC, Roupar DB, Ramos JC, et al. Automatic small bowel tumor diagnosis by using multi-scale wavelet-based analysis in wireless capsule endoscopy images. Biomed Eng Online. 2012;11:3.

50. Pasha SF, Hara AK, Leighton JA. Diagnostic evaluation and management of obscure gastrointestinal bleeding: a changing paradigm. Gastroenterol Hepatol (NY). 2009;5(12):839–50.

51. Zagorowicz ES, Pietrzak AM, Wronska E, et al. Small bowel tumors detected and missed during capsule endoscopy: single center experience. World J Gastroenterol. 2013;19(47):9043–8.

52. Flieger D, Keller R, May A, et al. Capsule endoscopy in gastrointestinal lymphomas. Endoscopy. 2005;37:1174–80.

53. Daum S, Wahnschaffe U, Glasenapp R, et al. Capsule endoscopy in refractory celiac disease. Endoscopy. 2007;39:455–8.

54. Baichi MM, Arifuddin RM, Mantry PS. Small-bowel masses found and missed on capsule endoscopy for obscure bleeding. Scand J Gastroenterol. 2007;42(9):1127–32.

55. Lewis BS, Eisen GM, Friedman S. A pooled analysis to evaluate results of capsule endoscopy trials. Endoscopy. 2005;37:960–5.

56. Hakim FA, Alexander JA, Huprich JE, et al. CT-enterography may identify small bowel tumors not detected by capsule endoscopy: eight years experience at Mayo Clinic Rochester. Dig Dis Sci. 2011; 56(10):2914–9.

57. Ohmiya N, Nakamura M, Tahara T, et al. Management of small-bowel polyps at double-balloon enteroscopy. Ann Transl Med. 2014;2(3):30.

58. Ross A, Mehdizadeh S, Tokar J, et al. Double balloon enteroscopy detects small bowel mass lesions missed by capsule endoscopy. Dig Dis Sci. 2008;53(8):2140–3.

59. Honda W, Ohmiya N, Hirooka Y, et al. Enteroscopic and radiologic diagnoses, treatment, and prognoses of small-bowel tumors. Gastrointest Endosc. 2012;76(2):344–54.

60. Liao Z, Gao R, Xu C, Li ZS. Indications and detection, completion, and retention rates of small-bowel capsule endoscopy: a systematic review. Gastrointest Endosc. 2010;71(2):280–6.

61. Riccioni ME, Urgesi R, Cianci R, et al. Current status of device-assisted enteroscopy: technical matters, indication, limits and complications. World J Gastrointest Endosc. 2012;4(10):453–61.

62. Tennyson CA, Lewis BS. Enteroscopy: an overview. Gastrointest Endosc Clin N Am. 2009;19(3): 315–24.

63. Islam RS, Leighton JA, Pasha SF. Evaluation and management of small-bowel tumors in the era of deep enteroscopy. Gastrointest Endosc. 2014;79(5):732–40.

64. Mensink PB, Haringsma J, Kucharzik T, et al. Complications of double balloon enteroscopy: a multicenter survey. Endoscopy. 2007;39(7):613–5.

65. Aktas H, de Ridder L, Haringsma J, et al. Complications of single-balloon enteroscopy: a prospective evaluation of 166 procedures. Endoscopy. 2010;42(5):365–8.

66. Partridge BJ, Tokar JL, Haluszka O, Heller SJ. Small bowel cancers diagnosed by device-assisted enteroscopy at a U.S. referral center: a five-year experience. Dig Dis Sci. 2011;56(9):2701–5.

67. Lee BI, Choi H, Choi KY, et al. Clinical characteristics of small bowel tumors diagnosed by double-balloon endoscopy: KASID multi-center study. Dig Dis Sci. 2011;56(10):2920–7.

68. Mitsui K, Tanaka S, Yamamoto H, et al. Role of double-balloon endoscopy in the diagnosis of small-bowel tumors: the first Japanese multicenter study. Gastrointest Endosc. 2009;70(3):498–504.

69. Cangemi DJ, Patel MK, Gomez V, et al. Small bowel tumors discovered during double-balloon enteroscopy: analysis of a large prospectively collected single-center database. J Clin Gastroenterol. 2013;47(9):769–72.

70. Chen W, Shan GD, Zhang H, et al. Double-balloon enteroscopy in small bowel tumors: a Chinese single-center study. World J Gastroenterol. 2013;19(23):3665–71.

71. Fry LC, Neumann H, Kuester D, et al. Small bowel polyps and tumors: endoscopic detection and treatment by double-balloon enteroscopy. Aliment Pharmacol Ther. 2009;29(1):135–42.

72. Bellutti M, Fry LC, Schmitt J, et al. Detection of neuroendocrine tumors of the small bowel by double balloon enteroscopy. Dig Dis Sci. 2009;54(5): 1050–8.

73. Pasha SF, Leighton JA, Das A, et al. Double-balloon enteroscopy and capsule endoscopy have comparable diagnostic yield in small-bowel disease: a meta-analysis. Clin Gastroenterol Hepatol. 2008;6(6): 671–6.

74. Hadithi M, Heine GD, Jacobs MA, et al. A prospective study comparing video capsule endoscopy with double-balloon enteroscopy in patients with obscure gastrointestinal bleeding. Am J Gastroenterol. 2006; 101:52–7.

75. Nakamura T, Terano A. Capsule endoscopy: past, present, and future. J Gastroenterol. 2008;43:93–9.

76. Gay G, Delvaux M, Fassler I. Outcome of capsule endoscopy in determining indication and route for push-and-pull enteroscopy. Endoscopy. 2006;38(1): 49–58.

77. Kaffes AJ, Siah C, Koo JH. Clinical outcomes after double-balloon enteroscopy in patients with obscure GI bleeding and a positive capsule endoscopy. Gastrointest Endosc. 2007;66:304–9.

78. Hendel JW, Vilmann P, Jensen T. Double-balloon endoscopy: who needs it? Scand J Gastroenterol. 2008;43:363–7.

79. Jones BH, Fleischer DE, Sharma VK, et al. Yield of repeat wireless video capsule endoscopy in patients with obscure gastrointestinal bleeding. Am J Gastroenterol. 2005;100:1058–64.

80. Lee H, Park JC, Shin SK, et al. Preliminary study of enteroscopy-guided, self-expandable metal stent placement for malignant small bowel obstruction. J Gastroenterol Hepatol. 2012;27(7):1181–6.

81. Fukumoto A, Manabe N, Tanaka S, et al. Usefulness of EUS with double-balloon enteroscopy for diagnosis of small-bowel diseases. Gastrointest Endosc. 2007;65(3):412–20.

82. Ivanova E, Fedorov ED, Budzinskiy S, et al. Which lesions found by balloon-assisted enteroscopy should undergo EUS examination and benefit from it? Gastrointest Endosc. 2013;77(5S):AB421.

83. Boudiaf M, Jaff A, Soyer P, et al. Small-bowel diseases: prospective evaluation of multi-detector row helical CT enteroclysis in 107 consecutive patients. Radiology. 2004;233:338–44.

84. Kamaoui I, De-Luca V, Ficarelli S, et al. Value of CT enteroclysis in suspected small-bowel carcinoid tumors. AJR Am J Roentgenol. 2010;194:629–33.

85. Van Weyenberg SJ, Meijerink MR, Jacobs MA, et al. MR enteroclysis in the diagnosis of small-bowel neoplasms. Radiology. 2010;254:765–73.

86. Brosens LAA, Jansen M, Giardiello FM, Offerhaus GJA. Polyps of the small intestine. Diagn Histopathol. 2011;17(2):69–79.

87. Culver EL, McIntyre AS. Sporadic duodenal polyps: classification, investigation and management. Endoscopy. 2011;43:144–55.

88. Jepsen JM, Persson M, Jakobsen NO, et al. Prospective study of prevalence and endoscopic and histopathologic characteristics of duodenal polyps in patients submitted to upper endoscopy. Scand J Gastroenterol. 1994;29(6):483–7.

89. Lépilliez V, Chemaly M, Ponchon T, et al. Endoscopic resection of sporadic duodenal adenomas: an efficient technique with a substantial risk of delayed bleeding. Endoscopy. 2008;40(10):806–10.

90. van Heumen BW, Mul K, Nagtegaal ID, et al. Management of sporadic duodenal adenomas and the association with colorectal neoplasms: a retrospective cohort study. J Clin Gastroenterol. 2012;46(5):390–6.

91. Murray MA, Zimmerman MJ, Ee HC. Sporadic duodenal adenoma is associated with colorectal neoplasia. Gut. 2004;53(2):261–5.

92. Arber N, Moshkowitz M. Small bowel polyposis syndromes. Curr Gastroenterol Rep. 2011;13(5):435–41.

93. Bulow S, Bjork J, Christensen IJ, et al. Duodenal adenomatosis in familial adenomatous polyposis. Gut. 2004;53:381–6.

94. Groves CJ, Saunders BP, Spigelman AD, et al. Duodenal cancer in patients with familial adenomatous polyposis (FAP): results of a 10 year prospective study. Gut. 2002;50:636–41.

95. Saurin JC, Gutknecht C, Napoleon B, et al. Surveillance of duodenal adenomas in familial adenomatous polyposis reveals high cumulative risk of advanced disease. J Clin Oncol. 2004;22:493–8.

96. Schulz AC, Bojarski C, Buhr HJ, Kroesen AJ. Occurrence of adenomas in the pouch and small intestine of FAP patients after proctocolectomy with ileoanal pouch construction. Int J Colorectal Dis. 2008;23(4):437–41.

97. Sampson JR, Jones N. MUTYH-associated polyposis. Best Pract Res Clin Gastroenterol. 2009;23(2):209–18.

98. Vasen HF, Möslein G, Alonso A, et al. Guidelines for the clinical management of familial adenomatous polyposis (FAP). Gut. 2008;57(5):704–13.

99. Utsunomiya J, Gocho H, Miyanaga T, et al. Peutz-Jeghers syndrome: its natural course and management. Johns Hopkins Med J. 1975;136:71–82.

100. Latchford AR, Phillips RK. Gastrointestinal polyps and cancer in Peutz-Jeghers syndrome: clinical aspects. Fam Cancer. 2011;10(3):455–61.

101. Giardiello FM, Brensinger JD, Tersmette AC, et al. Very high risk of cancer in familial Peutz-Jeghers syndrome. Gastroenterology. 2000;119:1447–53.

102. Boardman LA, Thibodeau SN, Schaid DJ, et al. Increased risk for cancer in patients with the Peutz-Jeghers syndrome. Ann Intern Med. 1998;128:896–9.

103. Hearle N, Schumacher V, Menko FH, et al. Frequency and spectrum of cancers in the Peutz-Jeghers syndrome. Clin Cancer Res. 2006;12:3209–15.

104. Beggs AD, Latchford AR, Vasen HF, et al. Peutz-Jeghers syndrome: a systematic review and recommendations for management. Gut. 2010;59(7): 975–86.

105. Koornstra JJ. Small bowel endoscopy in familial adenomatous polyposis and Lynch syndrome. Best Pract Res Clin Gastroenterol. 2012;26(3):359–68.

106. Saurin JC, Pilleul F, Soussan EB, et al. and the Capsule Commission of the French Society of Digestive Endoscopy (SFED). Small-bowel capsule endoscopy diagnoses early and advanced neoplasms in asymptomatic patients with Lynch syndrome. Endoscopy. 2010;42:1057–62.

107. Tulchinsky H, Keidar A, Strul H, et al. Extracolonic manifestations of familial adenomatous polyposis after proctocolectomy. Arch Surg. 2005;140(2):159–63. discussion 164.

108. Spigelman AD, Williams CB, Talbot IC, et al. Upper gastrointestinal cancer in patients with familial adenomatous polyposis. Lancet. 1989;2:783–5.

109. Mathus-Vliegen EM, Boparai KS, Dekker E, van Geloven N. Progression of duodenal adenomatosis in familial adenomatous polyposis: due to ageing of subjects and advances in technology. Fam Cancer. 2011;10(3):491–9.

110. Burke CA, Beck GJ, Church JM, van Stolk RU. The natural history of untreated duodenal and ampullary adenomas in patients with familial adenomatous polyposis followed in an endoscopic surveillance program. Gastrointest Endosc. 1999;49:358–64.

111. Matsumoto T. Natural history of ampullary adenoma in familial adenomatous polyposis: reconfirmation of benign nature during extended surveillance. Am J Gastroenterol. 2000;95:1557–62.

112. Mönkemüller K, Fry LC, Ebert M, et al. Feasibility of double-balloon enteroscopy-assisted chromoendoscopy of the small bowel in patients with familial adenomatous polyposis. Endoscopy. 2007;39:52–7.

113. Tajika M, Niwa Y, Bhatia V, et al. Risk of ileal pouch neoplasms in patients with familial adenomatous polyposis. World J Gastroenterol. 2013;19(40): 6774–83.

114. Brosens LA, Keller JJ, Offerhaus GJ, et al. Prevention and management of duodenal polyps in familial adenomatous polyposis. Gut. 2005;54:1034–43.

115. Alderlieste YA, Bastiaansen BA, Mathus-Vliegen EM, et al. High rate of recurrent adenomatosis during endoscopic surveillance after duodenectomy in patients with familial adenomatous polyposis. Fam Cancer. 2013;12(4):699–706.

116. Moussata D, Nancey S, Lapalus MG. Frequency and severity of ileal adenomas in familial adenomatous polyposis after colectomy. Endoscopy. 2008;40(2): 120–5.

117. Saurin JC, Napoleon B, Gay G, et al. Endoscopic management of patients with familial adenomatous

polyposis (FAP) following a colectomy. Endoscopy. 2005;37:499–501.

118. Wong RF, Tuteja AK, Haslem DS, et al. Video capsule endoscopy compared with standard endoscopy for the evaluation of small-bowel polyps in persons with familial adenomatous polyposis (with video). Gastrointest Endosc. 2006;64(4):530–7.

119. Burke CA, Santisi J, Church J, Levinthal G. The utility of capsule endoscopy small bowel surveillance in patients with polyposis. Am J Gastroenterol. 2005;100(7):1498–502.

120. Alderlieste YA, Rauws EA, Mathus-Vliegen EM, et al. Prospective enteroscopic evaluation of jejunal polyposis in patients with familial adenomatous polyposis and advanced duodenal polyposis. Fam Cancer. 2013;12(1):51–6.

121. Mata A, Llach J, Castells A. A prospective trial comparing wireless capsule endoscopy and barium contrast series for small-bowel surveillance in hereditary GI polyposis syndromes. Gastrointest Endosc. 2005;61(6):721–5.

122. Caspari R, von Falkenhausen M, Krautmacher C, et al. Comparison of capsule endoscopy and magnetic resonance imaging for the detection of polyps of the small intestine in patients with familial adenomatous polyposis or with Peutz-Jeghers' syndrome. Endoscopy. 2004;36(12):1054–9.

123. Tescher P, Macrae FA, Speer T, et al. Surveillance of FAP: a prospective blinded comparison of capsule endoscopy and other GI imaging to detect small bowel polyps. Hered Cancer Clin Pract. 2010;8(1):3.

124. Matsumoto T, Esaki M, Yanaru-Fujisawa R, et al. Small-intestinal involvement in familial adenomatous polyposis: evaluation by double-balloon endoscopy and intraoperative enteroscopy. Gastrointest Endosc. 2008;68(5):911–9.

125. Ruys AT, Alderlieste YA, Gouma DJ, et al. Jejunal cancer in patients with familial adenomatous polyposis. Clin Gastroenterol Hepatol. 2010;8(8):731–3.

126. Will OC, Man RF, Phillips RK, et al. Familial adenomatous polyposis and the small bowel: a locoregional review and current management strategies. Pathol Res Pract. 2008;204(7):449–58.

127. Mönkemüller K, Bellutti M, Fry LC, Malfertheiner P. Enteroscopy. Best Pract Res Clin Gastroenterol. 2008;22(5):789–811.

128. Bellutti M, Fry LC, Malfertheiner P, Mönkemüller K. Utility of double balloon enteroscopy for surveillance in intestinal polyposis syndromes. Tech Gastrointest Endosc. 2008;10(3):96–100.

129. Marmo C, Bizzotto A, Riccioni ME, et al. Multicentric italian study that compares diagnostic and prognostic capacity of balloon-assisted enteroscopy (BAE) and videocaspule endoscopy in patients with familial polyposis: preliminary results. Abstracts of the 20th National Congress of Digestive Diseases, Italian Federation of Societies of Digestive Diseases – FISMAD. Dig Liver Dis. 2014;46(S2):S130.

130. Groen EJ, Roos A, Muntinghe FL, et al. Extraintestinal manifestations of familial adenomatous polyposis. Ann Surg Oncol. 2008;15(9):2439–50.

131. Casillas J, Sais GJ, Greve JL, et al. Imaging of intra- and extraabdominal desmoid tumors. Radiographics. 1991;11:959–68.

132. Vandevenne JE, De Schepper AM, De Beuckeleer L, et al. New concepts in understanding evolution of desmoid tumors: MR imaging of 30 lesions. Eur Radiol. 1997;7:1013–9.

133. Hinds R, Philp C, Hyer W, Fell JM. Complications of childhood Peutz-Jeghers syndrome: implications for pediatric screening. J Pediatr Gastroenterol Nutr. 2004;39(2):219–20.

134. van Lier MG, Mathus-Vliegen EM, Wagner A, et al. High cumulative risk of intussusception in patients with Peutz-Jeghers syndrome: time to update surveillance guidelines? Am J Gastroenterol. 2011;106(5):940–5.

135. Parsi MA, Burke CA. Utility of capsule endoscopy in Peutz-Jeghers syndrome. Gastrointest Endosc Clin N Am. 2004;14(1):159–67.

136. van Lier MG, Wagner A, Mathus-Vliegen EM. High cancer risk in Peutz-Jeghers syndrome: a systematic review and surveillance recommendations. Am J Gastroenterol. 2010;105(6):1258–64.

137. Korsse SE, Dewint P, Kuipers EJ, van Leerdam ME. Small bowel endoscopy and Peutz-Jeghers syndrome. Best Pract Res Clin Gastroenterol. 2012;26(3):263–78.

138. Pennazio M, Rossini FP. Small bowel polyps in Peutz-Jeghers syndrome: management by combined push enteroscopy and intraoperative enteroscopy. Gastrointest Endosc. 2000;51(3):304–8.

139. Brown G, Fraser C, Schofield G, et al. Video capsule endoscopy in peutz-jeghers syndrome: a blinded comparison with barium follow-through for detection of small-bowel polyps. Endoscopy. 2006;38(4):385–90.

140. Ohmiya N, Taguchi A, Shirai K, et al. Endoscopic resection of Peutz-Jeghers polyps throughout the small intestine at double-balloon enteroscopy without laparotomy. Gastrointest Endosc. 2005;61(1):140–7.

141. Ohmiya N, Nakamura M, Takenaka H, et al. Management of small-bowel polyps in Peutz-Jeghers syndrome by using enteroclysis, double-balloon enteroscopy, and videocapsule endoscopy. Gastrointest Endosc. 2010;72(6):1209–16.

142. Gao H, van Lier MG, Poley JW, et al. Endoscopic therapy of small-bowel polyps by double-balloon enteroscopy in patients with Peutz-Jeghers syndrome. Gastrointest Endosc. 2010;71(4):768–73.

143. Sakamoto H, Yamamoto H, Hayashi Y, et al. Nonsurgical management of small-bowel polyps in Peutz-Jeghers syndrome with extensive polypectomy by using double-balloon endoscopy. Gastrointest Endosc. 2011;74(2):328–33.

144. Chen TH, Lin WP, Su MY, et al. Balloon-assisted enteroscopy with prophylactic polypectomy for Peutz-Jeghers syndrome: experience in Taiwan. Dig Dis Sci. 2011;56(5):1472–5.

145. Serrano M, Mão-de-Ferro S, Pinho R, et al. Double-balloon enteroscopy in the management of patients with Peutz-Jeghers syndrome: a retrospective color multicenter study. Rev Esp Enferm Dig. 2013; 105(10):594–9.

146. Lin TK. Enteroscopy in the pediatric population. Tech Gastrointest Endosc. 2013;15(1):36–40.

147. May A, Nachbar L, Pohl J, Ell C. Endoscopic interventions in the small bowel using double balloon enteroscopy: feasibility and limitations. Am J Gastroenterol. 2007;102(3):527–35.

148. Mathus-Vliegen EM, Tytgat GN. Intraoperative endoscopy: technique, indications, and results. Gastrointest Endosc. 1986;32(6):381–4.

Video Legends

Video 13.1 - Endoscopic biopsy of a large jejunal melanoma.

Video 13.2 - Very large jejunal polyp on DAE in a patient referred for OGIB.

Video 13.3 - Demonstration of endoscopic marking of SBT.

Video 13.4 - DAE with multiple endoscopic polypectomies in PJS.

Definition of Postoperative Anatomy and Placement of PEJ

Manuel Berzosa Corella and Frank Lukens

Postoperative Anatomy

The advanced endoscopist performing balloon enteroscopy has to be well acquainted with the postoperative anatomy. Understanding the different types of small bowel reconstructions will help the endoscopist troubleshoot any difficulties that arise from altered anatomy while performing enteroscopy.

Before starting the procedure, it is important to first get as much information as possible about the underlying postsurgical anatomy of your patient [1]. Ideally, the endoscopist should review the surgical report to determine what type of surgery was done, how much bowel has been resected, how long were the limbs, and what type of anastomosis was made. If not available, then the review of existing abdominal imaging posterior to the surgery (e.g., computed tomography or magnetic resonance enterography, small bowel

follow-through) might provide valuable information and be a road map before the endoscopy.

Before reviewing the most common postoperative anatomies encountered during small bowel enteroscopy, it is important to define the two main types of anastomoses: end-to-side and side-to-side. The type of anastomosis would depend on the method used to reconnect the bowel, for hand-sewn end-to-side and for stapled side-to-side.

End-to-side, also known as terminolateral anastomosis, is usually seen after laparotomy hand-sewn small bowel anastomosis (Fig. 14.1). In this situation, the endoscopist will encounter two openings (Fig. 14.2, Video 14.1). Side-to-side (Fig. 14.3), also known as laterolateral anastomosis, is commonly seen after laparoscopic stapled small bowel anastomosis. In this situation, the endoscopist will encounter three stomal openings (Video 14.2).

From an endoscopic view, it can be challenging to determine between the lumens of the anastomosed limbs. Usually the presence of a scar can aid with distinguishing between them. The efferent limb (limb used to reach the anastomosis) will have an intact mucosa on the contralateral portion of the small bowel wall to the anastomosis. This is different from the afferent limb, which would have a circumferential scar around the opening of the stoma. Therefore as a rule, to intubate the afferent limb, the anastomosis scar rim must be trespassed [2]. Careful observation of the peristaltic wave can also be

Electronic supplementary material: The online version of this chapter (doi: 10.1007/978-3-319-14415-3_14) contains supplementary material, which is available to authorized users. Videos can also be accessed at http://link.springer.com/chapter/10.1007/978-3-319-14415-3_14.

M.B. Corella, M.D. • F. Lukens, M.D. (✉)
Department of Gastroenterology, Mayo Clinic Florida, 4500 San Pablo Road, Jacksonville, FL 32224, USA
e-mail: manuelberzosa@hotmail.com; lukens.frank@mayo.edu

R. Kozarek and J.A. Leighton (eds.), *Endoscopy in Small Bowel Disorders*, DOI 10.1007/978-3-319-14415-3_14, © Springer International Publishing Switzerland 2015

199

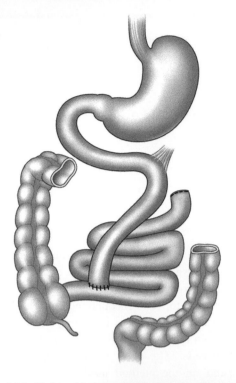

Fig. 14.1 End-to-side jejunoileal bypass. Reprinted with permission from Chousleb E, Rodriguez JP. Chapter 3. History of the Development of Metabolic/Bariatric Surgery. In: Nguyen NT, Rosenthal R, Ponce J, Morton J, Blackstone R (eds). The ASMBS Textbook of Bariatric Surgery, Vol. 1. New York, NY: Springer. 2014

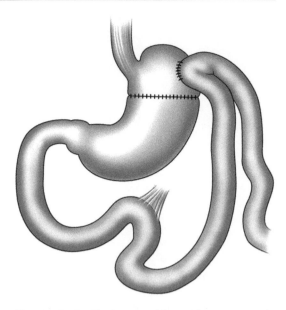

Fig. 14.3 Small bowel side-to-side anastomosis. Reprinted with permission from Chousleb E, Rodriguez JA, O'Leary JP. Chapter 3. History of the Development of Metabolic/Bariatric Surgery. In: Nguyen NT, Rosenthal R, Ponce J, Morton J, Blackstone R (eds). The ASMBS Textbook of Bariatric Surgery, Vol. 1. New York, NY: Springer. 2014

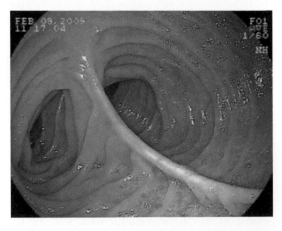

Fig. 14.2 Endoscopic view of an end-to-side anastomosis. Notice there are two stomal lumens

useful to differentiate between limbs. The efferent limb will have a peristalsis wave that will move away from the endoscope (natural down-stream peristalsis), but the afferent limb will have a peristaltic wave that would move toward the endoscope, which is also known as antiperistalsis (Video 14.3). In spite of these distinctions, the limbs are not always distinguishable, and in these cases the endoscopist will have to rely on fluoroscopic guidance to confirm the direction toward the desired quadrant (e.g., right upper quadrant if in need to reach the papilla on a Billroth II patient), or they will need to advance the scope as far as possible. If this latter strategy is followed, then we recommend marking the mucosa (e.g., biopsy or tattoo) of the limb to be examined. This might save time later upon withdrawal of the scope back to the anastomosis, as the scope can commonly fall back briskly upon withdrawal due to bowel fixation and angulation at the level of the anastomosis. If the limbs' openings are not clearly distinguishable (e.g., biopsy or tattoo), it can be difficult to determine which was the limb recently examined.

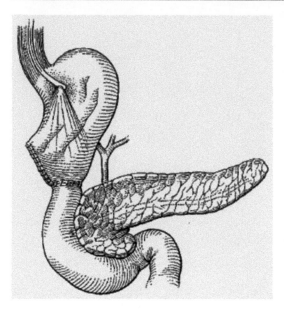

Fig. 14.4 Billroth I anastomosis diagram. Reprinted with permission Feitoza AB, Baron TH. Endoscopy and ERCP in the setting of previous upper GI tract surgery. Part II: post-surgical anatomy with alteration of the pancreaticobiliary tree. *Gastrointestinal endoscopy.* Jan 2002;55(1):75–79

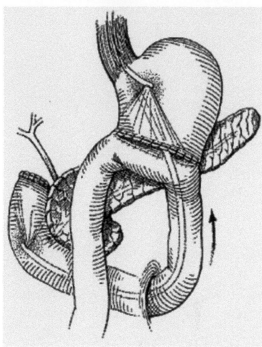

Fig. 14.5 Billroth II anastomosis diagram. Reprinted with permission Feitoza AB, Baron TH. Endoscopy and ERCP in the setting of previous upper GI tract surgery. Part II: postsurgical anatomy with alteration of the pancreaticobiliary tree. *Gastrointestinal endoscopy.* Jan 2002; 55(1):75–79

Billroth I

In Billroth I, the distal stomach is resected and the remaining stomach is anastomosed to the duodenum (Fig. 14.4) [1]. The endoscopist will encounter an intact esophagus and GEJ. The length of the stomach would vary depending on the extent of gastric resection. The endoscopist will find the anastomosis by following the greater curvature of the stomach. The bulb might be small or not present at all, and the duodenum will typically appear straightened [1].

Billroth II

In Billroth II, the distal stomach and first portion of the duodenum are resected. Different to a Billroth I, the duodenal stump is closed and instead the stomach is anastomosed to the jejunum in an end-to-side fashion, creating a gastrojejunostomy with two stomas—one each leading to the efferent and afferent limbs (Fig. 14.5 [1], Video 14.4). To reach the major papilla, the afferent limb should be intubated. The afferent limb will end as a blind

stump. The presence of bile and fluoroscopic confirmation of the direction of the scope toward the right upper quadrant or to cholecystectomy clips can help confirm the scope is within the afferent limb.

Braun Anastomosis

This is a side-to-side jejunojejunal anastomosis commonly seen during Billroth II reconstruction to divert bile from the gastric remnant by creating an anastomosis between both the efferent and afferent limbs (Fig. 14.6) [1].This means that the endoscopist would encounter a side-to-side anastomosis after intubating either opening of the gastrojejunal anastomosis. This Braun anastomosis is approximately 15 cm from the gastrojejunal anastomosis [1].

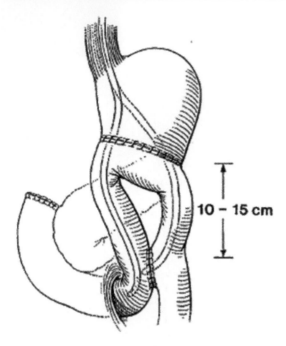

10 – 15 cm

Fig. 14.6 Braun anastomosis diagram. Reprinted with permission Feitoza AB, Baron TH. Endoscopy and ERCP in the setting of previous upper GI tract surgery. Part II: postsurgical anatomy with alteration of the pancreaticobiliary tree. *Gastrointestinal endoscopy*. Jan 2002;55(1):75–79

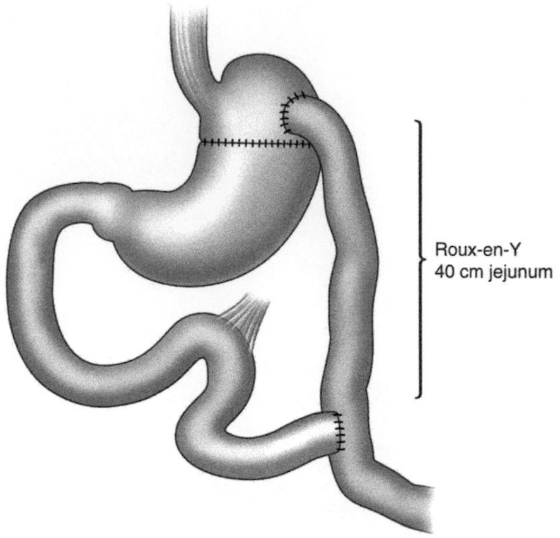

Roux-en-Y
40 cm jejunum

Fig. 14.7 Roux-en-Y limb for gastrojejunostomy. Reprinted with permission from Chousleb E, Rodriguez JA, O'Leary JP. Chapter 3. History of the Development of Metabolic/Bariatric Surgery. In: Nguyen NT, Rosenthal R, Ponce J, Morton J, Blackstone R (eds). The ASMBS Textbook of Bariatric Surgery, Vol. 1. New York, NY: Springer. 2014

Roux-en-Y Gastrojejunal Bypass

Roux-en-Y gastrojejunal bypass (RYGB) can be performed with gastrectomy (e.g., gastric cancer) or without gastrectomy (e.g., gastric bypass for weight loss) (Fig. 14.7). With either gastric bypass or partial distal gastrectomies, the endoscopist will encounter a normal esophagus and normal gastroesophageal junction. The gastric pouch will be connected distally to the jejunum in an end-to-side anastomosis. If the RYGB was performed for weight loss, the gastric pouch would be significantly smaller and will have a suture line or scar laterally [3]. This gastrojejunal anastomosis can have a length of 10–12 cm and will commonly have two small bowel limbs: a short blind limb and the efferent or Roux jejunal limb (Video 14.5) [3]. The length of the Roux limb can vary between 50 and 150 cm, with longer limbs used for weight loss surgeries and shorter ones for gastrectomy patients [3]. At the

end of the Roux limb, the endoscopists will find a jejunojejunal anastomosis. If the Roux-en-Y was performed for gastric bypass, the afferent limb will lead to the papilla and the stomach remnant can be entered in a retrograde fashion through an intact pylorus (Video 14.5). In a gastrectomy with Roux-en-Y, the limb will end in a blind stump similar to that seen on Billroth II anastomosis.

Biliopancreatic Diversion with Duodenal Switch

A biliopancreatic diversion with a duodenal switch consists of a partial gastrectomy (vertical sleeve gastrectomy) with preservation of the distal antrum, pylorus, and duodenal bulb; transection of the small bowel approximately half way between the ligament of Treitz and the ileocecal valve; and two enteroentero anastomoses—one

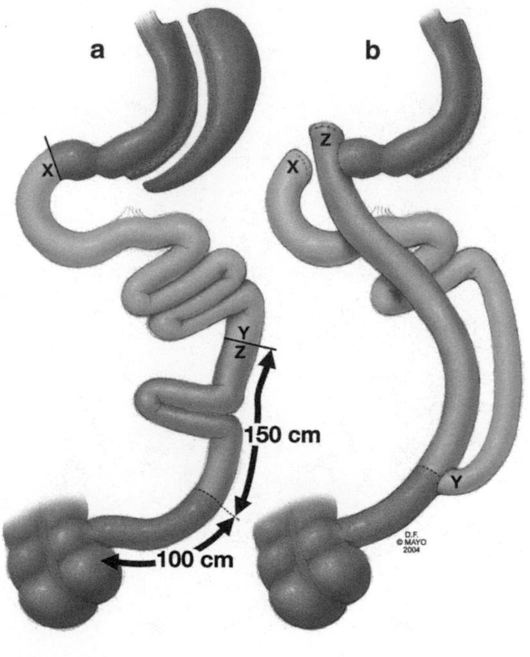

Fig. 14.8 Biliopancreatic diversion with duodenal switch diagram. From Decker GA, Swain JM, Crowell MD, Scolapio JS. Gastrointestinal and nutritional complications after bariatric surgery. Am J Gastroenterol 2007;102:2571–80. Used with permission of Mayo Foundation for Medical Education and Research, all rights reserved

between the duodenal bulb and the limb attached to the ileocecal valve (also known as the alimentary limb) and the second between the limb attached to the papilla (also known as the biliopancreatic limb) and the alimentary limb (Fig. 14.8) [4].

The endoscopist will encounter a normal esophagus and GEJ and then will find a stomach with a vertical sleeve gastrectomy. This means the lesser curvature will be intact and there will be a long vertical scar on the contralateral wall. The stomach would have a tubular shape but will have a preserved pylorus. Once the pylorus is transverse, the endoscopist will encounter the duodenal bulb and, soon after, an anastomosis with the alimentary limb. If the endoscopist continues down the alimentary limb, the endoscopist will reach a second enteroentero anastomosis. This anastomosis will have two open stomas: one into the biliopancreatic limb and the other into the common channel. Distal to the anastomosis

into the common channel limb, the endoscopist will reach the ileocecal valve. If the papilla needs to be reached, the biliopancreatic limb will have to be intubated. This limb is considerably longer when compared to Roux-en-Y gastrojejunal bypass.

Placement of Percutaneous Endoscopic Jejunostomy

Percutaneous endoscopic jejunostomy (PEJ) allows placement of a feeding tube directly into the jejunum. PEJ is an alternative to other direct methods of jejunal access, such as interventional radiology jejunostomy (IR-J) or surgical jejunostomy (SJ), and to the more commonly used technique for jejunal feedings, percutaneous endoscopic gastrostomy (PEG) tube with jejunal extension (PEG-J) [5]. There is no head-to-head study comparing these four techniques, but a recent review by Murphy et al. [6] summarizes the outcomes, adverse events, and reintervention rates published to date between these techniques (Table 14.1). PEJ allows jejunal access without the morbidities of surgery, but it does require sedation and in some cases general anesthesia, which is a disadvantage when compared to IR-J.

The most common indications for PEJ is the need for jejunal feedings due to previously failed PEG-J, previous gastrectomy, gastroparesis, recurrent aspiration, dysphagia, or poor nutritional status in patients with expected future foregut surgery (e.g., esophageal or gastric cancer resection) precluding PEG placement and gastric outlet or proximal small bowel obstruction [5].

The relative and absolute contraindications are similar to PEG. Absolute contraindications include uncorrected coagulopathy, thrombocytopenia or tense ascites, small bowel obstruction precluding distal scope passage, or intra-abdominal sepsis. Relative contraindications include obesity, small bowel dysmotility, eating disorders, functional nausea, vomiting, or abdominal pain. If it is uncertain that enteral feedings will be tolerated, a trial of nasojejunal feeding before PEJ placement can be considered [6].

Table 14.1 Outcomes of different methods of percutaneous jejunostomy placement

Procedure	First attempt success rate (%)	Overall adverse event rate (%)	Serious adverse event rate (%)	Reintervention rate (%)
PEG-J	88–93	35–56	0–3	22–56
IR-J	85–95	7.7–11.3	5–11	NA
PEJ	68–86	22–35	2–6.3	13.5–16.7
SJ	~100	12–35	0.6–4	1–8

Adapted from [6]

PEG-J percutaneous endoscopic gastrostomy tube with jejunal extension, *IR-J* interventional radiology jejunostomy, *PEJ* percutaneous endoscopic jejunostomy, *SJ* surgical jejunostomy

Placement Technique

PEJ placement uses the same principles and technique as a PEG placed by the pull technique [6]. Likewise, the use of an aseptic sterile technique and periprocedural antibiotics is recommended. To reach the jejunum, push enteroscopy with a pediatric colonoscope has been used most frequently, but there are also reports using balloon-assisted enteroscopy [7, 8].

Once the endoscope is advanced beyond the ligament of Treitz, the puncture site is selected by a combination of transillumination and finger indentation. If these two techniques fail to identify a clear window for needle puncture, one can consider the use of fluoroscopy [9], a long 15 cm needle [10], magnetic anchor [11], and/or transabdominal ultrasound guidance [12] as aids for successful bowel needle puncture:

1. After application of lidocaine within the desired needle tract, the needle is advanced with constant negative pressure suction until simultaneously air is aspirated and the needle is visualized within the lumen of the jejunum. If only air is suctioned and the needle is not visualized, then this suggests that the needle has entered another loop of bowel or hollow viscera at which point, the needle should be removed and a new puncture site selected.

2. The endoscopist will need to immediately secure the needle with a snare to avoid migration of the loop of bowel away from the abdominal wall (Fig. 14.9) [8]. This step is the major difference with conventional PEG

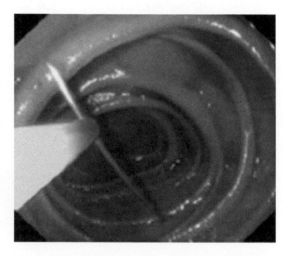

Fig. 14.9 Endoscopic view of the needle secured by snare after bowel puncture. Reprinted with permission from Aktas H, Mensink PB, Kuipers EJ, van Buuren H. Single-balloon enteroscopy-assisted direct percutaneous endoscopic jejunostomy. *Endoscopy*. Feb 2012;44(2):210–212

placement. The use of antispasmodics to reduce small bowel peristalsis has also been suggested as an aid to prevent migration of the small bowel [6].

3. A small incision is then made with a scalpel on the skin and subcutaneous tissue, which is followed by trochar introduction in the same tract as the needle. The trochar is then secured with the snare and the needle is removed (Fig. 14.10) [8]. The guidewire is fed through the trochar and then secured with the snare.

4. The scope is withdrawn and the guidewire is pulled through the patient's mouth. The feeding tube is attached to the guidewire and,

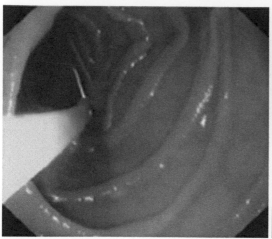
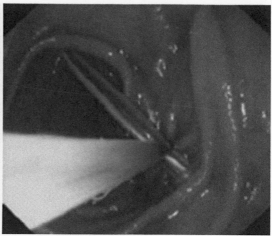
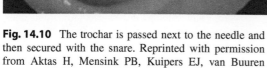

Fig. 14.10 The trochar is passed next to the needle and then secured with the snare. Reprinted with permission from Aktas H, Mensink PB, Kuipers EJ, van Buuren H. Single-balloon enteroscopy-assisted direct percutaneous endoscopic jejunostomy. *Endoscopy*. Feb 2012; 44(2):210–212

using the pull technique, the feeding tube is pulled through the abdominal wall and snug into the wall of the jejunum [6]. The scope can be reintroduced to confirm and photo document appropriate placement of the internal bumper of the feeding tube [6].

The success rate of PEJ placement can range from 68 to 86 % [5, 13–15]. The most common causes for failed PEJ placement include: absence or suboptimal transillumination and indentation, failure to reach the jejunum, and sedation complications [5, 13–15]. Increased success rates have been described in patients with previous gastric or esophageal resections, which are probably due to the shorter distance required to reach the jejunum and adhesions of the jejunum to the anterior abdominal wall that might facilitate bowel puncture. On the other hand, obesity has been described as cause for failed placement due to decreased transillumination and indentation from a thicker abdominal wall pannus [6, 15]. Complications rates range from 2 to 6.3 % for severe adverse events. See Table 14.2 [6].

Table 14.2 Adverse events reported in largest series of PEJ placement

Severe adverse events	Mild and moderate adverse events
Bleeding $n=4$	Infection $n=47$
Bowel perforation $n=8$	Pain $n=34$
Jejunal volvulus $n=6$	Chronic fistula $n=9$
Aspiration $n=1$	Aspiration $n=4$
Abscess $n=1$	Hematoma $n=1$
Necrotizing fasciitis $n=1$	Tube leak $n=13$
Jejunal obstruction $n=1$	Tube malfunction $n=3$
Sepsis $n=1$	Site ulceration $n=1$

Adapted from [6]

References

1. Feitoza AB, Baron TH. Endoscopy and ERCP in the setting of previous upper GI tract surgery. Part I: reconstruction without alteration of pancreaticobiliary anatomy. Gastrointest Endosc. 2001;54(6):743–9. Dec.
2. Moreels TG. Altered anatomy: enteroscopy and ERCP procedure. Best Pract Res Clin Gastroenterol. 2012;26(3):347–57. Jun.
3. Anderson MA, Gan SI, Fanelli RD, et al. Role of endoscopy in the bariatric surgery patient. Gastrointest Endosc. 2008;68(1):1–10. Jul.

4. Decker GA, Swain JM, Crowell MD, Scolapio JS. Gastrointestinal and nutritional complications after bariatric surgery. Am J Gastroenterol. 2007;102(11):2571–80. quiz 2581; Nov.

5. Maple JT, Petersen BT, Baron TH, Gostout CJ, Wong Kee Song LM, Buttar NS. Direct percutaneous endoscopic jejunostomy: outcomes in 307 consecutive attempts. Am J Gastroenterol. 2005;100(12):2681–8. Dec.

6. Murphy J, Fang JC. Direct percutaneous endoscopic jejunostomy: who, when, how, and what to avoid. Pract Gastroenterol. 2014;38(2):24–36.

7. Song LM, Baron TH, Saleem A, Bruining DH, Alexander JA, Rajan E. Double-balloon enteroscopy as a rescue technique for failed direct percutaneous endoscopic jejunostomy when using conventional push enteroscopy (with video). Gastrointest Endosc. 2012;76(3):675–9. Sep.

8. Aktas H, Mensink PB, Kuipers EJ, van Buuren H. Single-balloon enteroscopy-assisted direct percutaneous endoscopic jejunostomy. Endoscopy. 2012; 44(2):210–2. Feb.

9. Shetzline MA, Suhocki PV, Workman MJ. Direct percutaneous endoscopic jejunostomy with small bowel enteroscopy and fluoroscopy. Gastrointest Endosc. 2001;53(6):633–8. May.

10. Moran GW, Fisher NC. Direct percutaneous endoscopic jejunostomy: high completion rates with selective use of a long drainage access needle. Diagn Ther Endosc. 2009;2009:520879.

11. Yano T, Yamamoto H, Sunada K, et al. New technique for direct percutaneous endoscopic jejunostomy using double-balloon endoscopy and magnetic anchors in a porcine model. Dig Endosc. 2011;23(2):206. Apr.

12. Sharma VK, Close T, Bynoe R, Vasudeva R. Ultrasound-assisted direct percutaneous endoscopic jejunostomy (DPEJ) tube placement. Surg Endosc. 2000;14(2):203–4. Feb.

13. Fan AC, Baron TH, Rumalla A, Harewood GC. Comparison of direct percutaneous endoscopic jejunostomy and PEG with jejunal extension. Gastrointest Endosc. 2002;56(6):890–4. Dec.

14. Shike M, Latkany L, Gerdes H, Bloch AS. Direct percutaneous endoscopic jejunostomies for enteral feeding. Gastrointest Endosc. 1996;44(5):536–40. Nov.

15. Mackenzie SH, Haslem D, Hilden K, Thomas KL, Fang JC. Success rate of direct percutaneous endoscopic jejunostomy in patients who are obese. Gastrointest Endosc. 2008;67(2):265–9. Feb.

Video Legends

Video 14.1 - End-to-side anastomosis.

Video 14.2 - Side-to-side anastomosis. Small bowel anastomosis with 3 stomal openings.

Video 14.3 - Peristalsis and antiperistalsis at a small bowel anastomosis.

Video 14.4 - Billroth II anastomosis.

Video 14.5 - Roux-en-Y gastric bypass.

ERCP in Patients with Altered Anatomy

15

Adam Templeton and Andrew Ross

Introduction

The number of patients with surgically altered anatomy is rising due to the proliferation and success of bariatric surgery and liver transplant, as well as the improved detection of pancreatic and gastric neoplasms and their resultant surgical resection. Despite improved surgical technique, the inherent complication rate of these procedures as well as the baseline prevalence of stricture, stone, and the progression of unresected or metachronous malignancy provide a challenge to the endoscopist when treating patients with surgically altered anatomy [1].

This chapter will review the indications for and technical aspects associated with performing endoscopic retrograde cholangiopancreatography (ERCP) in patients with surgically altered anatomy.

Electronic supplementary material: The online version of this chapter (doi: 10.1007/978-3-319-14415-3_15) contains supplementary material, which is available to authorized users. Videos can also be accessed at http://link.springer.com/chapter/10.1007/978-3-319-14415-3_15.

A. Templeton, M.D.
Section of Gastroenterology, University of
Washington Medical Center, 1959 NE Pacific Street,
UW Box Number 356424, Seattle, WA 98195, USA
e-mail: templeaw@uw.edu

A. Ross, M.D. (✉)
Digestive Disease Institute, Virginia Mason Medical
Center, 1100 9th Ave, Mailstop C3-GAS, Seattle,
WA 98101, USA
e-mail: andrew.ross@vmmc.org

Surgically Altered Anatomy

There are at least eight commonly performed surgical procedures resulting in altered enteric anatomy that require nonstandard approaches to ERCP [1]. Patients with surgically altered anatomy are susceptible to both normal pancreaticobiliary pathology as well as adverse events related to their surgery such as anastomotic strictures, biliary stasis leading to stone formation, and retained stents [2–4]. From the perspective of the endoscopist, the resultant postsurgical anatomy can be categorized according to the length of the afferent limb and pancreatico-biliary enteric connection; i.e., "native" papilla or surgically altered biliary or pancreatic-digestive anastomosis. The length of the afferent limb dictates the type of endoscope used and this, in turn, dictates the available tools for performing endoscopic intervention. The presence or absence of a native papilla directly impacts ease of cannulation (Table 15.1). As such, it is imperative that the endoscopist has a keen sense of the patient's anatomy prior to embarking on endoscopy. Whereas cross-sectional imaging and contrast-enhanced radiography can provide some degree of useful information for preprocedure planning, the original operative report, past endoscopy notes, and a direct discussion with the surgeon are far superior.

Short afferent limbs are most commonly encountered in patients following a Billroth II gastrojejunostomy, as the afferent limb is

Table 15.1 Altered anatomy requiring nonstandard ERCP

Anatomy	Papilla intact?
Short afferent limb	
Bilroth II gastrojejunostomy	Yes
Long afferent limb	
Whipple's procedure	No
Gastrojejunostomy	Yes
Choledochojejunostomy/ hepaticojejunostomy	No
Total gastrectomy with esophagojejunostomy	Yes
Very long afferent limb	
Gastric bypass	Yes
Biliary diversion "duodenal switch"	Yes

anastomosed directly to the gastric remnant. In patients with retrocolic Billroth II anastomosis, the length of bowel that must be traversed can be as short as 30 cm [5]. These limbs can be traversed with a duodenoscope, though at times the acute angulation at the anastomosis may require a more flexible forward viewing endoscope or balloon-assisted enteroscopy (BAE) [5, 6]. The use of a side viewing duodenoscope has also been reported for patients with a gastrojejunostomy or pylorus-preserving Whipple procedure [6], though this mandates both a short afferent limb and an easy-to-navigate anastomosis.

More commonly, patients with a longer afferent limb such as those patients who have undergone a "standard" Whipple procedure or those with a Roux-en-Y anastomosis require the use of a long forward viewing endoscope or enteroscope [6, 7]. The lengths of Roux limbs are variable. Short afferent limbs (<50 cm) are commonly encountered in patients with oncologic, transplant, or biliary-diverting procedures such as total gastrectomy with Roux-en-Y esophagojejunostomy, Roux-en-Y choledochojejunostomy, or hepaticojejunostomy [8]. These limbs will have variable papillary anatomy depending on the original indication for surgery (see Table 15.1). Bariatric surgery typically results in a long Roux limb (>100 cm) to promote malabsorption as well as prevent bile reflux [9]. These longer limbs may require the use of overtube-assisted devices for deep enteroscopy, such as BAE or rotational enteroscopy (RE). In addition to particularly long

and tortuous Roux limbs, patients who have undergone a Roux-en-Y gastric bypass have a remnant stomach. This can allow for an additional access point (surgical gastrostomy, endoscopic-assisted gastrostomy) for performing ERCP. For the rare patient who has undergone pancreatico-biliary diversion ("duodenal switch") for obesity, the Roux-en-Y anastomosis can, in some cases, be reached with difficulty using the retrograde approach with BAE [5]. As with Billroth II anatomy, patients with gastric bypass or pancreatico-biliary diversion will generally have native papillary anatomy.

Technical Aspects of ERCP in the Surgically Altered Anatomy

There are three significant challenges to successful ERCP in altered anatomy: reaching the papilla or pancreatico-biliary anastomosis (enteroscopic success), identification and cannulation of the papilla or pancreatico-biliary anastomosis (diagnostic success), and finally, performing therapy if indicated (therapeutic success). A learning curve for successfully performing each of these three maneuvers has been described [10], and, although no single standardized approach exists, there are certain techniques which, when employed, can optimize the chances of overall endoscopic success.

Enteroscopic Success

Preprocedure Planning
With considerable variability in postsurgical anatomy, preprocedure planning is essential. When adequately prepared, the endoscopist can decrease the procedure duration, select the appropriate endoscope, and have the appropriate tools available at the time of endoscopy. Most importantly, the previous operative report should be obtained, recent cross-sectional imaging reviewed, and if possible, a discussion with the surgeon who performed the original operation [11]. Depending on operator expertise and difficulty of the procedure, the range of times reported

for ERCP in altered anatomy can vary from 24 to 150 min [12–14]. The increased complexity and longer procedure duration in patients with post-surgical anatomy may necessitate the use of an anesthesiologist, as adequate (and safe) sedation almost certainly plays a role in affecting the procedure outcome. Several groups have reported improved intubation depth, patient comfort, and decreased overall procedure duration with the use of CO_2 for procedures employing BAE [15, 16].

In patients with short afferent limbs, such as those with Billroth II gastrojejunostomy, a duodenoscope may suffice and provides the benefit of both an elevator and availability of standard ERCP tools. In patients with longer limbs, success has been reported with either the 164 cm long pediatric colonoscope or 240 mm long "standard" enteroscope [7, 17] both with and without the assistance of a gastric overtube. Gastric overtubes may reduce looping in the stomach and duodenum; in patients who have undergone gastrectomy, gastric overtubes are rarely needed. If a colonoscope is used, it is preferable to use one with a variable stiffness setting. Initial insertion is performed on the most flexible setting and the stiffness is increased once the endoscope is passed into the small intestine to reduce loop formation. In patients with longer intestinal limbs, it may be necessary to use the "hook and pull" technique to advance the endoscope deeper into the small intestine. The use of a colonoscope to place a wire into the pancreatico-biliary limb in patients with Roux-en-Y anatomy followed by advancement of a duodenoscope over the wire has been described [17]. More recently the advent of overtube-assisted enteroscopy (both BAE and RE) has allowed the endoscopist a means to navigate tight angulation at the anastomosis and very long Roux limbs to access the pancreatico-biliary tree.

Overtube-Assisted Enteroscopy

Several techniques are now available to perform overtube-assisted deep enteroscopy including the double balloon enteroscopy (DBE), single balloon enteroscope (SBE), and RE. In general, RE and balloon-assisted enteroscopy (BAE) consist of a forward viewing enteroscope that travels through a flexible overtube. As such, overtube-assisted enteroscopy is a term that can encompass both RE and BAE. RE utilizes a rotating overtube that sequentially reduces and pleats the small bowel over a standard enteroscope. In the case of BAE, there is either a balloon on the distal tip of the overtube (single balloon) or a balloon on both the overtube and the distal tip of the enteroscope (double balloon). The operator is able to inflate or deflate the balloons selectively. Using a push-pull technique, BAE works by pleating the bowel over the endoscope as it is advanced, using balloons to stabilize the device for both forward progress and reduction. With a double balloon, the endoscope is advanced and the balloon at the tip of the endoscope is then inflated, anchoring the scope tip. The overtube is then advanced over the endoscope and, once the overtube has reached the end of the scope, the overtube is inflated and either reduction can be performed or the endoscope balloon can be deflated and advanced further. The single balloon technology works in the same fashion, though without a balloon over the endoscope tip. This sacrifices a degree of stability but provides added flexibility, faster set-up time, and decreased complexity of balloon coordination [18].

Several authors have reported conceptualizing the overtube as a "large working channel" to assist ERCP [19–21]. Once the enteroscope is advanced to the ampulla or the pancreatic or biliary anastomosis, the balloon is inflated on the overtube and reduction is performed. This anchors the overtube and the enteroscope is then removed. In the case of longer overtubes, an incision can be made in the overtube just outside of the patient (taking care not to damage the balloon air channel) and a gastroscope or ultraslim gastroscope can be advanced to the ampulla. This allows passage of standard-biliary tools such as stents [20] that are precluded by the long and narrow working channel of the enteroscope, or direct cholangioscopy [21, 22].

Afferent Limb Intubation

Regardless of anatomy, selecting the appropriate limb to traverse can be the first challenge reached by the endoscopist. Selecting the wrong limb

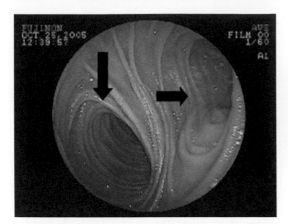

Fig. 15.1 Endoscopic image demonstrating the typical appearance of a jejunojejunostomy in a patient following a Roux-en-Y gastric bypass. The *vertical arrow* points to the typical location of the efferent limb whereas the *horizontal arrow* demonstrates the blind limb. The pancreaticobiliary limb cannot be seen in this image

adds time to an already lengthy procedure. In general, the endoscopist will encounter two or three potential lumens (Fig. 15.1) at the surgical anastomosis. If three lumens are visualized, invariably one of the openings is not a true opening, rather a "blind end," created by the end-to-side creation of the anastomosis. The passage visualized directly adjacent to this lumen is usually the efferent limb. Between these openings one should not see a surgical scar. If the efferent limb is entered and traversed for some distance the endoscopist will generally see multiple loops forming on fluoroscopy. Bile is not a reliable marker to indicate the afferent limb, though generally a greater amount of bile is found in the afferent limb. One group has reported improved identification of the afferent limb in patients with Roux-en-Y anatomy by injecting indigo carmine just beyond the stomach or the esophagojejunostomy. When the anastomosis is then reached, the afferent limb reportedly took up less indigo carmine and thus decreased time of procedure with little added expense or technical challenge [23].

It is not uncommon for endoscopists to become disoriented at the site of the anastomosis and, after accidentally traversing the efferent limb, reintubate the incorrect lumen. Once the appropriate limb has been determined, several groups advocate tattooing the afferent limb for improving ease of future access [24, 25]. Others recommend tattooing the limb that is initially intubated to prevent reintubation if this becomes the incorrect limb [26]. In either circumstance, clear documentation of which limb was tattooed is essential to expedite future endoscopy.

The second challenge to successful afferent limb intubation is navigating an often acute angulation. The afferent limb is generally located at 5–8 o'clock and should take off at a right angle—essentially an almost 180° turn once the endoscope is inserted into the Roux-en-Y anastomosis. If a variable stiffness colonoscope is used, making this turn should be attempted using the most flexible setting. Occasionally, changing the patient's position to left lateral decubitus or applying abdominal pressure can help navigate the turn. Fluoroscopy often can help confirm passage in the proper direction. If BAE systems are used, it is useful to reduce the scope as much as possible once the jejuno-jejunal anastomosis is reached (in the case of a Roux-en-Y anastomosis). Following reduction, the tip of the endoscope is advanced as deep as possible into the pancreatico-biliary limb. The balloon at the tip of the endoscope is then inflated and the endoscope tip is "hooked" into the limb using a combination of tip deflection and suction while the overtube is advanced through the anastomosis and into the pancreatico-biliary limb [5]. Despite these maneuvers, further advancement can be impossible. In these instances, a wire can be advanced downstream under fluoroscopy and a large balloon advanced over the wire. Using this balloon as an anchor, the enteroscope can be slowly inched forward [27].

Diagnostic Success

Once the proximal aspect of the pancreaticobiliary limb is reached, the next challenge lies in identifying the papilla, pancreatic, or biliary anastomosis and obtaining deep cannulation with the forward viewing endoscope. It is during cannulation and consideration of therapy that the lack of ERCP-specific tools, lack of an elevator, the altered vector forces, and abnormal anatomy

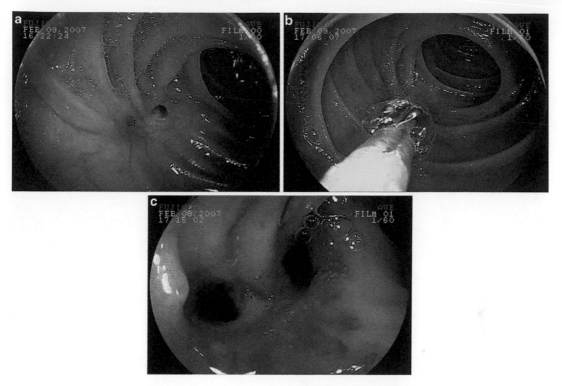

Fig. 15.2 (**a**) Typical endoscopic appearance of a hepaticojejunostomy. Note that the anastomosis is stenotic. (**b**) Balloon dilation of the hepaticojejunostomy using a con- trolled radial expansion balloon. (**c**) Postdilation appearance of the hepaticojejunostomy

(inverted orientation of the papilla) provide the greatest difficulty to providers accustomed to performing standard ERCP with a duodenoscope.

In patients with a choledochojejunostomy, hepaticojejunostomy, or pancreaticojejunostomy, cannulation is often relatively easy if the anastomosis can be found. Due to their small nature, the anastomosis may be difficult to find, either secondary to near complete stenosis or due to the positioning of intestinal folds or anatomic turns in the bowel (Fig. 15.2a). The hepaticojejunostomy is generally located 10–15 cm downstream from the blind end and is typically found in the lower left field of view. Administration of intravenous sincalide (Kinevac, Bracco Diagnostics, Princeton, New Jersey) at a dose of 0.02 μg/kg can be performed to stimulate the secretion of bile allowing identification of the biliary anastomosis. In patients with pancreaticojejunostomy, secretin (SecreFlo, Chesapeake Biologic Labs,

Baltimore, Maryland) administered intravenously as a 0.2 μg/kg bolus can help in a similar fashion. The use of a clear plastic cap (Olympus Co LTD, Japan) affixed to the tip of the endoscope can help improve visualization of biliodigestive anastomoses, as well as aid the visualization and cannulation of native papillae [19, 25]. The cap may also help anchor the endoscope during reduction via mucosal suctioning [12, 28]. Once found, cannulation is often amenable to forward viewing cannulation from the 6 o'clock accessory channel [18].

In patients with an intact "native" major papilla, a forward viewing endoscope will generally find the ampulla located at the 6 o'clock position [18] and "inverted." Cannulation of both native and anastomotic lumens is typically performed using a straight single or double lumen catheter after achieving wire guided access. The use of a clear plastic hood affixed

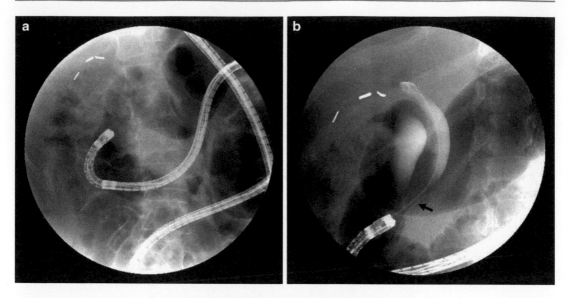

Fig. 15.3 ERCP performed using a double balloon enteroscope in a patient following RYGB. Note that biliary cannulation was achieved over a pancreatic duct stent (*arrow*)

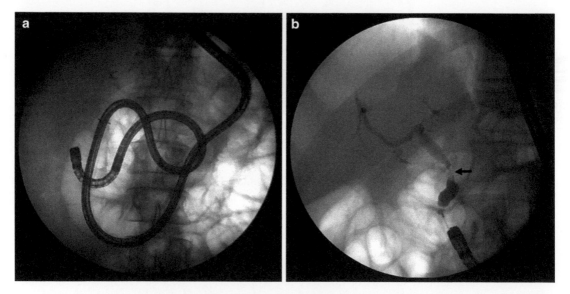

Fig. 15.4 ERCP performed following a Roux-en-Y esophagojejunostomy in a patient status post total gastrectomy for gastric cancer. Note the presence of a high-grade mid-common bile duct stricture (*arrow*)

to the endoscope tip may be useful in identification and cannulation of the native papilla. As with standard ERCP, in some instances where papillary anatomy preferentially results in pancreatic duct cannulation, biliary cannulation can be assisted by pancreatic duct stent placement and wire guided cannulation over the pancreatic duct stent (Fig. 15.3).

Therapeutic Success

After successful cannulation, the final step is delivery of therapy, often dilation of an anastomotic stricture, stone removal, bleeding treatment, or stent placement (demonstrated in Figs. 15.4, 15.5, and 15.6.). Forward viewing equipment provides the following challenges:

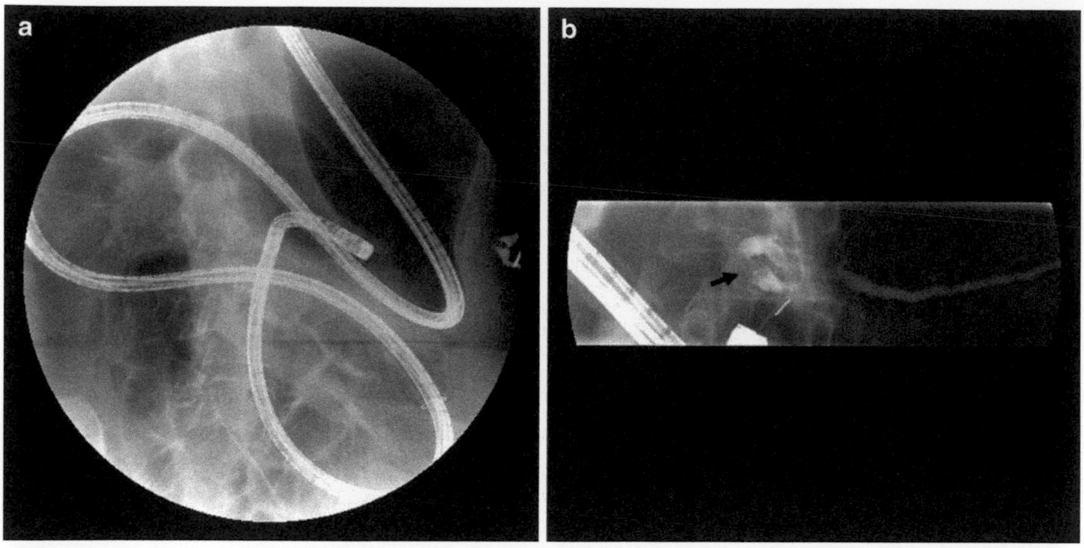

Fig. 15.5 ERCP performed in a patient following a central pancreactectomy with a Roux-en-Y pancreaticojejunostomy. Note the presence of a large pancreatic duct stone (*arrow*).

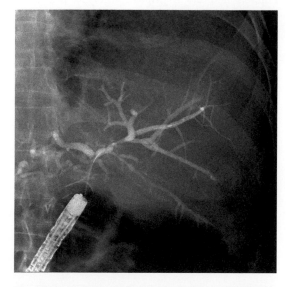

Fig. 15.6 Cholangiogram demonstrating a high-grade stricture of the common hepatic duct in a patient following a Whipple procedure for a cholangiocarcinoma of the distal common bile duct

lack of an elevator making wire exchanges tenuous, small diameter of working channel (generally a 2.8 mm channel compared to 4.2 mm standard duodenoscopes), and an increased length of the working channel precluding many standard ERCP tools. Lastly, due to the length of

the scope, the small diameter of the working channel, and the often multiple loops of the endoscope, there can be considerable resistance to wire and accessory passage. This last point can be improved with the use of a lubricant placed on the tip of the wire before advancement—either silicone or a spray oil such as PAM (ConAgra foods, Omaha, Nebraska). A review of available scope length and working channel diameters is provided in Table 15.2 (tools).

Sphincterotomy is typically performed by placement of a stent into either the pancreatic or bile duct followed by needle knife sphincterotomy over the stent (Fig. 15.7). Rotatable sphincterotomes have been reported [25] and some have reported success with limited sphincterotomy followed by controlled radial expansion (CRE) balloon dilation [19]. In general, the performance of other therapeutic maneuvers is relatively straightforward given the previously listed limitations. It should be noted that due to the long length of accessories, the assistant may "lose" the wire during exchange due to increased length relative to the wire guide being used. Whenever possible, the longest wire guide available should be used. If wire is "lost," use of a 60 mL syringe filled with water or saline affixed to the accessory in the

Table 15.2 Endoscopes used in altered anatomy

Endoscopes	Working channel (mm)	Working length (cm)	Distal end diameter (mm)	Overtube	Diameter (mm)	Length (cm)
Balloon-assisted endoscopes						
EN-450T5, Fujinon	2.8	200	9.4	TS-12140	13.2	145
EN-450P5, Fujinon	2.2	200	8.5	TS-12140	12.2	145
EC-450B15, EI-530B, Fujinon	2.8	152	9.4	TS-13101	13.2	105
SIF Q180, Olympus	2.8	200	9.2	ST-SB-1	13.2	140
SIF Q160Y, Olympus	2.8	200	8.4	ST-SB-1		
SIF-Y0004, Olympus	3.2	152	9.2	NR	NR	88
Spiral endoscopes						
Endo-Ease Discovery SB (DSB), Spirus	NA[a]				17.5	130

[a]Spirus is an overtube system compatable with standard enteroscopes

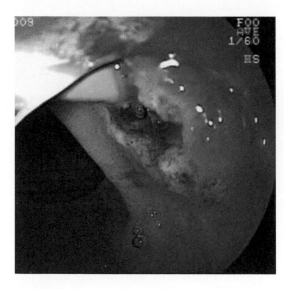

Fig. 15.7 Endoscopic image showing a needle knife biliary sphincterotomy performed over an indwelling pancreatic duct stent. Notice the direction of the cut is toward the 4 o'clock position on the inverted papilla

success using colonic length-CRE dilation balloons [18, 19] (Fig. 15.2b, c). A shorter double balloon enteroscope with a 2.8 mm working channel and 152 cm working length is available from Fujinon and an Olympus prototype has been reported with a 3.2 mm working channel and 150 cm working length. These endoscopes allow the use of shorter wires and standard ERCP implements, though they are still limited in working channel diameter size. As a workaround, several groups have reported using the overtube as a large working channel. Once the overtube is advanced to the pancreatico-biliary limb, anchored with balloon inflated, and wire guided cannulation is achieved, the endoscope is exchanged out leaving the wire or a long balloon inflated in the bile duct. A hole is cut in the overtube just outside the patient's mouth and shorter instruments such as self-expanding metal stents (SEMS) or ultraslim gastroscopes for direct cholangioscopy can then be utilized [12, 21, 22].

process of exchanging can be used to create a static column of water. This, along with gentle counter pressure, can help avoid losing duct access.

With the small diameter (2.8 mm) of most enteroscope or colonoscope working channels, a 7 Fr plastic stent is the largest caliber plastic endoprosthesis that can be used. Additional equipment such as enteroscopy-length sphincterotomes, needle knife, and extraction balloons and baskets are available. For balloon dilation, many have reported

Alternatives to PER OS Endoscopic Access and Failed Altered Anatomy ERCP

The approach to patients with altered anatomy and pancreatico-biliary pathology should be individualized to both the patient and the urgency/emergency of needed intervention as well as local institutional resources and operator experience. With the exception of Billroth II anatomy,

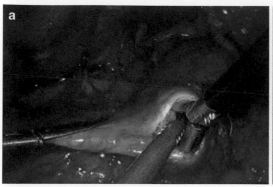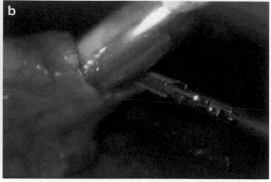

Fig. 15.8 A gastrostomy is made in the excluded stomach (**a**) in order to perform laparoscopic-assisted ERCP in a patient following Roux-en-Y gastric bypass surgery. A laparoscopic trocar is placed through the anterior abdominal wall into the excluded stomach (**b**) to allow for endoscope placement

until the advent of balloon-assisted technology, options for management of surgically altered anatomy were largely limited to surgical or percutaneous access. Percutaneous-biliary access via interventional radiology still remains a viable alternative when local gastrointestinal expertise or equipment is not available, or if endoscopic management is attempted without success. Additionally, percutaneous access may provide temporizing measures, allowing for patient transfer to an expert center with advanced enteroscopic specialty or allowing for decompression and rendezvous attempt with enteroscopy [29]. In some instances, such as nondilated bile ducts or pancreatic duct pathology, percutaneous access is also not a viable option.

Roux-en-Y gastric bypass surgery presents added difficulty for the endoscopist. In general, the afferent limb is very long (>100 cm), native papilla anatomy is expected, and, depending on weight loss, body habitus can provide further challenge. Almost uniformly, studies using balloon technology have lower success rates for both enteroscopic, diagnostic, and technical success (discussed later). Even if the papilla is reached, the procedure can be a failure due to the distance traveled and the lack of instruments adaptable for the 200 cm scope and 2.8 cm channel. As such, endoscopists have explored modified surgical options.

The first described report of surgical gastrostomy creation for ERCP in an excluded stomach was by Baron and Vickers in 1998 [30].

Subsequent reports have shown acceptable diagnostic and therapeutic success using this approach. Briefly, laparoscopic access to the gastric remnant is obtained and the duodenoscope is advanced through a gastrostomy or laparoscopic trocar and advanced to the duodenum in standard fashion [30, 31] (Fig. 15.8, Video 15.1). Following the procedure, if further intervention is thought likely, a gastrostomy tube can be left in place, otherwise the ports and gastrostomy site are closed. Several centers have also reported utilizing endoscopic ultrasound (EUS) for endoscopic transgastric PEG placement [32] or using BAE to reach the gastric remnant and subsequent placement of a self-expanding metal stent through a gastrostomy for same day ERCP [33].

The benefits of utilizing gastrostomy access include the ability to leave a tube for future access, the ability to perform EUS, the opportunity to perform cholecystectomy after ERCP or EUS if indicated, and the availability of standard equipment for diagnostic and therapeutic success. The limitations of this procedure are coordination between surgeon and endoscopist as well as the need and expense for an operating room and operating room staff. The cost effectiveness of laparoscopic access versus attempt at BAE was reviewed in a single center experience [31]. This study found that while ERCP success was much higher in the surgical arm and the time for the endoscopist shorter, the cost associated with surgical approach was considerably higher.

As such, the authors recommended that in patients with a known afferent limb <150 cm, a balloon-assisted enteroscopy be attempted first with surgical gastrostomy access as backup [31].

ERCP Failure

Despite improved equipment, anatomic and technical limitations can still preclude ERCP success. As with standard ERCP, if endoscopic means fail to gain access, interventional radiology can often assist to obtain percutaneous-biliary access, after which point a rendezvous procedure can be attempted. In the event of nondilated bile ducts, gallbladder cannulation followed by a wire placed through the cystic duct has also been reported [34]. More recently several centers have reported utilizing EUS to gain transgastric or transduodenal-biliary or pancreatic duct access for either primary drainage or for endoscopic rendezvous in patients with altered anatomy [35–38].

Systematic Review of Reported Literature

We performed a search of PubMed to identify the published literature of ERCP in altered anatomy with specific focus on ERCP after the advent of overtube-assisted technology. The following search terms were used: double balloon enteroscopy OR single balloon enteroscopy OR spiral enteroscopy AND ERCP. Eighty-one articles were identified with an additional ten articles identified by review of pertinent references. This search found 32 studies reporting retrospectively or prospectively collected data on operator experience with overtube-assisted technology. No randomized controlled trials were found and with few exceptions, these studies were single center, small series, and retrospective reviews.

In all, the case series represent more than 752 patients and 1,068 procedures performed on surgically altered anatomy. Of these, 9 studies reviewed SBE [12, 14, 18, 24, 39–43], 14 studies of DBE [1, 10, 12, 22, 44–53], 3 studies of RE [12, 13, 43], 2 studies of lap assisted [31, 54], 7

studies used "short" double balloon technology [25, 29, 55–59], and 5 studies had mixed modality instruments [19, 31, 60–62]. In general, enteroscopic and ERCP success rates were similar regardless of overtube-assisted technology and varied more by anatomy—enteroscopic and ERCP success decreased as limb length increased and if there was a native papilla. This search identified no head-to-head comparison studies of enteroscopes. However, several studies reported success of BAE after previous failures with forward viewing endoscopes, suggesting that BAE may be the preferable device for initial attempt in patients with long afferent limbs [1, 6, 51, 60].

Conclusion

Future Directions

The advent of overtube-assisted technology has greatly advanced the endoscopist's ability to perform minimally invasive and effective therapy for patients with surgically altered anatomy. In expert hands, if the papilla can be reached, the chance of diagnostic and therapeutic success is high. Shorter OAE systems and the conceptualization of the overtube as a large working channel have increased the armamentarium available, yet endoscopists are still limited by the lack of an elevator, poor accessory selection, and small diameter working channels within the endoscopes. Despite expert hands, the ability to reach the ampulla can still be a time intensive and difficult challenge, particularly in patients with very long Roux limbs. To work around failed ERCP, novel approaches with endoscopic ultrasound are increasingly described. Also promising are collaborative approaches between surgeons and endoscopists modifying long limb surgery to improve postoperative endoscopic treatment.

In the case of failed ERCP, several centers have reported success with transgastric or transduodenal EUS guided access [35, 38]. This can be for either definitive therapy such as decompression with stent, or can allow for wire placement and BAE rendezvous. The benefit of this approach is twofold: (1) the completion of the procedure can be accomplished without surgical or percutaneous drainage and (2) the ability to perform the procedure at the time of failed endoscopy. At the present point, techniques to prevent complication are still being worked out [63, 64], but hold promise for patients with surgically altered anatomy who may not be ideal candidates for surgical intervention and require definitive therapy.

In general, prevention is preferable to intervention and it may be possible to maintain the success of anatomic revision or bariatric or malignant intervention and improve the ability to endoscopically manage potential complications. The angulation and long length of Roux anatomy was initially postulated to provide patients with increased protection from bile reflux [9]. However, a recent study described using a short-limb (20 cm) Roux-en-Y reconstruction for gastric bypass. They also performed a submucosal tattoo of the afferent limb at the level of the jejunojejunostomy to help guide future endoscopy. The authors found that short limb Roux-en-Y hepaticojejunostomy (RYHJ) was both safe and associated with a low incidence of postoperative complications. Notably, those who required intervention were managed endoscopically in all cases [9].

ERCP in surgically altered anatomy is now both feasible and, in many cases, successful. Although time consuming and challenging, overtube-assisted technology is associated with fewer complications and decreased cost [31] when compared to surgical management. With the burgeoning population of patients with altered anatomy, particularly as a result of bariatric surgery, there will be further opportunities to determine optimal approaches to altered anatomy and how to manage the invariable failed ERCP.

References

1. Maaser C, Lenze F, Bokemeyer M, Ullerich H, Domaqk D, Bruewer M, et al. Double balloon enteroscopy: a useful tool for diagnostic and therapeutic procedures in the pancreaticobiliary system. Am J Gastroenterol. 2008;103:894–900.
2. Icoz G, Kilic M, Zeytunlu M, Celebi A, Ersoz G, Killi R, et al. Biliary reconstructions and complications encountered in 50 consecutive right-lobe living donor liver transplantations. Liver Transpl. 2003;9:575–80.
3. Saidi RF, Elias N, Ko DS, Kawai T, Markmann J, Cosimi AB, et al. Biliary reconstruction and complications after living-donor liver transplantation. HPB (Oxford). 2009;11:505–9.
4. Hamdan K, Somers S, Chand M. Management of late postoperative complications of bariatric surgery. Br J Surg. 2011;98:1345–55.
5. Haber GB. Double balloon endoscopy for pancreatic and biliary access in altered anatomy (with videos). Gastrointest Endosc. 2007;66(3 Suppl):S47–50.
6. Kawamura T, Mandai K, Uno K, Yasuda K. Does single-balloon enteroscopy contribute to successful endoscopic retrograde cholangiopancreatography in patients with surgically altered gastrointestinal anatomy? ISRN Gastroenterol. 2013. doi:10.1155/2013/214958.
7. Elton E, Hanson BL, Qaseem T, Howell DA. Diagnostic and therapeutic ERCP using an enteroscope and a pediatric colonoscope in long-limb surgical bypass patients. Gastrointest Endosc. 1998;47:62–7.
8. Moreels TG. Altered anatomy: enteroscopy and ERCP procedure. Best Pract Res Clin Gastroenterol. 2012;26:347–57.
9. Felder SI, Menon VG, Nissen NN, Margulies DR, Lo S, Colquhoun SD. Hepaticojejunostomy using short-limb roux-en-Y reconstruction. JAMA Surg. 2013;148:253–7. discussion 257–8.
10. Mehdizadeh S, Ross A, Gerson L, Leighton J, Chen A, Schembre D, et al. What is the learning curve associated with double-balloon enteroscopy? Technical details and early experience in 6 U.S. tertiary care centers. Gastrointest Endosc. 2006;64:740–50.
11. Stellato TA, Crouse C, Hallowell PT. Bariatric surgery: creating new challenges for the endoscopist. Gastrointest Endosc. 2003;57:86–94.
12. Shah RJ, Smolkin M, Yen R, Ross A, Kozarek RA, Howell DA, et al. A multicenter, U.S. experience of single-balloon, double-balloon, and rotational overtube-assisted enteroscopy ERCP in patients with surgically altered pancreaticobiliary anatomy (with video). Gastrointest Endosc. 2013;77:593–600.
13. Wagh MS, Draganov PV. Prospective evaluation of spiral overtube-assisted ERCP in patients with surgically altered anatomy. Gastrointest Endosc. 2012;76:439–43.
14. Tomizawa Y, Sullivan CT, Gelrud A. Single balloon enteroscopy (SBE) assisted therapeutic endoscopic retrograde cholangiopancreatography (ERCP) in patients with roux-en-y anastomosis. Dig Dis Sci. 2014;59:465–70.
15. Domagk D, Bretthauer M, Lenz P, Aabakken L, Ullerich H, Maaser C, et al. Carbon dioxide insufflation improves intubation depth in double-balloon enteroscopy: a randomized, controlled, double-blind trial. Endoscopy. 2007;39:1064–7.
16. Yamano HO, Yoshikawa K, Kimura T, Yamamoto E, Harada E, Kudou T, et al. Carbon dioxide insufflation for colonoscopy: evaluation of gas volume, abdominal pain, examination time and transcutaneous partial CO_2 pressure. J Gastroenterol. 2010;45:1235–40.

17. Wright BE, Cass OW, Freeman ML. ERCP in patients with long-limb roux-en-Y gastrojejunostomy and intact papilla. Gastrointest Endosc. 2002; 56:225–32.
18. Neumann H, Fry LC, Meyer F, Malfertheiner P, Monkemuller K. Endoscopic retrograde cholangiopancreatography using the single balloon enteroscope technique in patients with roux-en-Y anastomosis. Digestion. 2009;80:52–7.
19. Itoi T, Ishii K, Sofuni A, Itokawa F, Tsuchiya T, Kurihara T, et al. Long- and short-type double-balloon enteroscopy-assisted therapeutic ERCP for intact papilla in patients with a roux-en-Y anastomosis. Surg Endosc. 2011;25:713–21.
20. Skinner M, Gutierrez JP, Wilcox CM, Monkemuller K. Overtube-assisted placement of a metal stent into the bile duct of a patient with surgically altered upper-gastrointestinal anatomy during double-balloon enteroscopy-assisted ERCP. Endoscopy. 2013;45(Suppl 2 UCTN):E418–9. doi:10.1055/s-0033-1358806.
21. Koshitani T, Matsuda S, Takai K, Motoyoshi T, Nishikata M, Yamashita Y, et al. Direct cholangioscopy combined with double-balloon enteroscope-assisted endoscopic retrograde cholangiopancreatography. World J Gastroenterol. 2012;18:3765–9.
22. Monkemuller K, Popa D, McGuire B, Ramesh J, Wilcox CM. Double-balloon enteroscopy-ERCP rendezvous technique. Endoscopy. 2013;45 Suppl 2:E333–4. doi:10.1055/s-0033-1344329.
23. Yano T, Hatanaka H, Yamamoto H, Nakazawa K, Nishimura N, Wada S, et al. Intraluminal injection of indigo carmine facilitates identification of the afferent limb during double-balloon ERCP. Endoscopy. 2012; 44(Suppl 2 UCTN):E340–1. doi:10.1055/s-0032-1309865.
24. Saleem A, Baron TH, Gostout CJ, Topazian MD, Levy MJ, Petersen BT, et al. Endoscopic retrograde cholangiopancreatography using a single-balloon enteroscope in patients with altered roux-en-Y anatomy. Endoscopy. 2010;42:656–60.
25. Osoegawa T, Motomura Y, Akahoshi K, Higuchi N, Tanaka Y, Hisano T, et al. Improved techniques for double-balloon-enteroscopy-assisted endoscopic retrograde cholangiopancreatography. World J Gastroenterol. 2012;18:6843–9.
26. Ross AS, Semrad C, Alverdy J, Waxman I, Dye C. Use of double-balloon enteroscopy to perform PEG in the excluded stomach after roux-en-Y gastric bypass. Gastrointest Endosc. 2006;64:797–800.
27. Itoi T, Sofuni A, Itokawa F. Large dilating balloon to allow endoscope insertion for successful endoscopic retrograde cholangiopancreatography in patients with surgically altered anatomy (with video). J Hepatobiliary Pancreat Sci. 2010;17:725–8.
28. Shimatani M, Takaoka M, Okazaki K. Tips for double balloon enteroscopy in patients with roux-en-Y reconstruction and modified child surgery. J Hepatobiliary Pancreat Sci. 2014;21:E22–8.
29. Tsujino T, Isayama H, Sugawara Y, Sasaki T, Kogure H, Nakai Y, et al. Endoscopic management of biliary complications after adult living donor liver transplantation. Am J Gastroenterol. 2006;101:2230–6.
30. Baron TH, Vickers SM. Surgical gastrostomy placement as access for diagnostic and therapeutic ERCP. Gastrointest Endosc. 1998;48:640–1.
31. Schreiner MA, Chang L, Gluck M, Irani S, Gan SI, Brandabur JJ, et al. Laparoscopy-assisted versus balloon enteroscopy-assisted ERCP in bariatric post-roux-en-Y gastric bypass patients. Gastrointest Endosc. 2012;75:748–56.
32. Attam R, Leslie D, Freeman M, Ikramuddin S, Andrade R. EUS-assisted, fluoroscopically guided gastrostomy tube placement in patients with roux-en-Y gastric bypass: a novel technique for access to the gastric remnant. Gastrointest Endosc. 2011;74:677–82.
33. Baron TH, Song LM, Ferreira LE, Smyrk TC. Novel approach to therapeutic ERCP after long-limb roux-en-Y gastric bypass surgery using transgastric self-expandable metal stents: experimental outcomes and first human case study (with videos). Gastrointest Endosc. 2012;75:1258–63.
34. Okuno M, Iwashita T, Yasuda I, Mabuchi M, Uemura S, Nakashima M, et al. Percutaneous transgallbladder rendezvous for enteroscopic management of choledocholithiasis in patients with surgically altered anatomy. Scand J Gastroenterol. 2013;48:974–8.
35. Prachayakul V, Aswakul P. A novel technique for endoscopic ultrasound-guided biliary drainage. World J Gastroenterol. 2013;19:4758–63.
36. Fujii LL, Gostout CJ, Levy MJ. Single-scope endoscopic ultrasound-guided rendezvous-assisted biliary stent insertion. Endoscopy. 2012;44(Suppl 2 UCTN): E207–8.
37. Fujii LL, Topazian MD, Abu Dayyeh BK, Baron TH, Chari ST, Farnell MB, et al. EUS-guided pancreatic duct intervention: outcomes of a single tertiary-care referral center experience. Gastrointest Endosc. 2013; 78:854–64.
38. Shah JN, Marson F, Weilert F, Bhat YM, Nguyen-Tang T, Shaw RE, et al. Single-operator, single-session EUS-guided anterograde cholangiopancreatography in failed ERCP or inaccessible papilla. Gastrointest Endosc. 2012;75:56–64.
39. Dellon ES, Kohn GP, Morgan DR, Grimm IS. Endoscopic retrograde cholangiopancreatography with single-balloon enteroscopy is feasible in patients with a prior roux-en-Y anastomosis. Dig Dis Sci. 2009;54:1798–803.
40. Wang AY, Sauer BG, Behm BW, Ramanath M, Cox DG, Ellen KL, et al. Single-balloon enteroscopy effectively enables diagnostic and therapeutic retrograde cholangiography in patients with surgically altered anatomy. Gastrointest Endosc. 2010;71:641–9.
41. Itoi T, Ishii K, Sofuni A, Itokawa F, Tsuchiya T, Kurihara T, et al. Single-balloon enteroscopy-assisted ERCP in patients with billroth II gastrectomy or roux-en-Y anastomosis (with video). Am J Gastroenterol. 2010;105:93–9.
42. Kianicka B, Lata J, Novotny I, Dite P, Vanicek J. Single balloon enteroscopy for endoscopic

retrograde cholangiography in patients with roux-en-Y hepaticojejuno anastomosis. World J Gastroenterol. 2013;19:8047–55.

43. Lennon AM, Kapoor S, Khashab M, Corless E, Amateau S, Dunbar K, et al. Spiral assisted ERCP is equivalent to single balloon assisted ERCP in patients with roux-en-Y anatomy. Dig Dis Sci. 2012;57:1391–8.

44. Parlak E, Cicek B, Disibeyaz S, Cenqiz C, Yurdakul M, Akdogan M, et al. Endoscopic retrograde cholangiography by double balloon enteroscopy in patients with roux-en-Y hepaticojejunostomy. Surg Endosc. 2010;24:466–70.

45. Emmett DS, Mallat DB. Double-balloon ERCP in patients who have undergone roux-en-Y surgery: a case series. Gastrointest Endosc. 2007;66:1038–41.

46. Aabakken L, Bretthauer M, Line PD. Double-balloon enteroscopy for endoscopic retrograde cholangiography in patients with a roux-en-Y anastomosis. Endoscopy. 2007;39:1068–71.

47. Koornstra JJ. Double balloon enteroscopy for endoscopic retrograde cholangiopancreaticography after roux-en-Y reconstruction: case series and review of the literature. Neth J Med. 2008;66:275–9.

48. Kuga R, Furuya Jr CK, Hondo FY, Ide E, Ishioka S, Sakai P. ERCP using double-balloon enteroscopy in patients with roux-en-Y anatomy. Dig Dis. 2008;26:330–5.

49. Fahndrich M, Sandmann M, Heike M. A facilitated method for endoscopic interventions at the bile duct after roux-en-Y reconstruction using double balloon enteroscopy. Z Gastroenterol. 2008;46:335–8.

50. Moreels TG, Hubens GJ, Ysebaert DK, Op de Beeck B, Pelckmans PA. Diagnostic and therapeutic double-balloon enteroscopy after small bowel roux-en-Y reconstructive surgery. Digestion. 2009;80:141–7.

51. Pohl J, May A, Aschmoneit I, Ell C. Double-balloon endoscopy for retrograde cholangiography in patients with choledochojejunostomy and roux-en-Y reconstruction. Z Gastroenterol. 2009;47:215–9.

52. Patel MK, Horsley-Silva JL, Gomez V, Stauffer JA, Stark ME, Lukens FJ. Double balloon enteroscopy procedure in patients with surgically altered bowel anatomy: analysis of a large prospectively collected database. J Laparoendosc Adv Surg Tech A. 2013;23:409–13.

53. Park JH, Ye BD, Byeon JS, Kimdo H, Choi KD, Song TJ, et al. Approaching pancreatic duct through pancreaticojejunostomy site with double ballon enteroscope in patients with roux-en-Y anatomy. Hepatogastroenterology. 2013;60:1753–8.

54. Gutierrez JM, Lederer H, Krook JC, Kinney TP, Freeman ML, Jensen EH. Surgical gastrostomy for pancreatobiliary and duodenal access following roux en Y gastric bypass. J Gastrointest Surg. 2009;13:2170–5.

55. Choi EK, Chiorean MV, Cote GA, El Hajj II, Ballard D, Fogel EL, et al. ERCP via gastrostomy vs. double balloon enteroscopy in patients with prior bariatric roux-en-Y gastric bypass surgery. Surg Endosc. 2013;27:2894–9.

56. Shimatani M, Matsushita M, Takaoka M, Koyabu M, Ikeura T, Kato K, et al. Effective "short" double-balloon enteroscope for diagnostic and therapeutic ERCP in patients with altered gastrointestinal anatomy: a large case series. Endoscopy. 2009;41:849–54.

57. Sanada Y, Mizuta K, Yano T, Hatanaka W, Okada N, Wakiya T, et al. Double-balloon enteroscopy for bilio-enteric anastomotic stricture after pediatric living donor liver transplantation. Transpl Int. 2011;24:85–90.

58. Cho S, Kamalaporn P, Kandel G, Kortan P, Marcon N, May G. 'Short' double-balloon enteroscope endoscopic retrograde cholangiopancreatography in patients with a surgically altered upper gastrointestinal tract. Can J Gastroenterol. 2011;25:615–9.

59. Siddiqui AA, Chaaya A, Shelton C, Marmion J, Kowalski TE, Loren DE, et al. Utility of the short double-balloon enteroscope to perform pancreatico-biliary interventions in patients with surgically altered anatomy in a US multicenter study. Dig Dis Sci. 2013;58:858–64.

60. Chua TJ, Kaffes AJ. Balloon-assisted enteroscopy in patients with surgically altered anatomy: a liver transplant center experience (with video). Gastrointest Endosc. 2012;76:887–91.

61. Iwamoto S, Ryozawa S, Yamamoto H, Taba K, Ishigaki N, Harano M, et al. Double balloon endoscope facilitates endoscopic retrograde cholangiopancreatography in roux-en-y anastomosis patients. Dig Endosc. 2010;22:64–8.

62. Li K, Huang YH, Yao W, Chang H, Huang XB, Zhang YP, et al. Adult colonoscopy or single-balloon enteroscopy-assisted ERCP in long-limb surgical bypass patients. Clin Res Hepatol Gastroenterol. 2014;38(4):513–9.

63. Khashab MA, Kumbhari V, Kalloo AN, Saxena P. EUS-guided biliary drainage by using a hepatogastrostomy approach. Gastrointest Endosc. 2013;78:675.

64. Dhir V, Bhandari S, Bapat M, Maydeo A. Comparison of EUS-guided rendezvous and precut papillotomy techniques for biliary access (with videos). Gastrointest Endosc. 2012;75:354–9.

Video Legends

Video 15.1 - Transgastric access to biliary tree facilitated by laparoscopy in patient with Roux anatomy. Note contrast injection and unusual scope position.

The Future of Magnetic Guided Capsule Endoscopy: Designed for Gastroscopy, Does It Have a Role in Small Bowel Enteroscopy?

16

Jean-Francois Rey

Introduction

Capsule endoscopy has been introduced into gastroenterologic diagnostics primarily for small bowel imaging, where conventional endoscopy and radiology have traditionally failed to detect lesions, especially if they are small or discrete [1]. Attempts to expand indications for capsule endoscopy to the esophagus [2, 3] and colon [4, 5] have met several obstacles with regard to performance, bowel preparation, organization, and cost, which have prevented widespread capsule use in these areas. In the stomach, occasional lesions have been detected after esophageal capsule endoscopy or before small bowel imaging, but there has been consensus that the stomach is not a good target organ for passive capsule endoscopy.

Thus, there may be a need for guided capsule gastroscopy to allow for complete visualization of all areas of the stomach. After promising initial results using a capsule guided by a simple external magnet [5, 6] or by a more sophisticated magnetic guidance system [7–9], we carried out a prospective study in order to systematically evaluate the diagnostic accuracy of the latter system of capsule gastroscopy [10]. It was compared to conventional flexible gastroscopy in patients examined for upper gastrointestinal (GI) complaints.

How It Works

Material

The magnetically guided capsule endoscopy (MGCE) system has been developed as a joint project of Olympus Medical Systems Corporation and Siemens Healthcare to develop a prototype device that provides endoscopic visualization of the stomach. Olympus imaging technology has been combined with a guidance system from Siemens that is used to move the capsule in the gastric cavity. The guidance system is not used to move the capsule to the stomach. Passage through the esophagus occurs simply by gravity and esophageal motility. The Siemens guidance system, based on magnetic technology, was installed in the building used for computed tomography (CT) and magnetic resonance imaging (MRI) procedures, next to the endoscopy unit, at the Institut Arnault Tzanck in Saint Laurent du Var, France.

Electronic supplementary material: The online version of this chapter (doi: 10.1007/978-3-319-14415-3_16) contains supplementary material, which is available to authorized users. Videos can also be accessed at http://link.springer.com/chapter/10.1007/978-3-319-14415-3_16.

J.-F. Rey, M.D. (✉)
Department of Hepatology and Gastroenterology, Institut Arnault Tzanck, 116 Rue de Commandant Cahuzac, St. Laurent du Var 06700, France
e-mail: Jean.francois.rey@wanadoo.fr

Guidance System

The guidance system produces a very low level magnetic field (15 times smaller than the usual magnetic resonance used for radiological examinations). The capsule weighs 2.7 g and has a theoretical magnetic force of 50 mN (5.0 g); this is equivalent to a total of 7.7 g (approximately the same weight as a 1€ or 500¥ coin). The force required for navigation is very low and in a phantom stomach it is possible to stop the capsule with a minimal force. In a human stomach that means the capsule may be trapped by gastric mucus but on the other hand avoids any dangerous potential side effects for the patients. The system works silently in contrast to the conventional MRI machine.

The low magnetic field of the guidance system has a theoretical maximum of 100 mT; for comparison, this is 2,000 times greater than the Earth's magnetic field and 15 times smaller than the standard 1.5 T MRI field. The typical magnetic fields used for navigation (3–10 mT) are actually 60–200 times greater than the Earth's magnetic field and 150–500 times smaller than the 1.5 T MRI field. The low level of the magnetic field means that the equipment does not require a substantial cooling system and it is very quiet compared to the usual MRI machine. This also reduces the potential side effects for patients with any metallic internal medical devices (Fig. 16.1).

Capsule Maneuverability

The patient lies in the magnetic guidance equipment, with a stable stomach position allowing maximal force for navigation of the capsule. The capsule can be moved with five independent mechanical degrees of freedom: two rotational and three translational (i.e., in three dimensions) (Fig. 16.2). It can be tilted (equivalent to the large steering-wheel movements of an endoscope tip) and it can be rotated (equivalent to the small steering-wheel movements). The tilting command allows the position of the capsule at a fixed point to be oriented. The MGCE can be navigated at a water surface in the stomach or can be made to dive to the bottom of the stomach (Fig. 16.3). In close-up, a clear magnified view of the mucosal pattern is seen because of refraction by the water and the fixed-focus imaging. When the capsule is lying on the stomach wall, it can be

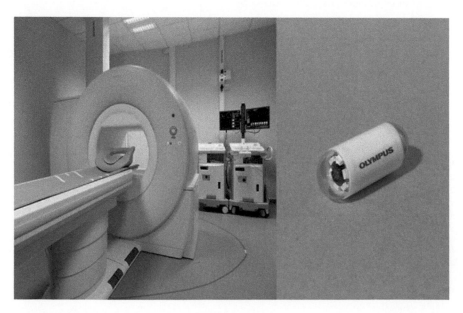

Fig. 16.1 Magnetic guided capsule endoscopy (MGCE) equipment

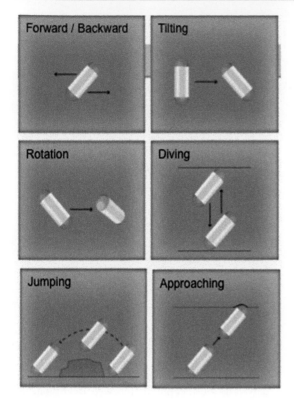

Fig. 16.2 Technical maneuverability

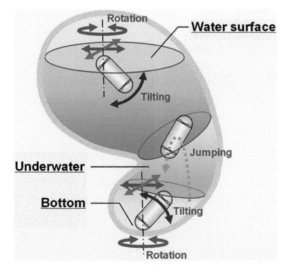

Fig. 16.3 Overall drawing of magnetic guided capsule endoscopy

made to crawl, and if the capsule is blocked between gastric folds it can be dislodged by being made to "jump" (Video 16.1).

Imaging System

As with the small bowel capsule, the patient is equipped with multiple antennas in order to record the images from the capsule. The MGCE capsule is 31 mm long and 11 mm in diameter, weighs 2.7 g and has two image sensors. The images are visualized and recorded at 4 frames/s. Standard imaging is done in real time. The images from both sensors are displayed simultaneously on a dual-monitor panel with one screen for each sensor.

MGCE Navigation

The practitioner stands in front of the dual monitors that show the images from both sensors and that display the possible capsule maneuvers and settings (forward, backward, rotating, diving, tilting, jumping). The physician responsible for guiding the device chooses which screen should be the "active" one for directing the capsule, and controls the motion of the capsule by means of two joysticks (Video 16.2).

Operator Learning Curve and Initial Pilot Study

Initially the operators gained in vitro experience in using the technology. The use of plastic "stomachs" with labeled areas or of pig stomachs allowed them to understand how the basic handling worked and to become familiar with the technical capability of the guided video capsule. This stage also provided information about the effectiveness of low level magnetic field guidance and its limitations as well as safety for patients. This stage was completed using simulation software as the practitioners were not familiar with joystick handling.

During the first month of the trial, 26 patients had been included in a pilot study that achieved 24 complete examinations of patients with conventional gastroscopy followed by capsule examinations. The capsule operators were aware of the gastroscopy findings and tried to identify the known lesions using the capsule. Initially, because of the unfamiliar appearance of the uninflated stomach, it was difficult to identify some structures, such as the closed cardia, for example. The operators also had to learn how to navigate through the human stomach, how to deal with gastric contractions and how to get rid of mucus that was stuck on the capsule sensors.

Studies Protocol

Clinical Protocol

Gastric examination with the MGCE was carried out using the following protocol. After overnight fasting, patients drank 500 ml of clear water at room temperature. One hour later, they drank another 400 ml of clear water at room temperature. Then after light exercise for approximately 15 min, in order to obtain a clean stomach, patients drank a further 400 ml of clear water near body temperature (35 °C). This was done to create enough space in the stomach for capsule navigation.

At that point, image-receiving antennae were attached to the patient's body and the patient was settled inside the magnetic guidance system. The patient position on the table was predetermined to allow for optimal gastric imaging and maximal magnetic force for capsule navigation. Capsule imaging was initiated and the patient ingested the capsule in a sitting position before lying down in the guidance system when the capsule had reached the stomach by esophageal gravity and esophageal motility.

MGCE Examination

At the beginning of the examination the position of the patient was left lateral; this was then changed to supine and finally right lateral. When it was difficult to move or navigate the capsule in a particular position, the patient was moved into another position. If necessary, additional water was ingested during the examination to create optimal conditions, as the MGCE requires an air–water interface for guidance. The visualization of the gastric surface in the antrum, body, and fundus, and identification of the two well-known landmarks of the cardia and pylorus were checked by the examiners. High definition gastroscopy under propofol sedation was considered as the "gold standard."

Evaluation of Outcomes and Data Analysis

The overall evaluations of stomach visualization, including all stomach areas, were documented immediately on a report sheet by the operator (Fig. 16.4). The examiner assessed these subjectively. Examination time and abnormal findings were also recorded.

The main outcome parameters were percentage of patients in whom there was complete visualization of the gastric surface in the antrum, body, and fundus, and identification of the cardia and pylorus. Further parameters were examination time, and the percentage of abnormal findings seen on gastroscopy that were reproducible by capsule endoscopy and vice versa.

Guided Capsule Data

Three Clinical Studies Have Been Performed

First Study
Twenty-four patients and 29 volunteers were included in order to assess the feasibility of a clinical trial comparing conventional gastroscopy and MGCE. Maneuverability of the two sensors' video capsule was obtained with water interface in the human stomach and a low level magnetic guidance equipment [7].

Second Study
Seventy-one patients were enrolled for the comparative blinded study and examinations were completed in 61 patients (39 men, 22 women; mean age 52.7 years, range 21–75). The capsule was swallowed and water ingested (overall

Fig. 16.4 Data collection chart

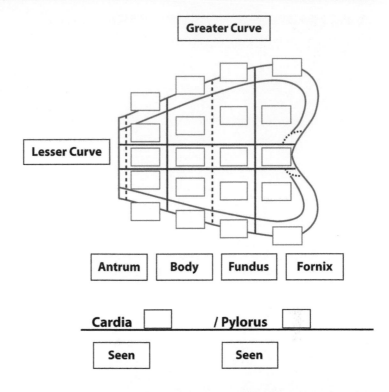

volume 1,300 ml as described in the protocol) without problem in all but two patients. A few patients ($n = 5$) needed to drink additional water at body temperature to keep the stomach distended. No technical defect occurred and we were able to analyze complete comparative examinations in 61 patients. No premedication was given or felt to be necessary for any patient. On follow-up, one patient had temporary abdominal pain, which subsided spontaneously and has not recurred. In another patient, left lower quadrant pain was diagnosed with recurrent sigmoid diverticulitis [8].

As mentioned, in close-up view, the mucosal pattern could be seen clearly as it was magnified because of refraction by the water and the fixed-focus imaging (Fig. 16.5). When the capsule was lodged between folds on the gastric wall, we could navigate the capsule using the jumping and floating functions. Impaired visualization caused by gastric mucus or remaining debris in the water could be overcome by turning the patient or in a few cases by further ingestion of water.

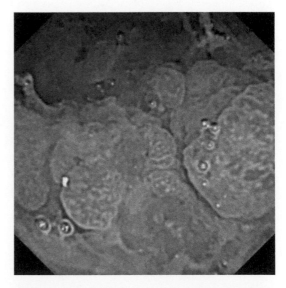

Fig. 16.5 Detailed aspect of abnormal gastric mucosa

Figures 16.5, 16.6, and 16.7 show various gastric images obtained by capsule navigation. Visualization of the gastric pylorus, antrum, body, fundus, and cardia was felt to be complete in 88.5 %, 86.9 %, 93.4 %, 85.2 %, and 88.5 % of

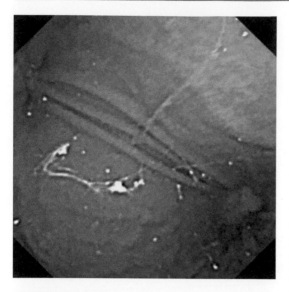

Fig. 16.6 Panoramic view of lesser curve with pylorus (*left*) and cardia (*right*)

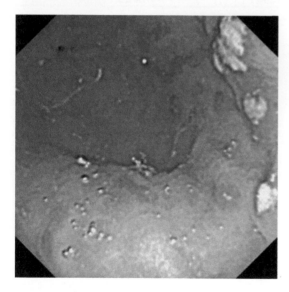

Fig. 16.7 Multiple antral ulcerations

patients, respectively (Fig. 16.8). Incomplete visualization was due to resistant mucus in 7 cases, excessive gastric motility in 2 cases, early pyloric passage of the capsule in 4 cases, and incomplete distension of gastric walls in 2. Capsule examination was achieved in a mean total examination time of 17.4 min (range 9.9–26.4). Capsule endoscopy examination time became shorter with increasing skill at navigation but also as new knowledge was gained such

as subsequent visualization of the lesser curve or closed cardia.

A total of 108 pathological findings were detected. Of these, 63 were identified by both conventional gastroscopy and capsule endoscopy: these included 44 cases of diffuse inflammation or erosion, 8 polyps, 3 ulcers (Figs. 16.5 and 16.7), 4 cases of atrophy, 2 cases of antral metaplasia, 1 case of external compression, and 1 case of fundic varices. Gastroscopy detected 14 additional lesions not identified at capsule endoscopy: 2 polyps, 1 case of inflammation, 2 angiodysplasias, 2 ulcers, 2 cases of atrophy, 1 case of important bile reflux, 2 cases of hypertrophic folds, and 2 of antral metaplasia. On the other hand, 31 lesions were detected only by capsule endoscopy and missed by conventional endoscopy: 11 polyps, 10 cases of inflammation, 1 angiodysplasia, 5 ulcers, 1 metaplasia, 2 bleeding lesions, and 1 hiatal hernia.

Third Study

The latter was blinded and randomized [10]: 215 patients were initially included, but 25 had to be excluded due to subsequent refusal for study participation ($n=14$), capsule impaction in the esophagus during scanning time ($n=3$), technical problems ($n=5$), protocol violation ($n=2$), and inability to swallow the capsule ($n=1$). The remaining 189 patients (105 males, 84 females, mean age 53.0 ± 13.7 years) with an indication for upper GI endoscopy such as upper abdominal pain and/or anemia were included into the study. Twenty-three major lesions were found in 21 patients and included 2 adenocarcinomas (tumor sizes 1.2 and 10 cm, both located in the gastric body), 4 submucosal lesions (size/location 1.5 cm, 0.8 cm in the gastric body, 0.9 cm in the cardia and 1.0 cm in the antrum), 9 gastric ulcers (mean size 0.8 cm, [0.5–1.5 cm], location: cardia $n=2$, fundus $n=1$, antrum $n=6$), 3 single hyperplastic polyps with a maximum size of 5 mm (location: fundus $n=2$, pylorus $n=1$), and 5 focal angiodysplasia (location: antrum$=2$, gastric body $n=2$, cardia $n=1$). Two patients were found to have 2 lesions (both cases with 1 ulcer and 1 hyperplastic polyp each). Minor lesions were marked inflammatory changes with erosions

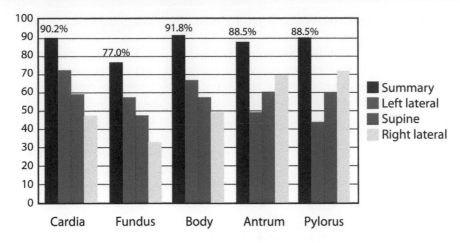

Fig. 16.8 Gastric visualization with overall results, and results related to patient position

Table 16.1 Accuracy values of capsule gastroscopy compared with gastroscopy as the final gold standard for the diagnosis of major lesions on a per-patient ($n=21$) and per-lesion ($n=23$) basis

	Per-patient (%)	95 % CI	Per-lesion (%)	95 % CI
Accuracy	90.5	85.4–94.3	89.5	84.3–93.5
Sensitivity	61.9	38.4–81.9	56.5	34.5–76.8
Specificity	94.1	89.3–97.1	94.1	89.3–97.1
PPV	56.5	34.5–76.8	56.5	34.5–76.8
NPV	95.2	90.7–97.9	94.1	89.3–97.1

CI confidence interval, *NPV* negative predictive value, *PPV* positive predictive value

($n=165$), multiple fundic gland polyps ($n=55$), gastric atrophy ($n=16$), and miscellaneous ($n=7$) (Table 16.1).

Examination times were a mean of 10.61 min (95 % CI 10.27–10.94) for capsule gastroscopy and 3.97 min (95 % CI 3.64–4.31) for blinded gastroscopy. With capsule gastroscopy, the examiners' subjective assessment rated 96.3 % of the 189 gastric capsule examinations as complete, with rates for pylorus, antrum, body, and cardia ranging from 93.0 % to 98.8 %, without significant differences between location. Subjective ratings for overall visibility, clarity, and absence of significant gastric contractile activity were 80.3 % (visibility VAS 1–2), 93.1 % (clarity 1–2 with 67.2 % completely clear), and 79.9 % (absence of contractile activity; an additional 12.7 % had mild contractile activity).

Whereas the two initial studies showed encouraging technical results, the blinded and randomized study was clinically disappointing, due to the technical limitations of the guidance system.

Pitfalls and Tricks

Because of the large size of the gastric cavity, complete gastric examination with a passive capsule seemed an impossibility. Thus, steering of capsule endoscopes has been a matter for intensive research [6, 11–14], and in fact, a self-experiment by the capsule pioneer Paul Swain has been reported [15, 16]. It is too early to assess the overall clinical benefit of MGCE compared with traditional endoscopy. However, these initial studies have defined the potential of gastric examination with MGCE and address potential technical difficulties. More recently, a new system has been introduced by Mirocam [17].

Stomach Preparation

The first hurdle for MGCE examination is to obtain a clean stomach distended with water. In the early phase, we used sparkling water for stomach distension but found that the bubbles impaired the visibility of the image. When participants drank still mineral water, in most cases the mucus remained minimal and could be moved out of the way by changing the patient's position. Subsequently, in the early phase of our experience, we found that an unexpectedly large amount of water remained in the stomach, for up to 45 min.

Patient Position

To obtain a complete stomach examination it was possible to move the patient from one position to another, allowing the water to fill the different gastric areas and facilitate MGCE movement. Patients were initially placed in the left lateral position, where in most cases, the cardia, fornix, fundus, and part of the antrum were visible; this part of the examination generally approximated 10 min. The patient was then moved to a supine position for a more complete examination of the fundus and antrum and finally to visualize the pylorus. The right lateral position was useful only for obtaining close-up appearances of the antrum and pylorus, but in many cases, it was also possible to navigate the MGCE back to the cardia.

Gastric Visualization

The first challenge was identification of gastric anatomical structures. MGCE images were recorded in various positions and without insufflation of the stomach. The capsule movement differs from that of the conventional endoscope as capsule guidance allows rotation in four directions with two views provided simultaneously from the sensors at each end of the capsule. Traditional gastroscopy is simpler with examination done in the forward direction in a distended stomach, or in retroflexion for observation of the cardia, fornix, or fundus. MGCE gives an excellent, new panoramic view of the lesser curve (Fig. 16.6). This is one of the main advantages, when the MGCE is made to dive near the greater curve in front of the angulus, giving an overview of the lesser curve anatomy for diagnosis and

orientation. The fundus and antrum are easy to assess in a larger or close-up view. The well-established differences in mucosal pattern were also a major aid to navigating the capsule. While the pylorus was easily identifiable, one needs to be aware that a cardia that is closed or only slightly open most of the time presents an unfamiliar aspect. In traditional endoscopy, this landmark is easily visible, seen with retroflexion with the gastroscope going through the cardia orifice; this is not the case with the MGCE. The overall results of the gastric examinations highlight the importance of overcoming some technical difficulties encountered during this initial clinical trial. The main drawback involved gastric mucus attaching to the MGCE, which impaired imaging. In most cases, the mucus could be removed from the lens using capsule movement; in several examinations this remained impossible.

Gastric motility was another difficulty as capsule forces were too low to counteract gastric movements. This was especially notable in the antrum where strong gastric contractions did not allow navigation to the area of the pylorus (Fig. 16.9). In a few cases, there was the opposite problem when antral motility moved the capsule forward to the duodenal bulb. Note that it neither proved impossible to traverse the pylorus by using the MGCE forces, nor when the MGCE

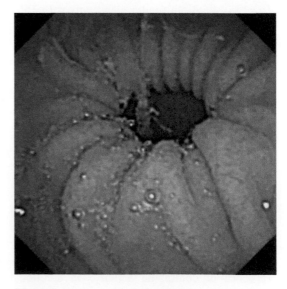

Fig. 16.9 Strong antral contractions

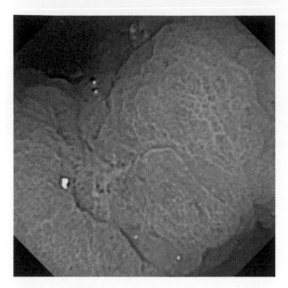

Fig. 16.10   Small antral ulceration

passed spontaneously through the pylorus could it be navigated back into the stomach. On the other hand, as the MGCE did not interfere with gastric motility, during the MGCE examination we were able to assess clear and strong fundal gastric contractions in two patients that were uncomfortable for the patients. This is a totally new field for studying gastric motility disorders. MGCE might be used to investigate this field as the current technology is limited.

Image Quality

Compared with conventional endoscopy, the video capsule images are comparable to those provided by endoscopes without high definition marketed in the early years of this century (Fig. 16.10). The brightness needs to be improved in order to extend the depth of field, but close-up views show excellent details of the gastric mucosal pattern. In some cases there was a foggy appearance at the beginning of examination, but this rapidly disappeared allowing a clear view of the gastric cavity. In some examinations, oral mucus stuck to the front of the MGCE lens; it was possible to remove it by using capsule movement or a special "capsule-shaking" command.

Adverse Effects

Impaction or retention is a concern with capsule gastroscopy as it has been with capsule endoscopy in general. Reports in patients, mostly studied for obscure bleeding, have described a low risk. In our trials it may be that a transient bowel obstruction was the cause of pain in one patient, which subsided spontaneously after some hours. Further studies will show what the overall risk of capsule gastroscopy will be. It may be wise, however, to exclude those patients with suspected or known strictures from initial trials as well as those with previous small-bowel surgery. No side effects were reported due to the low intensity magnetic field.

Future

Our third study is the first large study that systematically evaluated guided capsule gastroscopy in patients with upper abdominal symptoms [10]. We defined the accuracy of capsule gastroscopy in the diagnosis of major lesions as the main outcome, since these lesions would require subsequent conventional endoscopy for biopsy and/or therapy, such as endoscopic removal of (early) tumors, endoscopic ultrasound for suspected submucosal tumors, biopsy including *Helicobacter* testing for ulcers, and thermal coagulation for angiodysplasias. Our findings of 11 % major lesions in an average gastroscopy setting is likely realistic, and the poor sensitivity of only 61 % is unlikely to become substantially better with more lesions, since examiner experience and case load did not play a role as shown in our multivariate analysis (Table 16.1). Thus it has to be concluded that at the present stage of development, guided capsule gastroscopy is not sufficiently sensitive to even be considered as a filter test to stratify patients for conventional gastroscopy or clinical follow-up alone, irrespective of cost issues. Previous studies with a different technology involved only a small number of volunteers in feasibility trials [11, 12] or—using the same capsule in a pilot trial and prestudy testing—did not systematically evaluate a patient population of comparable size [8, 9].

The limited capsule sensitivity was generally felt to be related to several factors including both stomach characteristics and capsule technology. Among the former, limited expansion of the stomach by drinking water to fill the gastric cavity compared to air expansion during gastroscopy was probably the most important one. Sufficient intragastric volume of clear fluid is required for good visualization and capsule maneuvering [8, 9], but ingested water left the stomach too quickly; adding water during the examination did not substantially improve the results, since outflow was similarly quick. The fact that visibility rating by examiners yielded excellent results, yet detection of focal lesions was poor, points toward the fact that the subjective impression of examiners of visibility probably represents an over judgment of their own performance. This conclusion is also supported by the low detection rate of isolated major lesions versus the high detection rate of minor ones, which were usually multiple, and thus would limit the importance of incomplete inspection of the stomach. That the visualization of minor lesions was significantly better in the proximal stomach was mostly due to antral motility leading to a pushback of the capsule, which could not be counteracted by capsule maneuvering.

Therefore, future technical requirements for capsule gastroscopy include addition of a lens cleaning system as with conventional endoscopy, and a stronger guidance system, which currently appears too weak and should be delivered at faster speed and with stronger force, as well as a better capability to keep the capsule in place when needed. More force would probably also help to pass the pylorus intentionally and to keep the capsule in the esophagus, since esophageal endoscopy, searching for reflux erosions, Barrett esophagus, and varices, has to be an integral part of upper GI endoscopy performed by guided capsules in the future. A technical dream would be a capsule endoscopy able to visualize the entire digestive tract from the esophagus to the rectum and certainly a steerable capsule has some potential for application in assessing the small intestine in the future [7].

Conclusion

Current models of steerable capsules do not appear to provide sufficient accuracy to be further studied as a filter test in clinical routine for gastric examination, such as for gastric cancer screening in Japan, nor do they play an imminent role for the evaluation of small bowel disorders. Only with the substantial improvements mentioned previously, would it make sense to discuss cost issues including equipment and time needed for performance and reading. A new system is currently being tested in Japan. Further refinements are expected, which will require subsequent studies using similar methodology to include outcome studies that have to be done to define the role of guided upper GI capsule endoscopy in a variety of clinical settings.

Acknowledgements These trials have involved multiple physicians:

- *Department of Gastroenterology, Institute Arnault Tzanck, St. Laurent du Var, France*: Jean-Francois Rey, I. Pangtay, Michel Greff, Bilal Hoytat, Mohammed Abdel-Hamid.
- *Keio University School of Medicine, Tokyo, Japan*: Haruiko Ogata, Naoki Hosoe, Toshifumi Hibi.
- *Showa University Northern Yokohama Hospital, Yokohama, Japan*: Kazuo Ohtsuka, Noriyuki Ogata, Shin-El Kudo.
- *Jikei University School of Medicine, Tokyo, Japan*: Keiichi Ikeda, Hiroyuki Aihara, Hisao Tajiri.
- *Department of Interdisciplinary Endoscopy, University Hospital Hamburg-Eppendorf, Hamburg, Germany*: Ulrike Denzer, Thomas Rösch, Andras Treszl, Karl Wegscheider.
- *Department of Gastroenterology, Centre Hospitalier Universitaire and University of Nice Sophia Antipolis, Nice, France*: Xavier Hebuterne, Geoffroy Vanbiervielt, Jerome Filippi.

Technical Acknowledgements: These trials have been supported by excellent technical teams from Olympus endocapsule system and Siemens Healthcare, and by all the nursing team of Institut Arnault Tzanck.

We are grateful to our Japanese colleagues who accepted to spend time in St. Laurent Du Var for the achievement of the trial.

References

1. Ladas SD, Triantafyllou K, Spada C, Riccioni ME, Rey JF, Niv Y, et al. ESGE Clinical Guidelines Committee. European Society of Gastrointestinal

Endoscopy (ESGE)/Recommendations (2009) on clinical use of video capsule endoscopy to investigate small-bowel, esophageal and colonic diseases. Endoscopy. 2010;42:220–7.
2. Sharma VK, Eliakim R, Sharma P, Faigel D, ICCE. ICCE consensus for esophageal capsule endoscopy. Endoscopy. 2005;37:1060–4.
3. Waterman M, Gralnek IM. Capsule endoscopy of the esophagus. J Clin Gastroenterol. 2009;43:605–12.
4. Spada C, Hassan C, Galmiche JP, Neuhaus H, Dumonceau JM, Adler S, et al. European Society of Gastrointestinal Endoscopy. Colon capsule endoscopy: European Society of Gastrointestinal Endoscopy (ESGE) Guideline. Endoscopy. 2012;44:527–36. Epub 2012 Mar 2.
5. Spada C, Hassan C, Marmo R, Petruzziello L, Riccioni ME, Zullo A, et al. Meta-analysis shows colon capsule endoscopy is effective in detecting colorectal polyps. Clin Gastroenterol Hepatol. 2010; 8(6):516–22.
6. Ciuti G, Donlin R, Valdastri P, Arezzo A, Menciassi A, Morino M, et al. Robotic versus manual control in magnetic steering of an endoscopic capsule. Endoscopy. 2010;42:148–52. Epub 2009 Dec 16.
7. Rey JF. Future perspectives for esophageal and colorectal capsule endoscopy: dreams or reality? In: Niwa H, Tajiri H, Nakajima N, Yasuda K, editors. New challenges in gastrointestinal endoscopy. Japan: Springer; 2008. p. 55–64.
8. Rey JF, Ogata H, Hosoe N, Ohtsuka K, Ogata N, Ikeda K, et al. Feasibility of stomach exploration with a guided capsule endoscope. Endoscopy. 2010;42(7):541–5. Epub 2010 Jun 30.
9. Rey JF, Ogata H, Hosoe N, Ohtsuka K, Ogata N, Ikeda K, et al. Blinded nonrandomized comparative study of gastric examination with a magnetically guided capsule endoscope and standard videoendoscope. Gastrointest Endosc. 2012;75(2):373–81. Epub 2011 Dec 9.
10. Denzer UW, Rosch T, Hoytat B, Abdel-Hamid M, Hebuterne X, Vanbiervielt G, et al. Magnetically guided capsule versus conventional gastroscopy for upper abdominal complaints. A prospective blinded study. J Clin Gastroenterol. 2014; Mar 10 (Epub ahead of print)
11. Keller J, Fibbe C, Volke F, Gerber J, Mosse AC, Reimann-Zawadzki M, et al. Remote magnetic control of a wireless capsule endoscope in the esophagus is safe and feasible: results of randomized clinical trial in healthy volunteers. Gastrointest Endosc. 2010;72(5):941–6. Epub 2010 Sep 19.
12. Keller J, Fibbe C, Volke F, Gerber J, Mosse AC, Reimann-Zawadzki M, et al. Inspection of the human stomach using remote-controlled capsule endoscopy: a feasibility study in healthy volunteers (with videos). Gastrointest Endosc. 2011;73(1):22–8. Epub 2010 Nov 9.
13. Menciassi A, Valdastri P, Quaglia C, Buselli E, Dario P. Wireless steering mechanism with magnetic actuation for an endoscopic capsule. Conf Proc IEEE Eng Med Biol Soc. 2009;2009:1204–7.
14. Valdastri P, Quaglia C, Susilo E, Menciassi A, Dario P, Ho CN, et al. Wireless therapeutic endoscopic capsule: in vivo experiment. Endoscopy. 2008;40:979–82. Epub 2008 Dec 8.
15. Swain P. History and future. In: Faigel DO, Cave DR, editors. Capsule endoscopy. Philadelphia, PA: Saunders Elsevier; 2008. p. 3–11.
16. Swain P, Toor A, Volke F, Keller J, Gerber J, Rabinovitz E, et al. Remote magnetic manipulation of a wireless capsule endoscope in the esophagus and stomach of humans. Gastrointest Endosc. 2010; 71:1290–3.
17. Rahman I, Pioche M, Shim CS, Sung IK, Saurin J-C, Patel P. 219 Magnet Assisted Capsule Endoscopy (MACE) in the upper GI tract is feasible: first human series using the novel Mirocam-Navi System. Gastrointest Endosc. 2014;79(5 Suppl):AB122.

Video Legends

Video 16.1 - Showing how the MGCE can be maneuvered.

Video 16.2 - MGCE navigation. Using dual monitors that show images from both sensors of the capsule, the physician controls the motion of the capsule by means of two joysticks.

Improved Capsule Hardware and Software

17

Felice Schnoll-Sussman and Fouad A. Otaki

Introduction

The prospect of endoscopically visualizing the small bowel is a medical breakthrough. Significant technological advancements are pushing the frontier even further: improved optics, maneuverable capsules, and the possibility of simultaneous sampling and localized treatment. The field has also witnessed software advancements. The majority revolve around improving the experience of viewing the exhausting wealth of visual recordings [1, 2].

Capsule endoscopy in its entirety is time consuming. Although the administration and setup need only a few minutes, the equipment must be worn for 10–12 h and the study generates 14,400–72,000 frames. These need to be meticulously reviewed as pathology might be limited to a single frame. The goal of software augmentations is to make the analysis easier whilst maintaining the highest level of accuracy.

Given Imaging (Covidien) developed and released the first small bowel capsule for clinical use in 2001. Since then they have released various models. A handful of capsules have also been developed by competing companies. In addition to variations in the image sensory, dimension, data transmission, angle of view, battery life, and light exposure, each pill offers unique software packages and features.

Patient registration, data download, study analysis, and report generation are the four major components of any software package. In tandem with the proprietary hardware each major manufacturer has attempted to provide an intuitive system. Moreover, various modules of these packages are available including patient, online, mobile, workstation/reader, and live feedback stations. Some also embed a safety mechanism to account for battery life deterioration at around 400 charge cycles.

This chapter will give a basic overview of the current manufacturers capsule endoscopy hardware and software with a major emphasis on the technological improvements since initial release into the marketplace.

Resolution

A key technological advancement that ushered in capsule endoscopy was the miniaturization of the wireless transmitter. An oscillating electromagnetic radiation in the microwave range

F. Schnoll-Sussman, M.D. (✉)
Department of Medicine, Gastroenterology,
New York Presbyterian Hospital/Weill Cornell
Medical College, 1315 York Avenue, 1st Floor,
New York, NY 10021, USA
e-mail: fhs2001@med.cornell.edu

F.A. Otaki, M.D.
Department of Gastroenterology, Weill Cornell/
New York Presbyterian Hospital, 1305 York Avenue,
GI Department, 4th Floor, New York, NY 10021, USA
e-mail: foo9006@nyp.org

R. Kozarek and J.A. Leighton (eds.), *Endoscopy in Small Bowel Disorders*,
DOI 10.1007/978-3-319-14415-3_17, © Springer International Publishing Switzerland 2015

(0.3–300 GHz) was deemed to be safe and reliable [3]. As data transmission drains the majority of the limited onboard batteries, the image quality of capsules is poorer than conventional endoscopy. Compared to the standard solution of image compression, more innovative technology includes electric field propagation (MiRo capsule, IntroMedic, Seoul, Korea) to transmit data independent of radiofrequency transmitters. This proprietary technology relies on the use of the human body's natural conductive capacity to transmit images to the recorder. Moreover, dynamic images of a higher resolution are also necessary as the frontier is advancing toward therapeutic capsules.

Recording a Video

Not limited to the analysis, some newer-generation recorders are able to trigger appropriate alerts in reference to predefined instructions. These include dietary restriction, and termination notices. In the near future, prompts for prokinetic "boosters" could rely on real-time data regarding capsule mobility.

Viewing a Video

Automatic Modes

A number of algorithms have been developed to eliminate or stack similar images; Quickview (Given Imaging) and Express-Selected and Auto-Speed-Adjusted mode (Olympus Imaging) are examples. Such developments preceded dynamic frame rates and aimed to minimize images captured during periods of capsule stagnation, hence shortening the study duration and highlighting pathology.

In a retrospective analysis of 70 patients, the Express-Selected mode resulted in a significantly quicker read time with minimal drop in sensitivity [4]. Authors were cautious to recommend larger multicenter trials. Comparatively, the 2012 review by Kyriakos et al. [5] of 100 wireless capsules using Quickview had a diagnostic miss rate of 12 %, but reduced the reading time of manual mode, at 10 frames per second, by a factor of 4. The authors recommended the abbreviated mode as a safe diagnostic tool in larger or diffuse lesions. Others have used Quickview confidently in the analysis of obscure gastrointestinal bleeding (OGIB) with sensitivity, specificity, and positive and negative predictive values exceeding 90 % [6].

Other augmented diagnostic modalities have been developed. Analyzing colors and contours, first-generation image-processing software have limited sensitivity but have the potential to significantly shorten reading time [7]. Some more promising models in development are specific for Crohn's disease lesions [8].

Another strategy to shorten duration is the automatic elimination of images of poor quality or bubbles and debris that might interfere with mucosal evaluation (Endocapsule 10 System, Olympus Imaging, Japan).

Overview Methods

Upon importing, most video capsule software systems provide an overview of the recording time overlaid with average color representation from each image. This allows for an approximation of the various anatomic locations, a comprehensive representation of the entire video, and an alternative method of navigation via a moving slider or pointer.

The ability to identify anatomic locations is paramount to analyzing images, putting them into perspective, and highlighting pathology. Moreover, landmarks are needed for various software augmentation and report generation including localization and GI segment passage times, both discussed later.

Various landmarks have been suggested. In addition to the conventional, esophageal, gastric, duodenal, and cecal images, some manufacturers recommend identifying the Z-line, ileocecal valve, and hepatic and splenic flexures depending on the capsule being used.

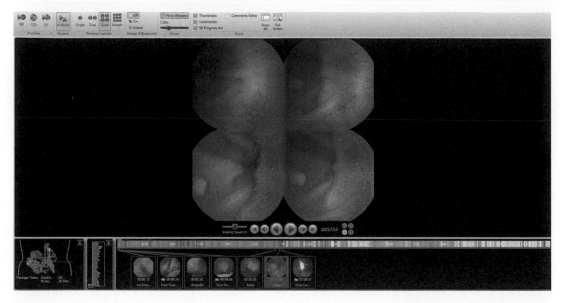

Fig. 17.1 A sample of Quadview image overview

Single, Double, and More Advanced Viewing Modes

Users are able to adjust the rate of view of various software systems. To increase efficiency whilst maintaining the highest yield for pathology, the viewing layout has advanced from a single frame on screen, to two, and four frames. The four-frame view, Quad View (Given Imaging, Yokenam) (Fig. 17.1), displays four consecutive images in a clockwise fashion. Other formats are specific to each company, including mosaic view, which displays 18 consecutive frames, collage view, and 360, which generates a panorama from the four cameras on the CapsoCam model (Capsovision, CA) (Fig. 17.2). All these methods increase the number of images at one time but paradoxically decrease the individual image change rate.

There are limited comparative data assessing the diagnostic outcome of the various image-viewing options. Zheng et al. compared detection rates of 24 clips analyzed by 23 experienced endoscopists in four different modes. Single view at 15 and 25 frames per second (fps) in addition to Quad view at 20 and 30 fps. With the exception of the single view at 25 fps,

overall detection rate was not affected by viewing mode or speed, and was independent of endoscopist experience. The authors recognize the limited pathology in their sample, the absence of surgical or endoscopic confirmation, and small sample size [9].

Given PillCam Progress Indicator

Upon identification of the duodenal and cecal landmarks, the Progress Indicator (Fig. 17.3) allows for a graphical indication of the percentage of small bowel that has been viewed at any point. It also estimates a degree of image similarity based on pixel redundancy between adjoining images, which aims to reflect the variable speed of transit of the capsule at various anatomic locations.

Size Estimation

Various tools have been developed to approximate the size of lesions visualized on VCE. Validation of such systems is limited to specific lesions and cannot be generalized (e.g., Given's Polyp Size

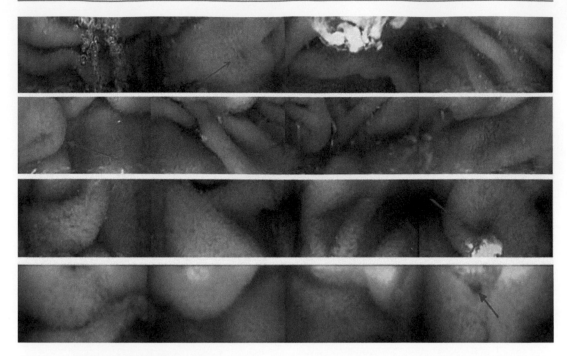

Fig. 17.2 Panoramic images from the CapsoCam capsule. *Blue arrows*, sample duodenal papillas. Reprinted with permission from Friedrich K, Gehrke S, Stremmel W, Sieg A. First clinical trial of a newly developed capsule endoscope with panoramic side view for small bowel: a pilot study. J Gastroenterol Hepatol. 2013;28(9):1496–501

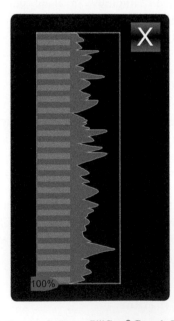

Fig. 17.3 Progress Indicator, PillCam® Capsule Endoscopy

Estimation tool). Most companies emphasize these tools as research platforms that should not be used in clinical decision-making.

Software Augmentation—Blood Indicators

Both Given and Olympus have developed software algorithms that highlight images containing red pixels. Indicative of suspected bleeding or angioectasias, they allow the interpreter to rapidly review sequences when capsules are utilized for obscure gastrointestinal bleeding.

At best complimentary, these features do not replace a thorough evaluation of all the images. There has been a conflicting wealth of literature regarding the accuracy of blood indicator software. The strongest evidence comes from active small bowel bleeding. Accuracy was higher in patients who required larger amounts of blood transfusion [10]. In a retrospective review of 109 lesions from a single center, the blood-indicating algorithm had a sensitivity, positive predictive value, and accuracy of 81.2 %, 81.3 %, and 83.3 % respectively [11], whereas other groups have deemed the technology to have no timesaving utility and limited clinical value [12].

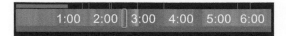

Fig. 17.4 Blood Indicator, PillCam® Capsule Endoscopy

Supporting that view, Signorelli et al. found an overall and per-patient sensitivity of 28 % and 41 % in their retrospective review of 95 patients [13]. Experimental ex-vivo models indicate that yield is greatly affected by background color and capsule velocity [14].

To avoid mislabeling images, such features can only be activated once the anatomic landmarks have been identified. Moreover, the threshold for degree of redness and number of pixels can be adjusted. In the Given system the suspected bleeding is displayed as red "ticks" overlying the time bar (Fig. 17.4). A review method is available allowing easy navigation between the suspected images.

Blood detection is currently only available for small bowel capsules, but the technology should be easily exportable to colonic and esophageal systems with limited tweaking.

Resolution and Image Adjustment

Moving away from electronic parts designed for general consumer use, biomedical engineering collaborators have developed capsule technology further. This includes, but is not limited to, photo recording chips with greater dynamic range that can switch between linear and logarithmic to better emulate the natural accommodation and range of the human eye. Such capsules are advancing the frontier with images of greater resolutions, captured at faster frame rates, with minimal power consumption [15].

Some manufacturers include proprietary technology to enhance images by altering sharpness, color, brightness, and contrast [16]. One such innovation, virtual chromoendoscopy, employed by Fujinon's Intelligent Chromoendoscopy and Given's FICE (versions 1, 2 and 3) and Blue Mode, use spectral estimation to narrow the bandwidth of conventional endoscopy. These filters are analogous to digitized formats of the narrow band imaging of conventional endoscopy. There are widely discrepant results in the literature regarding the utility of these modalities. In a review assessing the validity of FICE or Blue mode, improvement ranged from 7.7 % to 87.7 % depending on the indication and mode of FICE. Moreover, in the same review FICE false positivity was increased with poor bowel preparation [17].

Olympus's Contrast Image Capsule has combined hardware and software changes which utilizes a blue enhanced white light emitting diode. In addition to white light images, contrast images are generated by extracting the green and blue wavelengths from the spectrum [18]. A feasibility study limited to a few patients suggests that this technology enhances visibility in polyposis syndromes [19].

In an editorial, Spada and associates reviewed the discordant literature and concluded that virtual chromoendoscopy visually enhanced lesions which had been previously identified, but did not improve upon the detection rate [20].

Panoramic and 3D Modeling

Panoramic segmental images of the small bowel can be captured by positioning cameras on the side of the capsule (CapsoCam, Capsovision, CA). Similar images can also be generated via mathematical modelling. Moreover, algorithmic manipulation of a series of two-dimensional images has generated a three-dimensional model of the small bowel as reported by Fan et al. [21]. Such software reconstruction significantly enhances vascular lesions but has been shown to have limited yield in inflammatory and protruding lesions [22].

Localization

Triangulation by utilizing the variable strength of signals reaching the various leads allows for the approximation of the location of the capsule in the small bowel, which can be modeled on a two-dimensional chart. The belt and sensor array can be used for the location of the Given PillCam small bowel and colon (Fig. 17.5) and the

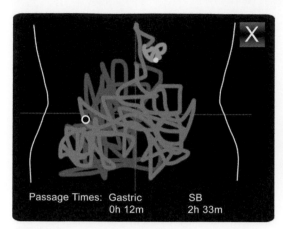

Fig. 17.5 Localization, PillCam® Capsule Endoscopy

Olympus Endocapsule systems. Localization is of greatest yield in anatomical anchored segments of the bowel.

Some software systems allow for the segmentation of the figure to include various anatomical locations, usually reported by a number of colors. Under development, feature tracking [23], contraction pattern analysis [24], and locality-preserving projections [25] have generated a precision of 95 %, 51 %, >90 % respectively in automatic localization of images relative to gastrointestinal organs.

Other modalities include the use of embedded magnetoresistive arrays and ultrasonic localization.

Reporting

Most software packages have sophisticated reporting modules. Results are documented alongside indications and performance parameters.

Many reporting systems include templates and dictionaries linked to prepopulated and customizable databases that aim to simplify data and create a more efficient report generation process.

In addition to including text, most systems allow the operator to include representative images, markings (including circles and arrows), size estimation, and comments. They also have the option to link various images with anatomic pictorial illustrations for ease of interpretation.

Master video files are frequently exportable. This creates a platform to share videos for the purpose of consultation or academic discussion/analysis. Moreover, many systems allow for the generation of a "findings" file that can be exported independent of either the master video or report. Moreover, most programs are well integrated with existing electronic health records.

Lewis Score

The Lewis Score [26] is a scoring system based on quantitative and qualitative descriptors—of endoscopic variability in villous edema, ulceration, and stenosis—that measure extent of mucosal damage. It provides a standardized score that is highly reproducible, which provides a common language to quantify small bowel inflammatory changes.

Once the tertiles (three equal segments of the small bowel evaluation) are defined, the three endoscopic parameters are measured and inputted into the software package for each tertile segment.

The edema component includes the appearance (relationship of the width to the height of the villi), longitudinal extent, and distribution. Ulcers are defined as mucosal breaks with a white or yellow base surrounded by a red or pink color, this parameter incorporates the number, longitudinal, and circumferential extent of visualized ulcers. In addition to identifying the number of stenotic lesions, the presence or absence of ulcerating features and ability to be traversed are also documented. Numbers are recorded as single, few, or multiple, while distribution is localized, patchy, or diffuse in nature. Finally, longitudinal extent is judged as short, long, or whole segment.

Total scores of 135 and less, 135–790, and greater than 790 are consistent with clinically insignificant findings, mild inflammatory changes, and moderate to severe mucosal inflammation, respectively.

Atlas

The rapid utilization of capsule endoscopy to diagnose an expanding list of gastrointestinal illness, notably in the small bowel, has generated an ever-growing resource of images. These have been grouped into various disease categories based on correlative conventional endoscopy, surgical resections, postmortem analysis, and pattern similarities with other disease entities.

The grouping of such images into conventional atlases has generated reference texts that are essential to every practice. They provide an overview of normal anatomy, acceptable variants, and pathophysiological patterns. Moreover, they are essential in the training of any endoscopic capsule interpreter.

Most software now includes digital atlases. Unique features include the ability to compare selected thumbnails side-by-side with the atlas, and online atlases that are constantly updated. They are frequently indexed based on anatomy and pathophysiology.

Conclusion

Video capsules have allowed us to explore the black box of endoscopy: the small bowel. Just as with any medical innovation the frontier is advanced on a nearly daily basis by ongoing development in both hardware and software. A significant portion of the software development comes from other fields. Its success is the product of collaborations between physicians, engineers, mathematicians, and physicists. This chapter attempts to highlight some of the key developments in the field, and shed light on upcoming technology.

References

1. deFranchis R, Lewis BS, Mishkin DS, editors. Capsule endoscopy simplified. Thorofare: SLACK Incorporated; 2010.
2. Koulaouzidis A, Rondonotti E, Karargyris A. Small-bowel endoscopy: a ten-point contemporary review. World J Gastroenterol. 2013;19:3726–46.
3. Gong F, Swain P, Mills T. Wireless endoscopy. Gastrointest Endosc. 2000;51:725–9.
4. Subramanian V, Mannath J, Telakis E, Ragunath K, Hawkey CJ. Efficacy of new playback functions at reducing small-bowel wireless capsule endoscopy reading times. Dig Dis Sci. 2012;57:1624–8.
5. Kyriakos N, Karagiannis S, Galanis P, Liatsos C, Zouboulis-Vafiadis I, Georgiou E, et al. Evaluation of four time-saving methods of reading capsule endoscopy videos. Eur J Gastroenterol Hepatol. 2012;24:1276–80.
6. Koulaouzidis A, Smirnidis A, Douglas S, Plevris J. Quick-view in small bowel capsule endoscopy is useful in certain clinical settings, but quick-view with blue mode is of no additional benefit. Eur J Gastroenterol Hepatol. 2012;24:1099–104.
7. Gan T, Wu JC, Rao NN, Chen T, Liu B. A feasibility trial of computer-aided diagnosis for enteric lesions in capsule endoscopy. World J Gastroenterol. 2008;14:6929–35.
8. Kumar R, Zhao Q, Seshamani S, Mullin G, Hager G, Dassopoulos T. Assessment of Crohn's disease lesions in wireless capsule endoscopy images. IEEE Trans Biomed Eng. 2012;59:355–62.
9. Zheng Y, Hawkins L, Wolff J, et al. Detection of lesions during capsule endoscopy: physician performance is disappointing. Am J Gastroenterol. 2012;107:554–60.
10. Gross SA, Schmelkin IJ, Kwak GS. Relationship of suspected blood indicator and blood transfusions in wireless capsule endoscopy. Am J Gastroenterol. 2003;98:S288.
11. Liangpunsakul S, Mays L, Rex DK. Performance of given suspected blood indicator. Am J Gastroenterol. 2003;12:2676–8.
12. D'Halluin PN, Delvaux M, Lapalus MG, Sacher-Huvelin S, Ben Soussan E, Heyries L, et al. Does the "Suspected Blood Indicator" improve the detection of bleeding lesions by capsule endoscopy? Gastrointest Endosc. 2005;61:243–9.
13. Signorelli C, Villa F, Rondonotti E, Abbiati C, Beccari G, de Franchis R. Sensitivity and specificity of the suspected blood identification system in video capsule enteroscopy. Endoscopy. 2005;37:1170–3.
14. Park SC, Chun HJ, Kim ES, Keum B, Seo YS, Kim YS, et al. Sensitivity of the suspected blood indicator: an experimental study. World J Gastroenterol. 2012;18:4169–74.
15. Valdastri P, Simi M, Webster RJ. Advanced technologies for gastrointestinal endoscopy. Advanced Gastrointestinal Endoscopy 2012. Annu Rev Biomed Eng. 2012;14:397–429.
16. Imagawa H, Oka S, Tanaka S, Noda I, Higashiyama M, Sanomura Y, et al. Improved visibility of lesions of the small intestine via capsule endoscopy with computed virtual chromoendoscopy. Gastrointest Endosc. 2011;73:299–306.
17. Krystallis C, Koulaouzidis A, Douglas S, Plevris JN. Chromoendoscopy in small bowel capsule endoscopy: Blue mode or Fuji Intelligent Colour Enhancement? Dig Liver Dis. 2011;43:953–7.
18. Aihara H, Ikeda K, Tajiri H. Image-enhanced capsule endoscopy based on the diagnosis of vascularity when using a new type of capsule. Gastrointest Endosc. 2011;73:1274–9.
19. Hatogai K, Hosoe N, Imaeda H, Rey JF, Okada S, Ishibashi Y, et al. Role of enhanced visibility in evaluating polyposis syndromes using a newly

developed contrast image capsule. Gut Liver. 2012; 6:218–22.

20. Spada C, Hassan C, Costamagna G. Virtual chromo-endoscopy: will it play a role in capsule endoscopy? Dig Liver Dis. 2011;43:927–8.

21. Fan Y, Meng MQ, Li B. 3D reconstruction of wireless capsule endoscopy images. Conf Proc IEEE Eng Med Biol Soc. 2010;2010:5149–52.

22. Koulaouzidis A, Karargyris A, Rondonotti E, Noble CL, Douglas S, Alexandridis E, et al. Three-dimensional representation software as image enhancement tool in small-bowel capsule endoscopy: a feasibility study. Dig Liver Dis. 2013;45:909–14.

23. Bulat J, Duda K, Duplaga M, Fraczek R, Skalski A, Socha M, et al. Data processing tasks in wireless GI endoscopy: image-based capsule localization & navigation and video compression. Conf Proc IEEE Eng Med Biol Soc. 2007;2007:2815–8.

24. Lee J, Oh JH, Shah SK, Yuan X, Tang SJ. Automatic classification of digestive organ in wireless capsule endoscopy. SAC'07 March 11–15, 2007

25. Azzopardi C, Hicks YA, Camilleri KP. Exploiting gastrointestinal anatomy for organ classification in capsule endoscopy using locality preserving projections. Conf Proc IEEE Eng Med Biol Soc. 2013;2013:3654–7.

26. Gralnek IM, Defranchis R, Seidman E, Leighton JA, Legnani P, Lewis BS. Development of a capsule endoscopy scoring index for small bowel mucosal inflammatory changes. Aliment Pharmacol Ther. 2008;27:146–54.

New Designs in Balloon Enteroscopes

Hironori Yamamoto and Tomonori Yano

Introduction

It has been more than 10 years since the release of the first model of the double-balloon endoscopy (DBE) system (EN-450P5) in the autumn of 2003 [1]. Ten years later, in 2013, a new model was released: EN-580T. This new enteroscope has a larger accessory channel of 3.2 mm instead of 2.8 mm while at the same time maintaining the same outer diameter of the endoscope (9.4 mm) as the previous model (EN-450T5). The larger channel will improve therapeutic intervention capability. In addition, the image quality is much improved, providing near focusing with a longer focus range. This chapter will review recent developments in DBE including its application for other uses in addition to standard enteroscopy.

Electronic supplementary material: The online version of this chapter (doi: 10.1007/978-3-319-14415-3_18) contains supplementary material, which is available to authorized users. Videos can also be accessed at http://link.springer.com/chapter/10.1007/978-3-319-14415-3_18.

H. Yamamoto, M.D., Ph.D. (✉) • T. Yano, M.D., Ph.D.
Department of Medicine, Division of
Gastroenterology, Jichi Medical University,
3311-1 Yakushiji, Shimotsuke, Tochigi
329-0498, Japan
e-mail: ireef@jichi.ac.jp

Characteristics of DBE

The remarkable features of DBE are not only its ability to intubate deep into the small intestine but also the ability to maintain good control of the endoscope tip during deep intubation. In addition, the accessory channel has allowed for endoscopic interventions such as biopsy, polypectomy, hemostasis, and balloon dilation in the deep small intestine. The endoscopic capabilities, along with the ability to deliver endoscopic therapy for a wide range of small intestine disorders, have definitely helped to revolutionize the management of small intestinal diseases.

Endoscopic Treatments in the Small Intestine

Most of the endoscopic treatments available in colonoscopy have become feasible in the small intestine using DBE. However, endoscopic treatments in the small intestine should be performed with special care because the intestinal wall is thin and soft, making it more vulnerable to perforation than other segments of the gastrointestinal tract. To prevent perforation, submucosal injection of normal saline at the site of treatment should be considered whenever such a risk is noted. Moreover, because the lumen of the small intestine is narrow and control of the endoscope is sometimes difficult, it is best to avoid over insufflation, which can make endoscopic treatment difficult. Attachment of a transparent hood at the tip of the endoscope is useful to maintain an adequate endoscopic view without insufflation (Fig. 18.1). Use of CO_2 instead of room air is also useful for avoiding over insufflation (Fig. 18.2).

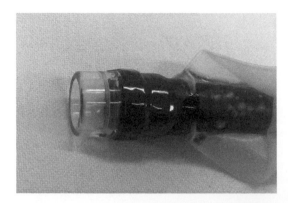

Fig. 18.1 A transparent hood (D201-10704, Olympus, Tokyo, Japan) attached to the tip of the endoscope

Desire for a Larger Accessory Channel

The therapeutic DBE with a 2.8 mm accessory channel (EN-450T5) can accommodate most of the accessory devices for endoscopic treatment, such as clip devices and balloon-dilation catheters. However, the insertion of these accessory devices can be difficult at times because the channel is tight and the endoscope shaft is long and often intricately looped. Moreover, suctioning of intestinal fluid or blood is almost impossible while accessory devices are in the channel. Therefore, a therapeutic DBE with a larger accessory channel has been long desired.

Development of New Therapeutic DBE (EN-580T)

The distinctive feature of the double-balloon scope is the effective transmission of endoscopic control to the tip from the proximal endoscope shaft through the balloon overtube (Video 18.1).

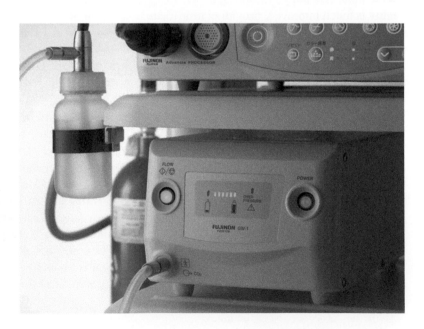

Fig. 18.2 CO_2 insufflation device (GW-1, Fujifilm, Tokyo, Japan)

Table 18.1 Specification of the double-balloon endoscopes

	Diagnostic type		Therapeutic type		Short type	
	EN-450P5	EN-580XP	EN-450T5	EN-580T	EC-450BI5	EI-530B
Outer diameter (mm)	8.5	7.5	9.4	9.4	9.4	9.4
Accessory channel (mm)	2.2	2.2	2.8	3.2	2.8	2.8
Working length (mm)	2,000	2,000	2,000	2,000	1,520	1,520
Viewing angle (°)	120	140	140	140	140	140
Minimum focus distance (mm)	5	2	3	2	3	3

Fig. 18.3 Comparison of the accessory channel sizes between EN-450T5 and EN-580T

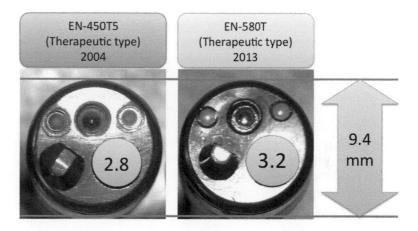

The transmission of the control does not rely on the stiffness of the shaft. Therefore, a thin and soft endoscope can be inserted and controlled in the deep small intestine. In order to intubate the soft and tortuous small intestine safely and effectively, the endoscope shaft should be thin and soft. Therefore, the manufacturer kept the same outer diameter of the endoscope even though the size of the accessory channel is increased to 3.2 mm. The new therapeutic EN-580T has a larger 3.2 mm accessory channel, but its outer diameter is the same at 9.4 mm (Table 18.1 and Fig. 18.3). As a result, this new model has improved intervention capability while maintaining the same ability to insert deeply into the small bowel.

Features of EN-580T

Improved Interventional Capabilities

With the large accessory channel, insertion of accessory devices is easier because of less friction between the channel and the devices. This is

especially notable for the balloon-dilation catheter because with the smaller channel there was significant friction at the tip of the catheter.

Endoscopic hemostasis for bleeding lesions is one of the more common therapeutic interventions performed during deep enteroscopy. Argon plasma coagulation, injection therapy, and clip placement are all available with DBE. When attempting control of hemostasis, it is important to identify the bleeding point and precisely apply the endoscopic treatment to the appropriate blood vessel. In order to identify the bleeding point, washing and suctioning the blood at the area of bleeding is very important. Once the bleeding point is identified, an accessory device for hemostasis is inserted through the accessory channel. However, because of the long shaft of the double-balloon scope, and the time it takes to insert the device, the bleeding point is often covered by blood before the device is fully inserted. In such cases, the bleeding point could be difficult to identify and withdrawal of the device is then required to wash the blood again. Using the new therapeutic EN-580T, water infusion for washing and suctioning is possible while keeping the hemostatic device in the channel because there remains enough space between the channel and the device. This feature makes the hemostatic procedure much easier and reliable.

For the infusion of water through the accessory channel while keeping the accessory devices in place, BioShield irrigator (US Endoscopy, Mentor, OH, USA) is a useful tool (Fig. 18.4). Water can be infused through the irrigator using a syringe or a water pump. The BioShield irrigator is also useful for adding contrast medium during balloon dilation of an intestinal stricture. Balloon dilation is performed under fluoroscopy guidance after the stricture is visualized with contrast medium (Fig. 18.5a). However, after the first dilation with the balloon dilator, the contrast medium in the intestinal lumen often disappears distally down the intestine (Fig. 18.5b). In such cases, it was previously necessary with the 2.8 mm accessory channel to withdraw the balloon dilator to delineate the stricture again with additional contrast medium. Using the 3.2 mm accessory channel, however, contrast medium can be added through the BioShield while the balloon dilator is kept in the channel (Fig. 18.6a). Because the stricture can be delineated clearly again (Fig. 18.6b), the second dilation can be performed properly and safely (Fig. 18.6c).

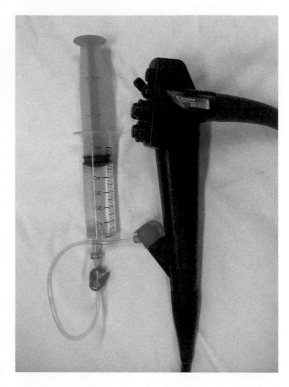

Fig. 18.4 BioShield irrigator (US Endoscopy, Mentor, OH, USA)

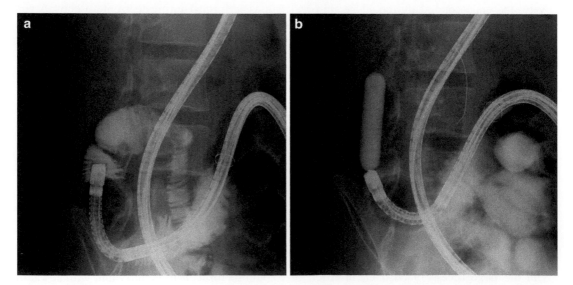

Fig. 18.5 (**a**) Fluoroscopic image of the stricture visualized with contrast medium. (**b**) Fluoroscopic image of the first balloon dilation

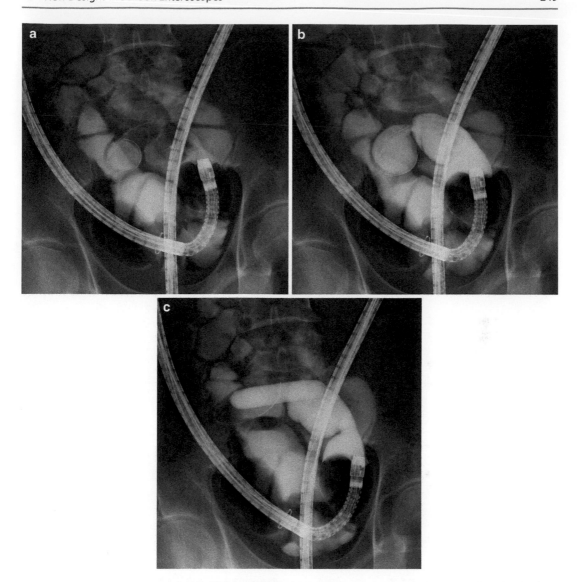

Fig. 18.6 (**a**) Fluoroscopic image before the second dilation. The contrast medium in the intestinal lumen has disappeared distally down the intestine. (**b**) Fluoroscopic image of the stricture revisualized with additional infusion of contrast medium through the BioShield irrigator. (**c**) Fluoroscopic image of the second balloon dilation

Improved Image Quality

Despite the limited space for image capturing units due to the larger accessory channel, the image quality of EN-580T has actually improved significantly. The EN-580T enteroscope has a new Charge Coupled Device (CCD), which is smaller but has a higher resolution than the previous model. The new CCD is very compatible with Flexible Spectral Imaging Color Enhancement (FICE). Small intestinal villi can be clearly visualized using FICE with EN-580T (Fig. 18.7). This new model also added a newly designed lens, which has a long focus range of 2–100 mm. Due to the clear image with the near focus of 2 mm, small intestinal villi can be observed clearly with a magnified image. Because of the long focus range, both the close-up view and the distant view are clear enough for a detailed examination (Video 18.2).

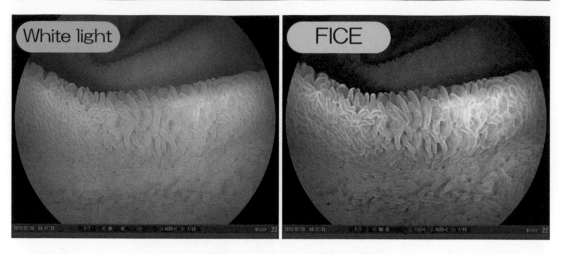

Fig. 18.7 Endoscopic images of small intestinal villi with white light and FICE

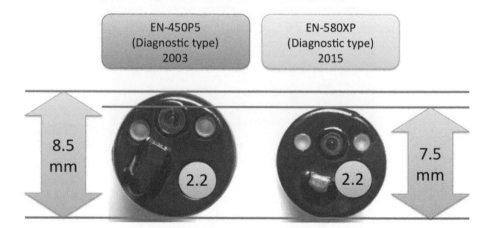

Fig. 18.8 Comparison of the outer diameter sizes between EN-450P5 and EN-580XP

Desire for a Thinner DBE

Even with the double-balloon enteroscope, deep enteroscopy can be challenging. The reasons for the difficulty include sharp angulations due to adhesions, narrowing of the intestinal lumen, and/or active inflammation of the intestine. Because the insertion principle of DBE does not rely on the rigidity of the endoscope shaft, a thinner scope should work as well. A thinner DBE could overcome the aforementioned difficulties and should be gentler and safer. This would be a particular advantage in the pediatric population where the usefulness of deep enteroscopy has been reported [2]. Therefore, a smaller diameter enteroscope would have clear advantages.

Development of New Diagnostic DBE (EN-580XP)

Expecting a gentler and less invasive insertion, a new diagnostic DBE scope (EN-580XP) has been developed. This DBE is even thinner and softer than the current DBE model, EN-450P5 (the outer diameter: 7.5 mm versus 8.5 mm). The diameter of the overtube for EN-580XP is also 1 mm smaller than the one for EN-450P5. The size of the accessory channel is the same as the current model (2.2 mm) (Fig. 18.8).

This new diagnostic DBE has the same optical units as EN-580T. Therefore, it has an excellent image quality that is similar despite the very small diameter.

Expected Utility of EN-580XP

This new diagnostic enteroscope is especially useful for pediatric patients and patients with Crohn's disease. Because of the less invasive insertion procedure expected with this new model, it could be used for evaluating inflammation in the small intestine. The image quality with a clear close-up view is also an attractive feature for investigation of morphological changes of the villi in various small intestinal diseases.

Other Applications of DBE

The improved features of DBE, including improved performance in insertion and stabilization, can be applied to other procedures in addition to standard enteroscopy. It has been reported that DBE is useful for exploring segments of intestine in patients with surgically altered anatomy, such as intubation into the afferent limb of a Roux-en-Y reconstruction [3]. DBE can therefore be used for ERCP in patients who have undergone total gastrectomy, pancreaticoduodenectomy, or living-donor liver transplantation [4, 5].

DBE is also useful for patients with a history of difficult colonoscopy. In some cases, complete colonoscopy is not possible with a conventional colonoscope. One reason is adhesions in the sigmoid colon or transverse colon, which prevent straightening of that region and complicate deep insertion of the endoscope. Without straightening, the curved segment of the colon is stretched by the shaft of a colonoscope in attempts to insert the scope. However, the double-balloon scope can prevent stretching of the curved colon by gripping the colon with the overtube balloon. Force can thus be transmitted to the tip of the endoscope effectively in endoscopic insertion. This feature of DBE enables total colonoscopy even in such difficult cases. The success rate for total colonoscopy using DBE for difficult colons has been reported as 88–100 % in the literature [6–9].

DBE is also useful in stabilizing the endoscopic control for complicated treatments such as endoscopic submucosal dissection (ESD) in the colon. Maintaining a stable position can be difficult at times with paradoxical movement in some parts of the colon. Using the double-balloon scope, however, the overtube balloon can grip and stabilize colon, enabling a more stable position with straightforward movements of the endoscope tip.

A short version of the double-balloon endoscope, the EC-450BI5 and EI-530B, with a working length of 152 cm and accessory channel of 2.8 mm is useful for the aforementioned purposes. Most of the standard accessories for ERCP and some accessories for colonoscopic therapies are too short for the 200 cm DBE, but can be used with the 152 cm DBE.

An Overtube Holder for DBE

Double-balloon endoscopy usually requires an assistant to hold the overtube for conducting the procedure. However, during therapeutic procedures, the overtube is mainly used for stability and does not require active insertion or withdrawal. In such circumstances, an overtube holder (Fig. 18.9) is useful, allowing the assistant to help with the therapeutic procedure instead of holding the overtube. We use the overtube holder for all the ESD and ERCP procedures [10].

Conclusion

Future Perspective

It is clear that deep enteroscopy now has a high success rate due to improvements in technology. It clearly has revolutionized the management of small intestinal diseases. The accessory channel has enabled endoscopic treatments for many difficult disease conditions such as small intestinal polyps in Peutz–Jeghers syndrome and small intestinal strictures in Crohn's disease. The new therapeutic DBE should make endoscopic therapy easier and safer and it could expand the application of endoscopic therapies in the small intestine. The improved image quality will also

Fig. 18.9 A handmade
overtube holder

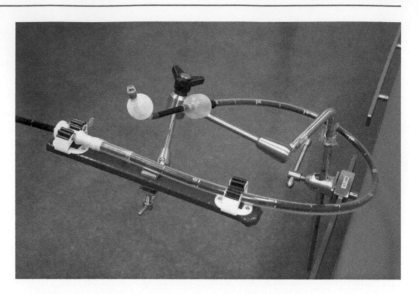

enhance the ability to examine the mucosa more thoroughly. In the future, it is hoped that this technology will lead to the development of an automated insertion device.

References

1. Yamamoto H, Yano T, Kita H, Sunada K, Ido K, Sugano K. New system of double-balloon enteroscopy for diagnosis and treatment of small intestinal disorders. Gastroenterology. 2003;125(5):1556. author reply 1556–7.
2. Nishimura N, Yamamoto H, Yano T, Hayashi Y, Arashiro M, Miyata T, et al. Safety and efficacy of double-balloon enteroscopy in pediatric patients. Gastrointest Endosc. 2010;71(2):287–94.
3. Kuno A, Yamamoto H, Kita H, Sunada K, Yano T, Hayashi Y, et al. Double-balloon enteroscopy through a Roux-en-Y anastomosis for EMR of an early carcinoma in the afferent duodenal limb. Gastrointest Endosc. 2004;60(6):1032–4.
4. Haruta H, Yamamoto H, Mizuta K, Kita Y, Uno T, Egami S, et al. A case of successful enteroscopic balloon dilation for late anastomotic stricture of choledochojejunostomy after living donor liver transplantation. Liver Transpl. 2005;11(12):1608–10.
5. Shimatani M, Matsushita M, Takaoka M, Koyabu M, Ikeura T, Kato K, et al. Effective "short" double-balloon enteroscope for diagnostic and therapeutic ERCP in patients with altered gastrointestinal anatomy: a large case series. Endoscopy. 2009;41(10):849–54.
6. Hotta K, Katsuki S, Ohata K, Abe T, Endo M, Shimatani M, et al. A multicenter, prospective trial of total colonoscopy using a short double-balloon endoscope in patients with previous incomplete colonoscopy. Gastrointest Endosc. 2012;75(4):813–8.
7. Gay G, Delvaux M. Double-balloon colonoscopy after failed conventional colonoscopy: a pilot series with a new instrument. Endoscopy. 2007;39(9):788–92.
8. Kaltenbach T, Soetikno R, Friedland S. Use of a double balloon enteroscope facilitates caecal intubation after incomplete colonoscopy with a standard colonoscope. Dig Liver Dis. 2006;38(12):921–5.
9. Pasha SF, Harrison ME, Das A, Corrado CM, Arnell KN, Leighton JA. Utility of double-balloon colonoscopy for completion of colon examination after incomplete colonoscopy with conventional colonoscope. Gastrointest Endosc. 2007;65(6):848–53.
10. Hayashi Y, Sunada K, Yamamoto H. A prototype holder adequately supports the overtube in balloon-assisted ESD. Dig Endosc. 2014;26(5):682.

Video Legends

Video 18.1 - A video showing the effective transmission of endoscopic control to the tip from the proximal endoscope shaft through the balloon overtube. The rotation and in-and-out motions are effectively transmitted through the overtube even with a looping of the shaft.

Video 18.2 - A video showing clear image of intestinal villi with EN-580T. Both the close-up and distant images are well focused because of the long focus range.

Index

R. Kozarek and J.A. Leighton (eds.), *Endoscopy in Small Bowel Disorders*,
DOI 10.1007/978-3-319-14415-3, © Springer International Publishing Switzerland 2015

CPI Antony Rowe
Chippenham, UK
2017-01-18 10:04